More praise for *Creating Sanctuary*,
by Dr. Sandra Bloom:

"This is a valuable, inspiring book. Dr. Bloom compels us to look at the society in which we live and helps us see how we can create a world in which we can grow, a world truly supportive of life."

–Ervin Staub, author of
*The Roots of Evil: The Origins of
Genocide and Other Group Violence*

"*Creating Sanctuary* places abuse and trauma squarely in the realm of social problems, calling for solutions at the individual, community, and societal levels. Dr. Bloom presents a clear, pointed, and much-needed call to action–action by every one of us to change the devastation of human potential wrought by interpersonal violence."

–Laurie Anne Pearlman, co-author of
*Trauma and the Therapist: Countertransference
and Vicarious Traumatization in Psychotherapy
with Incest Survivors*

"Dr. Bloom...revisit[s] some of the forgotten roots of modern social psychiatry. *Creating Sanctuary* serves as a potent integration for all psychotherapists of where they have been, where they are, and where they are going."

–Dr. Mark Schwartz, Clinical Director,
Masters & Johnson Clinic

For further information about The Sanctuary, please contact:

The Sanctuary
C/o The Alliance for Creative Development
1110 N. West End Blvd.
Quakertown, PA 18951

(888) 538-3124

Creating Sanctuary

Toward the Evolution of Sane Societies

Sandra L. Bloom, M.D.

ROUTLEDGE
New York and London

Reprinted 2010 by Routledge

Routledge
Taylor & Francis Group
270 Madison Avenue
New York, NY 10016

Routledge
Taylor & Francis Group
2 Park Square
Milton Park, Abingdon
Oxon OX14 4RN

Library of Congress Cataloging-in-Publication Data

Bloom Sandra L., 1948–
Creating sanctuary : toward the evolution of sane societies / Sandra L. Bloom.
p.   cm.
Includes bibliographical references and index.
ISBN 0–415–91568–6 (cloth). — ISBN 0–415–91858–8 (pbk.)
1. Adult child abuse victims—Rehabilitation.   2. Adult child abuse victims—Rehabilitation—
Case studies.   3. Psychic trauma—Social aspects.   4. Social psychiatry.   5. Clinical sociology.
I. Title.
RC569.5.C55B56   1997
616.85'82239—dc21   96–37298
CIP

This book is dedicated to the staff and patients
of 2 Main South, 2 West, and The Sanctuary

and

to Roy Stern, M.D.,
teacher and friend

Contents

Acknowledgments

Much of what I understand and write about concerns the mysterious web of connection that surrounds each of us, from birth to death. The writing of this book has provided me with an opportunity to traverse time and thank those who have served as nodal points for the way I think and the truth I know today. My thanks go first to my parents, Dorothy E. Treen and Charles W. Treen Jr., for providing me with enough of a sanctuary growing up that I am able to recognize love and safety when I feel it. Second to Edith Shapin, my guide through the rough spots, who did not live to see this job completed. In honoring the past, I must also say thank you to the memory of Arthur Shannon, who did so much to confirm my sense of self, to Craig Bloom, who taught me about vision and hope and provided me with the safety to untie so many knots.

I first learned about the power of groups and the unconscious at Temple University Hospital and am forever grateful especially to Roy Stern, Jack Benson, Alan Krystal, and David Soskis for all they taught me about the mysteries of mental illness in individuals and in systems. Thomas Fleming and James Crawford helped to provide my first opportunity to create a psychiatric unit from scratch, without which none of this would have happened. For more than ten years, Quakertown Hospital provided the backdrop and support for the evolution of the Sanctuary concepts and I am grateful for all of the people there who enabled us to prosper, and most particularly for the fine nursing staff that we had to leave behind. From 1991 to 1996, Northwestern Institute provided us with a home, and I am appreciative of the staff there who made our continuing survival possible and to Gary Hoyes, who gave us shelter from the storm.

I would never have had the courage to put these ideas down in writing had it not been for the unflagging friendship, encouragement, and support of a community of women, most particularly Elizabeth Kuh and Lyndra Bills, my special buddies, along with Francia White, Lou Naue, Marda Smith, Sara Steele, Susan Arnett, and Bette Van der Kolk. Gloria Steinem has been particularly supportive of my ideas, and her encouragement, as well as the example she sets, has meant a great deal to me. And had it not been for Peter Tear, my dear friend and personal catalyst for change, I would never have taken up the challenge of putting pen to paper in the first place. It was through late-night conversations with Peter and with Simon Green in London that I learned about the inside world of the theater and was led to see the wisdom of Shakespeare's astute observation about stage and world.

Thanks to Natalie Goldberg who taught me about "writing practice" and convinced me that I did not have to be Dostoevsky to have something worth saying. Lloyd DeMause has been taking unpopular positions his entire life and in doing so has made a significant contribution to the historical body of knowledge, constantly challenging established ideas. He published my first paper and has been unflagging in his support ever since. Charlie Boren has willingly shared his store of knowledge from serving so many years at the Institute for Living. Stan Gorski, as friend and librarian, has unfailingly supplied me with the research material I need, along with John Gach, who supplied me with all the out-of-print books I needed in my attempt to preserve a piece of the psychiatric past.

My friends in Great Britain offered me the opportunity to test out my ideas in a completely different context. It was Salley Brown, who in the guise of an Oxford tutor, encouraged me to write for the first time since college. Brett Kahr, Valerie Sinason, Ann Scott, Gordon Turnbull, Kate White, and John Southgate have provided much encouragement for my teaching and writing as well as extending the hands of friendship across the Atlantic.

Judith L. Herman and Bessel A. Van der Kolk were the teachers who "turned the lights on" in my head. I love and admire them both for their intellectual prowess and their unflagging integrity, their willingness to remain connected to the bigger picture, even though it would have been far easier to bury their heads in the proverbial sand. I am grateful to them both for their friendship and support. Without them, *The Sanctuary* would never have been created.

Studying the effects of traumatic experience is painful and difficult. It has been made unsurpassingly easier for me by a community of scholars who have generously shared their time and wisdom. Donald Nathanson walked onto *The Sanctuary* a few years ago and decided that he wanted to learn more. His affirmation of our achievements was critical. Without him, this book would not have become a reality. Christine Courtois, Louis Tinnin, Mark Schwartz, and Lori Galprin have freely offered their insights, experience, wisdom, and friendship. Bob Dobyns and I met when he too declared publicly that America suffers from cultural post-traumatic stress disorder and we have been laughing together ever since. Gillian Templeton, Michelle Hess, and David Wright brought *The Sanctuary* to Canada, and it has been a privilege to work with them.

The *International Society for Traumatic Stress Studies* has provided me with a collegial home among a group of clinicians and researchers I admire and respect. And Sandy Dempsey, Martha Davis, Joel Chinitz, Rob Garfield, Michael Reichert, Ellen Berman, Paul Fink and others at Philadelphia *Physicians for Social Responsibility* have provided me with a local home to put into practice what I preach. Douglas Coopersmith has been our legal adviser and I am grateful to him for all the years of sound advice. Marti Loring got me to Routledge via Philip Rapapport and I am grateful to both of them. Thanks too to Alan Miller and Tom Bender of *Universal Health Services* for their belief and investment in our work and to Gary Gottlieb and *Friends Hospital* for providing us with a new home.

But the greatest share of my gratitude, love, respect, and pride goes to all of the nursing staff, the support staff, and the clinical staff—past and present—of *The Sanctuary*, and the Alliance for Creative Development, most importantly my co-creators and my family, Joseph Foderaro, Ruth Ann Ryan, Beverly Haas, Bobbi Bliss, Marlene Finkelstein, Jean Vogel, and Joel Lerman of whom I can state, along with W. H. Auden that, "*Among those whom I like or admire, I can find no common denominator, but among those whom I love, I can: all of them make me laugh.*"

And finally with profound respect, I give my thanks to our patients, who have taught us so much over these years, most especially to "Dawn."

introduction

Dawn

It seemed to me imperative that there be somewhere, somehow established a sane asylum, however inadequate temporarily, and accordingly it was the aim of my associates and myself voluntarily to commit ourselves wholeheartedly to the opportunity afforded by such an experimental social set-up.

—Trigant Burrow, 1937, *The Biology of Human Conflict*

This is our major problem in social psychiatry: to learn how to keep these United States from becoming in long periods of peace a conglomeration of disunited states of mind and heart.

—Lawrence Kubie, M.D., 1943, *Psychiatry and the War*

In the field of mental health, most attention has been given to psychotherapy; some to mental hygiene, but very little as yet to the design of a whole culture which will foster healthy personalities.

—Maxwell Jones, 1953, *The Therapeutic Community*

For most of us, life runs like an invisible thread through time, each day connected to the next, indistinguishable from the one before, changes blending into more or less smooth transitions. But then along come days or moments that stand out as markers, abrupt rifts in the otherwise seamless fabric of day-to-day life. I am going to describe to you one of those rifts in my life, one of those events that prompted a voice in my head to whisper, "You will never be the same again."

In 1985 my life was going reasonably well. I was running a psychiatric practice and a hospital psychiatric unit that was a success. I was doing well financially, had a lovely home in the country, drove only fifteen minutes to work in the morning, and was a member of a small community. I was completely insulated from professional politics and had even less interest in national or global politics. Like so many Americans, I blocked out the unpleasant realities of my fellow countrymen, the alarming reports about the escalating national debt, the growing fear of some impending doom that seemed to lie beneath the Reaganomic hypomania. After all, I had no idea what the underlying causes were for all these problems, and I had no idea what to do about any of them. I did my part to be a good person, a good psychiatrist, and a good boss. What else could anyone expect of me?

I had first met Dawn as I will call her, in 1980, when she was only eighteen. She was a college student on a Philadelphia campus. She had falsely accused a man of raping her, and when confronted with the obvious evidence of his innocence, she broke down emotionally. Her mother, whom I had known from a previous job, asked me to see her, and I agreed.

Dawn was a beautiful young woman. Bright, funny, warm, and engaging, she was the ideal patient. Her "false memory" initially appeared to be a fluke, an anomaly in an otherwise unremarkable life. As we probed, however, it became apparent that Dawn had always had trouble with the men in her life. Her teen-age relationships were more chaotic than the average, and she seemed predisposed to become involved with men who manipulated, seduced, and exploited her. She had sexual problems, gaps in her memory which she took as a matter of course and inexplicable bouts of depression alternating with anxiety that would come and go for no apparent reason. Her self-esteem was relatively poor, and despite her obvious abilities she felt worthless. Sometimes she had difficulties giving an accurate account to me of her experiences, particularly if these involved men. Her father had been an abusive, sick, and troubled man who had died a few years before. He had beaten and humiliated her mother and her brother, but Dawn denied that she had ever had much difficulty with him.

Her recall of the events that had precipitated her visits to me were hazy at best, and she avoided much discussion about it, managing to steer me off course quite successfully on any number of occasions. In those days I was much more likely to just go where the patient directed, not choosing to probe troubled spots on my own initiative—good therapy was supposed to be "non-directive." I saw her regularly, and then more sporadically, for two or three years, helping to guide her through the crises of young adulthood. She graduated college and moved to Boston with her mother, but she stayed in touch with me. Eventually, she started therapy again, this time with a very competent feminist therapist, because of the recurrence of anxiety, depression, and difficulties with relationships. Still, I was surprised one day in 1985 when I received a panicked call from her mother. Dawn was using drugs for the first time in her life and had become suicidal. She desperately needed hospitalization to keep her safe, and her mother asked if I would admit her to our psychiatric unit. I spoke to her therapist, who agreed with this plan, and I advised her mother to bring Dawn back to Philadelphia immediately.

On the day that Dawn was admitted I remember experiencing profound shock and revelation, but I had no idea where this revelation would lead. I walked into the examining room expecting to see a depressed version of the young woman I knew. I expected that she would shamefully explain to me her recent misadventures and that together we would struggle to make some sense of it all. I expected that she would be embarrassed and hopeful that I would not be angry with her, a scenario we had run through many times in the past.

When I walked into the examining room the person I saw before me was Dawn—but not Dawn. This person was sitting cross-legged on the couch and greeted me not with the sob and plea for a hug that I had expected, but with a shy little mischievous grin, not entirely appropriate to the current situation. Most striking was her voice, which was tiny and childlike, and her physical mannerisms, which demonstrated the indescribable sense of movement one associates only with children. Had a camera been on, I could have received a special Emmy nomination for my overt composure, which bore no relationship to what I was feeling inside. I smiled back and simply asked "Who are you?" That is how striking the difference in the two was—I actually had the sense that I was with another person, different in a substantial way from the one I knew so well. She responded that she was "Little Dawn" and, when asked, gave the address and phone number of her family home when she was seven, a fact I later confirmed.

This was simply not possible. Oh, sure, I had read *The Three Faces of Eve* and I had seen *Sybil*—both representing the most well-known presentations of multiple personality disorder. But that was Hollywood. This was a small town in Pennsylvania. I was sure that I would never see a case of multiple personality disorder, and certainly not in someone I knew as well as I thought I knew Dawn.

Over the course of the next three weeks I learned a great deal. Dawn's child "alter" already felt safe with me because unbeknownst to me, we had spoken many times in the past. As I thought back, I remembered that Dawn occasionally called me at a time of personal crisis, outside of our usual therapeutic hour. When she first got on the phone, her voice would sound childlike, but I always assumed that this was simply "regression" and that she was voluntarily adopting a little-girl voice because of some emotion she was experiencing. Actually, that gives me far too much credit—I really never reflected on why she was doing it. She did it, and I was responding to her as a mother might to a little child. As she calmed down, her voice changed, she sounded more in control of herself, and that was the signal that we could end the conversation. I never asked her at our next meeting whether she remembered the content of the phone call—it never occurred to me that she didn't. I assumed continuity of consciousness because I really was not aware of any alternative.

My training experience had been a good one. As psychiatric residents in the late 1970s, we became very proficient at getting histories and learning about childhood experiences and family dynamics. Family therapy was gaining a great deal of credibility in those days, and we had come to recognize that the family system was the crucial context for understanding the patient. We knew that childhood and family experience had some kind of direct connection to adult dysfunction and yet we did not really understand.

No theoretical model was available to pull together the biological, the psychological, the social, and the philosophical/spiritual into one comprehensive framework. There were only fragments of knowledge—a piece here, a piece there. I knew about child abuse from my work in the emergency room and in pediatrics. But I never really thought about those abused children grown up. Incest was certainly known to exist, but was said to be exceedingly rare. I had heard about "dissociation" and "hysteria" but I associated them more with faking and attention-seeking than with responding to overwhelming life events. I understood a little about the personal oppression of violent homes but made no larger connections to racial, sexual, or political oppression. I had heard of the repetition compulsion, but *why* people would continually repeat the past never really made sense to me even though I could daily see the evidence with my own eyes.

We rarely if ever asked people about their history of abuse assuming, perhaps, that any major traumatic experience would be volunteered willingly by the patient. We knew that repression existed, but believed that people repressed what they felt guilty about, all those putative sexual fantasies and longings for the parent of the opposite sex. The idea that people could be "forgetting" memories of actual experiences of rape, molestation, and physical abuse simply did not go across the screen of our minds. We were never told that these things *did not* happen. In fact, there was often clear evidence that they had. But the real traumatic events in our patients' lives were not emphasized. Instead we overlooked, denied, or minimized their importance. And the patients colluded with this denial because they were no more eager than we were to open up the Pandora's box of their own childhood experiences.

What I hope I am getting across to the reader is that the particular kind of blindness I had experienced was really a sort of figure-ground problem. If you have ever puzzled over an optical illusion picture, you know what I mean. You only can see the old hag or the vase, and no matter how hard you try there just isn't anything else there. Suddenly your eyes blink and there is the beautiful young girl in a big hat or the two faces staring at each other. In retrospect, the facts of Dawn's case seem blatantly obvious. But back then I had no way to understand the facts, no context within which they would make sense.

As I asked questions that demonstrated my willingness to hear, the child alter revealed a history of paternal incest, brutality, and emotional abuse about which I had been totally unaware, and yet which helped to make so much more sense out of the symptoms that had always plagued Dawn. It also helped to explain the earlier "false" memory. Her memory had not been as much false as it was distorted and displaced. She had superimposed a stranger's face on that of the true perpetrator, her father, because it was less shocking to her conscious mind. But the lie had led not to relief, but a worsening of symptoms. Dawn's mother confirmed, as best she could, the reality of Dawn's experience, and it was consistent with a pattern of abusive behavior that her father had imposed on other family members. I gently explained to the adult Dawn, who would be brought back "out" at the behest of the child, what the difficulty was and then received permission from both Dawns to make a videotape of the child alter.

I sat with Dawn while she watched this unknown part of her, in her body, the me-but-not-me, on the television screen communicating directly with her. This helped to substantially decrease her understandable anxiety about her sanity and within a few sessions they were communicating internally. I stayed with her while she re-experienced the rape. Reexperience is not quite the right word because the adult part of her experienced it for the first time with me. It was the child part that had taken care of the memories and feelings of that awful night. Putting together the missing pieces of her life helped Dawn enormously. She had spent most of her life being haunted by events she could not remember, and they had left their imprints on every relationship she had tried to have. Before she left the hospital, she had integrated herself into one identity. Out of the hospital, she began to show dramatic improvement in every aspect of her life as more memories returned. A decade later, she now leads a productive and worthwhile life as a teacher and mother, although depression, one of the common chronic symptoms of childhood trauma, continues to periodically dog her heels.

Dawn's diagnosis, though perhaps the best thing that had happened to her as an adult because it led to better treatment, marked in my own life a personal and professional crisis: I was a mess!! I thought I was a pretty good diagnostician. I thought I was very skilled at formulating an understanding of a person after I had gotten to know them. But now I felt as though I didn't know anything, or at least I was no longer sure what I did know and what I didn't. My assumptive world had shifted and knocked me off my pins. After all, Dawn was someone I had thought I knew well. What other secrets were lying in the dark closets of memory for which we held no key? What was most humbling about the experience was the recognition that the information had not even been that well hidden. The problem was that I had no mental schema within which the information would make sense and therefore, I simply failed to see it. I had been taught to believe that multiple personality disorder was extremely rare, if it existed at all, and therefore it did not exist for me. I had been told that incest does not occur in nice families, and therefore Dawn could not have been an incest victim—after all, I knew and liked her mother. Caught in the middle of my own personal earthquake, I realized only later that I had experienced some of the first tremors of an intellectual quake that was going to shake the entire psychiatric profession, the aftershocks of which are still with us today. Once the lid is off the box, there is no putting the hobgoblins safely back in.

Naturally, I started wondering about what I was missing in my other patients. This experience had a similar impact on the other members of my treatment team. Our scientific curiosity was aroused. How many more stories were unheard? How many others among our patients had childhood histories of severe trauma, of overwhelming experiences that were more than a child could safely bear? Many patients, when asked, simply volunteered the information about abuse and other traumas in their backgrounds, and when we asked why they hadn't told us before they replied, "You never asked!" Others responded that they had told us, and to our horror we reviewed some of their charts going back through the years, and, sure enough, they were right. We had obtained the history, carefully recorded it, and then behaved as if it had absolutely no bearing on their mental state. The information had played little if any role in our case formulations or treatment decisions. Other patients denied any history of abuse or trauma and talked about the ideal nature of their families of origin and their childhood experiences. They would then promptly fall apart with an exacerbation of symptoms, an increase in self-destructive behavior, and what we considered, at the time "acting out" and manipulation. This seemed an odd response to relatively straightforward questions, and we began wondering what that behavior meant. As we gently probed further, these patients would often tell us—no, show us—their memories of horrifying childhood experiences, often at the hands of someone who professed to love them.

This was awful. Oh, yes, from a scientific point of view it was fascinating. A mental iceberg we had never seen before, an entirely new intellectual landscape. There was some of the associated thrill of the explorer, I suppose, but that thrill was largely overwhelmed by the fear and horror of it all. *I did not want to know this information.* It scared me, as it did the rest of my team. How could this be true? How could there be so much child abuse? What were we supposed to do with something we knew virtually nothing about—the effects of child abuse on adult behavior? Worst of all, it made us sick—sick at heart, sick in our souls, and sick to our stomachs. When you read accounts of people "remembering" childhood trauma, the implication is often that the patient sits quietly on some couch, gently whimpering perhaps, but calmly remembering events as if it were you remembering what you ate for breakfast yesterday. This is not what it is like. When people "remember" previous trauma, or abreact, as it is called in psycholingo, they relive it, or more often, as in Dawn's case, live it for the first time. It is terrible for them, extremely painful, embarrassing, and disgusting. But at least, deep inside, they know the secret they have been unwittingly carrying for a long time, and afterward they usually feel a kind of relief at the shedding of this burden.

The participant-observer is completely unprepared for what is coming and inevitably experiences some kind of secondary or "vicarious" traumatization at witnessing the horror and trauma of a past time intruding into the present. Trauma shatters assumptions (Janoff-Bulman 1992); it destroys the wall of safety and invulnerability that we use to shield ourselves from harsh realities, from recognizing our essential vulnerability. Witnessing trauma produces a similar effect on the bystander. Since that time I have not been puzzled by why the psychiatric profession has turned its back repeatedly on the reality of victimization (Herman 1992). It is too painful to bear. Blaming the victims for their problems and thereby allying oneself with the powerful perpetrator is far easier than emotionally containing the raw pain of innocent suffering and helplessness. Compassion for the victim leads to the need to take action to stop perpetration, and this means directly challenging the holders of power. It's a scary business.

We were unable to return to our former position of the three monkeys, "Hear no evil, see no evil, speak no evil." The smoking gun of child abuse lay all around us. We began to carefully explore what has been called "the black hole of trauma" (Pitman and Orr, 1990). Our body of knowledge grew as we academically and clinically surveyed this strange, terrifying, and yet oddly empowering landscape. Previously, psychiatry—and its primary focus, the human mind—had appeared to be a fragmented, often confusing and confused area of endeavor. So many of the reasons we had offered for why people do crazy things always seemed fragmented, circular, inconclusive, or just patently wrong. Implicitly, underlying many of our psychiatric notions and our psychiatric jargon was the concept of "original sin"—that somehow the patients were ultimately to blame for the troubles they got themselves into and if they would only do as they were told, they would get better. Biological psychiatry countered this implicit judgmental attitude by attributing the cause of mental disturbance to impaired neurotransmitter function and genetic vulnerability, but in doing so it often veered in the direction of a dangerous and foolish reductionism, attempting to explain very complex problems with simplistic and unproven answers.

Just as confusing was the fact that mental *health* was never actually defined. What does a healthy person look like? How does he or she behave? It has become increasingly clear over the last forty years that the definition of health is profoundly influenced by cultural and social mores, but there are certain aspects of human health that are grounded in universal human needs. And if human health and ill health is so influenced by the social matrix within which we all function, then what about us? The participant role of the society and its representatives, in this case us, was never fully clarified and often simply ignored. Whenever a patient was unresponsive to our particular interventions we would deny or minimize our frustration or lack of accomplishment and call it resistance or manipulation, or some similar term whose purpose was to convince us that their lack of improvement was their fault, not ours.

As we studied the effects of psychological trauma, what began to emerge was the beginning hazy outlines of a field theory of human nature, a biopsychosocial philosophy within which all the fragmented pieces of knowledge about human biology, behavior, and inner life could begin to form a cohesive whole. Through an understanding of how trauma affects the whole human being we were able to see the interconnected and mutually interacting web of biology, individual psychology, and social behavior, as well as philosophical, religious, and spiritual beliefs. Gradually, we awakened to the fact that our patients do not, by virtue of their psychiatric symptomatology, comprise a separate and discrete category of human experience. Rather, they march along the far end of a very long continuum of traumatic adaptation that chains us all together in our common—and often tragic—humanity.

As we deepened our understanding of the manifestations and effects of psychological trauma, we came to understand that the trauma itself does not determine outcome. Rather, the response of the individual's social group plays a critical role in determining who becomes a psychiatric casualty, who pursues a life of criminal behavior, and who is spared. Although as therapists we had previous contact with the ideas of family therapy and systems theory, we were still working from the premises of an individual model, in which problems are seen as being caused by the individual person or, at most, by "communication problems." In this view of the world, which characterizes such a fundamental aspect of Western philosophy, psychology, and politics, attachment behaviors are always slightly suspect, easily merging into the pathological and called neediness and dependency, regression or manipulation.

The entire experience with trauma provoked disturbing insights that have shaken us out of our complacency. The insight that humans have a predisposition to repeat traumatic experience has led to the eruption of a profound and disturbing fear: Our society appears to be in the grips of a post-traumatic deterioration that could also end in self-destruction, just as it does with patients who remain locked in the patterns of the past. We have become convinced that trauma is not an unusual or rare experience, but that it is in fact normative. Just as a traumatic experience can become the central organizing principle in the life of an individual victim, so too is trauma a *central organizing principle of human thought, feeling, belief, and behavior* that has been virtually ignored in our understanding of human nature. Without this understanding we cannot hope to make the sweeping changes we need to make if we are to halt a universal post-traumatic deterioration.

This was yet another blow to our sense of secure knowledge. If other people are that critical in determining outcome, then we were bound to reexamine the basic assumptions that inform our therapeutic environment, the social sphere within which patients are plunged when they are at their most vulnerable. About this time, Dr. Steven Silver published a chapter about his experience in treating Vietnam War veterans in which he described "sanctuary trauma" as that which occurs when an individual who has suffered a severe stressor next encounters what was expected to be a supportive and protective environment and discovers only more trauma (Silver, 1986). We thought about the many patients who had come into psychiatric facilities expecting help, understanding, and comfort but found instead rigid rules, humiliating procedures, conflicting and often disempowering methods, and inconsistent, confusing, and judgmental explanatory systems. This led to a rethinking of the basic assumptions upon which we base treatment and a formulation of our treatment approach as "The Sanctuary Model of Inpatient Treatment" (Bloom 1994a, 1994b, 1994c).

A "sanctuary" is a place of refuge and protection. For our purposes the word connotes a place of temporary refuge, where some of the rules of our present everyday society are suspended to allow for a different kind of social experience. A concrete description of the place we call *The Sanctuary*® is fairly easy. It is a discrete unit in a psychiatric hospital that can house twenty-four people with plenty of space for group meetings, private consultations, and various activities. The furnishings are attractive, the colors soft, warm, and inviting. There are pictures on the wall, some professionally done, some by people who have contributed a message of their own after their stay. The unit has televisions, a lounge space, a small kitchen. Ideally, people live in this environment for two to three weeks, although that rarely happens in these days of restricted care. Within the confines of these walls, a special program has been created to address the needs of adults who were traumatized as children. They all suffer from a psychiatric or psychophysiological problem severe enough to compromise their level of function and necessitating hospitalization. This usually means that they pose enough threat to themselves or others that intensive treatment is vital.[1]

The Sanctuary is, of course, exactly what it says it is—a program to treat traumatized adults. But from another perspective a parallel agenda is visible. The truth is, we did not create *The Sanctuary* for the sole purpose of treating patients. We wanted to create a relatively sane environment for us as well, an environment that would satisfy some important needs of the people who work in and manage the program.[2]

This book is the story of how a group of friends and clinicians came to a better understanding of some of the mysteries of life. People who consider themselves patients or victims of trauma may certainly find the information contained within these pages of benefit. But I am not as much interested in writing about how we taught our patients as I am in sharing what they taught us. These lessons have been personally and professionally transformative and if properly understood could contribute to transformative changes in the concentric series of social systems of which we all are a part.

In chapters 1 and 2, I will focus on what traumatic experience does to the body, the mind, the relational network, and the ontology of the victim and those close to the victim. Learning about the effects of trauma is not as simple as learning a new body of information. Traumatic experience forces us to develop new categories, new ways of thinking about our past, our present, and our future. Trauma theory challenges, reinterprets, expands, and even demolishes many of our existing paradigmatic structures—the underlying rules and practices that give form and meaning to our lives. These rules are partly or wholly unconscious, undefined, simply accepted as the way things are. They define the way we perceive reality.

In the practice of psychiatry, nature and nurture have run as parallel and often warring etiologic positions. Just as today, other times in our past have witnessed efforts by biological reductionism and genetic determinism to drown out the voices of nurture, environment, and development (Kirshner and Johnston 1982). In Chapter 3 we hear again a few of those insistent voices arguing for the essentially social construction of human existence. One of the most important lessons we have learned is that honoring and learning from the past is the only way of guaranteeing safety in the present and ensuring that we have a future. It is profoundly true, as Santayana reminds us: *"Those who cannot remember the past are condemned to repeat it."* We cannot hope to integrate the biological, the psychological, the social, and the philosophical without learning from the wisdom of the past.

In Chapter 4, I pick up the threads of my story and recount how we were changed by—and changed—our small experimental society as a result of what we learned about trauma. We called the physical and psychological result of this change *The Sanctuary,* and in this section I will describe our experience of creating and maintaining a therapeutic milieu that is designed to address the needs of adults who were traumatized as children.

For years the inpatient setting has been considered a laboratory for social change.[3] But before we had an understanding of trauma it was difficult to generalize from the microcosm of a psychiatric inpatient unit to the larger social sphere in any significantly relevant way. No commonly shared language could adequately express our insights. Psychiatric disorder was constituted of basic "otherness" that bore little if any causal relationship to the outside world.

Trauma theory has taught us that this perception is nonsense, that most psychiatric disorder is the culmination of "normal reactions to abnormal situations," situations largely created by the failure of our social systems to provide traumatized children with the protection and care to which they have a right. As this recognition grew, the implications became enormous.

Our tiny inpatient community was a small system embedded in a series of concentric systems that failed us in the same way that we were failing our patients, and that they had been failed as children. In fact, the degree of health in those "parent" systems was a limiting ceiling on how healthy we could make our own, not at all unlike the situation in which children find themselves when confronted with impaired parents.

We realized clearly that without reverberating change in the hierarchy of systems, we would continually find ourselves fighting to maintain the safety and security of the unit, forced to mount psychic and corporate battles to protect the state of health we had achieved. This drain of energy, consequently, took its toll on the development of further progress. This has been an extremely useful lesson in graphically detailing the necessity of total system change and the difficulties involved in attempting to fix a part without fixing the whole. It was humbling to discover that our system and the systems around us are as *resistant* to change, *manipulative,* and *stubborn* as any of the psychiatric patients we were treating. This was another example of the dawning recognition that the wall we establish between *them* and *us* is an arbitrary one, born out of our need to distance ourselves from our own shortcomings rather than out of any sense of absolute reality.

I have come to believe that we have had a number of experiences with victims of trauma that may have a great deal of relevance for the social systems within which we all must function. In Chapter 5, I speculate about the potential for social reconnection. Everyone seems to recognize that we presently are in need of change. Argument abounds, however, about what form that change should take. Powerful forces in our society are pushing for a movement backward in an attempt to undo the perceived damage that has been wrought by the profound changes of the last half century. Other forces are pushing us forward into a "new age," which is described either in dark forecasts of apocalyptic doom or idyllic utopianism. Community life has broken down dramatically, and we are only beginning to recognize how important to our daily survival is the web of connection that a community provides.

But there are relatively few voices talking about *how* we get from "here" to "there." Part of the problem may be that we do not yet have any kind of a clear vision about where "there" is. We do not spend a great deal of time envisioning a better future for ourselves and our children and even less time figuring out how to make that future a reality. Nor have we had available to us an understanding of how "complex adaptive systems" function. Only now is a model for systems change being developed (Holland 1995). We have, however, learned a great deal about the human elements within any system that create the most chaos and disorder. That is why I think I have something to share with you. I have been a part of a better system for the last fifteen years. It is not idyllic or utopian. It does not work flawlessly. But it is more responsive to human well-being than any other system I have ever encountered. As a result, we have learned a great deal about what is important to human beings—all human beings—and some important lessons about how human systems succeed and how they fail.

My world view has changed almost entirely as a result of what I have learned about what happens to human beings who are exposed to overwhelming stress. These changes have been alternately terrifying and exciting, frustrating and gratifying, infuriating and pleasurable. At times I seek out new knowledge, a new way of looking at the world. At other times, I regress, harking back to old and timeworn explanations for puzzling feelings and behaviors. This new way of viewing the world is far more personally demanding and draining than the old. In the last ten years, my life has totally and unexpectedly changed both personally and professionally. I now have bigger areas of clarity about things that were in a muddle before and this understanding has brought with it more compassion for myself, for other people, and for our sad, struggling world. But there is no longer any place to hide. I see what is meant by the saying "Ignorance is bliss." Now that I know more about the ways of the world and how the pieces fit together, I cannot bear the silence that gives consent. Suffering demands a voice, a witness, and that means giving up the freedom to be a bystander. This book is a call for more company out here, on the edge, on the firing line, speaking out against tyranny in all its forms, including the tyranny of a dying and deadly vision.

We are on the threshold of a new millennium. Signs of social strain are manifest all around us. Our existing paradigmatic structures no longer adequately hold us. We appear to lack adequate methods to solve problems that are global, interconnected, ecological, and biopsychosocial. We lack an alternative vision for the future, and as the Bible says, without a vision a people perish. When Thomas Kuhn (1970) talked about a "paradigm shift" he noted that it is impossible for an old paradigm to be overturned until a new paradigm is born. I believe that our work with some of the most injured and socially alienated of human beings provides us all with important information about what we need to do to reconnect to each other and to the natural world that sustains us. These patients have provided us with some vital pieces of a new paradigm, the still hazy outlines of a new way of thinking, relating, and behaving, and a new way of defining reality. I have used the phrase "creating sanctuary" as a way of illustrating the verb-noun, process-object, ever-changing organic nature of what *The Sanctuary* means. A sense of safety, wholeness, life, caring, and home is something each of us actively creates—or destroys—every moment of our lives. It is the ultimate choice of every human being, of every human community. It is my hope that the insights we have gained from our work with some of the most injured warriors in the battle of life can contribute to an interdisciplinary, interracial, transgendered, global conversation leading to a new, more humane and attainable vision for the centuries to come.

one

Trauma Theory
Deconstructing the Social

And truly, now we see through a glass darkly, not face to face.
—*The Confessions of St. Augustine*, Saint Aurelius Augustine, 401 A.D.

THROUGH A GLASS DARKLY: THE THEORY OF TRAUMA

In ways vastly more complicated than any computer, the human organism is designed to function as a unity, an integrated and interconnected whole. Unfortunately, our ability to think clearly, logically, and in an integrated way is vulnerable to a multitude of stresses. These stresses can be biological, psychological, social, or moral, or any combination of these. Regardless of the kind of stress, our capacity for clear thinking is constantly jeopardized by physiologically based bodily and emotional reactions over which we have little control and about which we often have little awareness. Any kind of overwhelming stress produces fragmentation, and, like Humpty-Dumpty, the pieces often elude reunion.

It is when we are severely stressed, when the expected routine of daily life is disturbed by traumatic events, that our bodies respond in primitive ways and we find ourselves in the midst of a storm of emotional and physical reactions that we cannot understand or control. In many ways, we are not the same people when we are terrified as when we are calm. Our bodies change in remarkable ways, as do our perceptual abilities, our emotional states, our thought processes, our attention, and our memory. When under this kind of stress it is as if we become another person, no longer able to respond to others as we would under less threatening circumstances.

Compared with other animals, humans are astonishingly vulnerable to their environment. We cannot run very fast, our fingernails are poor substitutes for claws, our skin offers little resistance to the vicissitudes of weather, we have no poisonous fangs. We are, however, "set" internally to respond to situations of danger more readily than situations that evoke feelings of contentment, satisfaction, or joy. Like other animals, we are biologically equipped to protect ourselves from harm as best we can. But even with our superior brains, an early human standing alone against a dangerous foe had very little defense. Our ability to form attachments to each other and form social groups has been our best defense and has guaranteed our survival. Attachment to our social group is a deeply ingrained structure that derives from our primate heritage.

In the next two chapters I will lead the reader through a condensed process of re-education similar to the one my colleagues and I experienced over the course of several years. We are still looking "through a glass darkly" because there is yet so much to be learned.

I am going to look at what happens to the body, the mind, the emotions, the social identity, the behavior, and the meaning system of people who are exposed to experiences of terror, most particularly terror that is unrelenting, repeated, severe, or secret. Then, I am going to begin building a case for the "antidote"—the capacity of human relatedness to provide the healing integration that is necessary if the victim is to transform suffering into victory.

BACKGROUND

The most persistent sound which reverberates through man's history is the beating of war drums.

—Arthur Koestler, 1978, *Janus*

Accounts of the effects of overwhelming stress on the body, mind, and soul of the victim go back at least as far as Ancient Greece, whose writers had a great deal to say about combat, traumatic death, grief, horror, guilt, betrayal and tragedy (Shay 1994, 1995). Likewise, women have described experiences with domestic violence and child abuse since at least the twelfth century (McLennan 1996). Shakespeare knew well the signs and symptoms of states of terror, and in 1666, Samuel Pepys described post-traumatic stress disorder in depicting people's reactions to the great fire of London. Over the years, post-traumatic stress disorder has had many names—hysteria, soldier's heart, psychic trauma neurosis, shell shock, physioneurosis, combat fatigue, railway spine disorder, battle fatigue, traumatic neurosis, survivor's syndrome, rape trauma syndrome, battered child syndrome, battered wife syndrome (Meichenbaum 1994).

In the last century, knowledge of the effects of psychological trauma has twice surfaced in public consciousness and been lost again (Herman 1992). Each time awareness has grown, it has been in connection with a sociopolitical movement that gave it support. The first emergence was the study of hysteria in the late nineteenth century and grew out of the republican, anticlerical political movement of late nineteenth century France. Freud and his colleagues noted a strong connection between the psychiatric symptoms of "hysterical" women and a personal history of sexual molestation. But he became increasingly concerned about the sociopolitical implications of his observations. It was not credible that there could be so many adults molesting children. In place of the real events of women's lives he substituted sexual fantasy. As Dr. Herman summarizes, "Sexuality remained the central focus of inquiry. But the exploitative social context in which sexual relations actually occurred became utterly invisible" (Herman 1992). As a result the connection between childhood sexual abuse and adult psychiatric disorder was buried for another century.

The study of trauma reemerged as a result of the first and second world wars when so many soldiers and POWs returned with what was called "shell shock" in W.W. I and "combat fatigue" or "combat neurosis" in W.W. II. Just after W.W. II, researchers asserted that 200–240 days of combat was enough to break anyone (Herman 1992). Despite this, combat fatigue was still considered to be a result of individual weakness on the part of the soldier. Not until the 1970s did the reality of violence and its effects become central to our culture. This centrality derived largely from the problems of Vietnam War veterans who organized themselves outside of official governmental systems, paralleling a similar movement among American and Western European feminists whose concerns focused on violence toward women and children.

In 1980, the diagnosis of "post-traumatic stress disorder" or PTSD, entered the formal psychiatric lexicon of the *Diagnostic and Statistic Manual*.[1] In 1985, the *International Society for Traumatic Stress Studies* was founded to provide a forum for the sharing of research, clinical strategies, public policy concerns and theoretical formulations on trauma in the United States and around the world.[2]

The result of this resurgence of interest in traumatic experience is trauma theory, a knowledge base that serves as an anchor for the integration of various psychological theories, techniques, and points of view, a possible "unified field theory" of human behavior. We cannot formulate effective strategies to deal with violence unless we have a common knowledge base that explains to us what violence actually does to the body, mind, and soul of the individual and how that affects the group.

THE PHYSICAL RESPONSE TO DANGER

Fight or Flight

The basic internal protective mechanism is called "the fight-or-flight" response (Cannon 1939). This is not a planned, deliberately thought-out reaction, but a rapid-fire, automatic, total body response that we share with other animals. Whenever we perceive that we are in danger our bodies make a heroic and rapid response. Numerous neurotransmitters and hormones produce massive changes in every organ system (Van der Kolk 1994). The brain sends instantaneous signals to the adrenal glands to secrete epinephrine or, as it is also called, adrenaline. At the same time the brain releases a kindred substance, norephinephrine, which affects only the brain itself. Likewise, increased amounts of steroids flood into the bloodstream, as well as opioid substances that are pain relievers.

Heart rate, blood pressure, and respiratory rate increase along with alertness and vigilance. Simultaneously a decrease occurs in feeding, reproductive activity, and immune response. This radical adjustment is in the service of survival, preparing us to make an immediate response to the dangerous situation. When this reaction is a response to a real danger, is time-limited, and is effective, it is life-saving and highly adaptive. Problems arise only when this reaction is evoked in the absence of any threat, when the threat is prolonged, or when the organism can do nothing to protect itself from the threat.

Chronic Hyperarousal

Under conditions of chronic stress, something goes wrong as the body attempts to cope with this massive overload of responses. The effectiveness of the response diminishes, and the body becomes desensitized to some of the effects of the neurohormones. The entire system can become dysregulated in many different ways. This results in a set of highly dysfunctional and maladaptive brain activities (Perry and Pate 1993). The person experiences this as a state of chronic hyperarousal.

We all have a "volume control" over our level of arousal. If we are in a lecture hall and hear a noise at the back, we cease paying attention to the speaker and swivel our heads to appraise the source of the noise. Once we are assured that the noise was just a latecomer and that there is nothing to fear, our level of arousal rapidly returns to normal and we are able once again to attend to the lecturer. Our reaction is quite different if we hear a sound, turn our heads and see a man with a gun heading toward the front of the room. In this case we become hyperaroused. This is a clear and present danger, and the fight-or-flight response is triggered within each of us.

People who have been severely or repeatedly traumatized may lose this capacity to modulate their level of arousal. Their reaction to the benign latecomer is quite similar to their reaction to the threatening stranger. They stay hyperaroused and guarded; they are unable to calm themselves down even when they see that there is no danger. They feel embarrassed by their response, while at the same time, they are irritable, angry, and frightened for no apparent reason. They are prepared to fight or flee, even though there is no apparent danger. They may also become flooded with memories, images, and sensations that are overwhelming. As a result, they are likely to feel they are "crazy."

This reaction can be triggered by almost anything. Once we have experienced a stimulus that evokes fear we become "fear-conditioned," a state that is incredibly powerful and difficult for the logical centers of the brain to override (Le Doux 1992; 1994). Because of the vast associational network of our brains, we can pair fear with virtually anything. This happens at the time of the fear, beyond conscious control, and very quickly. Later the person is usually not consciously aware of the connection between the fear-provoking stimulus and the fear-response.

Each episode of danger connects to every other episode of danger in our minds, so that the more danger we are exposed to, the more sensitive we become to danger. With each fight-or-flight experience, our mind forms a network of connections that is triggered by every subsequent threatening experience or stimulus. Because we are so intelligent, these connections can be very widely linked to any stimulus that is paired with the dangerous experience.

An example can help us to understand this phenomenon. A man is in a car crash in which his wife is severely injured. We would not be surprised if he subsequently developed hyperarousal when driving or as a passenger in a car. But why would he become hyperaroused whenever he sees a woman's *wristwatch*? Only with great difficulty does he become *aware* of the fact that he is being triggered by wristwatches, and only with help and careful questioning, or even more specific therapy, does he finally recall that the last thing he laid eyes on before the crash was the watch on his wife's wrist. His brain has made the connection without his conscious knowledge. Not only will he unconsciously and self-protectively resist identifying the stimulus of the watch, but he will even more strongly resist remembering the actual event because the memory is so horrifying. Instead, the triggering will continue with a widening network of associations. Wristwatches may associate to clocks, or women's bracelets, or arms. The man may reach the point where even leaving his house becomes an impossibility because he is too easily triggered by stimuli he can neither identify nor control. Meanwhile, every experience of hyperarousal further compromises and resets his central nervous system.

Now if this same man discovers something that helps calm down this uncontrollable sense of hyperarousal—even temporarily—would we fault him for utilizing it? Would it be so very hard for us to understand his dilemma? Alcohol, drugs, sexual activity, violent acting out, risk-taking behavior, eating excessively, inducing vomiting, purposely hurting the body, exercising, overinvolvement in work—all of these behaviors can temporarily produce some relief from the hyperarousal. The problem, of course, is that the relief is only temporary. After withdrawal from alcohol or other drugs, or other behaviors, the agitation rebounds with even greater ferocity. All of these behaviors can become habitual, even addictive, in such a situation (Van der Kolk and Greenberg 1987; Van der Kolk 1996a, b).

If this man seeks treatment, he will likely get treated for the complicating and exacerbating symptom—perhaps anxiety, a substance abuse problem, depression, or physical symptoms—and the underlying cause is missed. Even if a clinician or friend does make the connection, it is just as likely that the man will remain totally unaware of the connection, and in fact, that he will protect himself from knowing, and experiencing the initial trauma all over again.

Children who experience trauma may be more dramatically affected by chronic hyperarousal than adults. Trauma in childhood occurs before the brain has developed normal modulation of arousal. One of the most essential functions of parenting is to provide children with external modulation for their internal states. To develop normally, children require exposure to environmental stress sufficient to promote skills development and mastery experiences combined with sufficient buffering to prevent them from becoming overwhelmed. Only gradually and with the responsive care of adults do children develop the ability to modulate their own level of emotional response to both events that come from outside and events that originate within their own bodies. Children cannot always soothe themselves and therefore the capacity of adults to soothe frightened, angry, or shamed children is essential to their development. Without such help, children become chronically hyperaroused and will develop a panoply of destructive symptoms and behaviors in attempts to diminish this insupportable state.

Failure to provide children with sufficient modulation by not protecting them or by exposing them to overwhelming stress appears to cause actual impairments in normal brain development. The majority of individual cell growth and specialization in the brain occurs after birth. The brain development proceeds in response to complex and critical neurohormonal cues (Perry and Pate 1993). There are critical times in brain development when the brain cells are especially sensitive to certain signals which must be properly received for normal function. The brains of children exposed to severe or repeated stress are exposed to abnormally high concentrations of critical neurotransmitters that play vital roles in neurodevelopment and early evidence suggests that this exposure is having long-term detrimental effects on basic brain and body function (Perry 1994, Perry and Pate 1993). Researchers in the area of childhood posttraumatic stress believe that childhood stress and trauma may be the common link between many medical and psychiatric conditions related to the immune system, the cardiovascular system and the neuroendocrine system (Perry 1994).

Stress-related Physical Symptoms and Disease

Stress is a major contributor to the development of physical illness. The growing fields of psychosomatic medicine, psychoendocrinology, and psychoimmunology are increasingly providing information about the relationship between external events, brain biochemistry, the body, and the way the mind interprets all these events (Moyers 1993).

Researchers at Duke University have become interested in a cluster of biobehavioral characteristics that seem to account for an increased risk for somatic disease and earlier death. These characteristics include: 1) depressed mood; 2) increased anger/irritation; 3) increased sympathetic nervous system reactivity; 4) decreased parasympathetic nervous system function; 5) increased smoking; 6) increased eating; and 7) increased alcohol consumptions. All of these characteristics have also been associated with chronic stress (Williams 1995).

In study after study, chronic stress appears to play an important etiologic role in many disease processes (Brown 1993). Biochemical messengers that are released during the stress response including adrenaline, corticosteroids, and endorphins, all play a role in suppressing immune function. Chronic stress results in repeated activation of the autonomic nervous system, and this can result in psychosomatic disorders including hypertension, asthma, headaches, and some forms of ulcers. This biochemical aspect of the stress response may also help to explain the decreased immune function found in socially isolated people.

THE COGNITIVE RESPONSE TO DANGER

Learned Helplessness

Self-efficacy, the term used to describe our belief about what we are capable of doing in any given situation, is influenced by experience and the actions of others, and it is put to the test when we are caught in dangerous situations (Bandura 1982). If we are able to master the situation of danger, to successfully run away or win the fight, or we are able to successfully recruit help, then the risk of long-term physical and psychological changes are lessened. But if we can do nothing to prevent ourselves or someone else from sustaining harm, we experience helplessness. Human beings deplore feeling helpless. We will do almost anything to avoid experiencing our own impotence. Children are especially prone to post-traumatic stress because they are helpless in most situations.

Important animal and human research confirms that powerful physiological forces are at work in the phenomenon called "learned helplessness." It has been repeatedly demonstrated that in an environment in which some important outcome is beyond control, an animal will give up trying to alter its situation and will come to expect that nothing it can do will change the outcome. The animal learns to be helpless and this helplessness persists even when conditions change and the animal could regain control in the environment.

The normal response of a dog, cat, rat, or human is to escape from any situation that evokes fear. When the animal successfully escapes, it learns to escape from similar situations quite rapidly and suffers no long-term effects from the experiment. This normal response is altered when an organism has previously been exposed to fear-evoking stimuli, like electric shocks, from which escape is physically impossible. Under such circumstances, the animal learns that nothing it can do alters the inevitability of the fear-provoking stimuli. Then, when presented with situations that are similar, except for the fact that now the animal can escape, it fails to do so, acting as if it were blind to the fact that an escape route lies before it. Even when it does respond effectively and the fear-evoking stimuli cease as a result, it has trouble learning, perceiving, and believing that the response worked. Repeated experiences with such helplessness produces learning, motivational, and emotional problems in animals and humans (Seligman 1992). Physically, the immune response is altered and the animals are more susceptible to tumors and to infections (Shavit 1991). Helplessness has also been associated in humans and animals with increased risk of death not as a result of the overwhelming fear, but as a result of passivity, of giving up and giving into death (Seligman 1992). According to Seligman's findings, only one third of animals tested were resistant to these effects and behaved normally and we have much yet to learn about the factors which may produce such resilience.

People who are traumatized have been exposed to an acute experience of impaired self-efficacy and helplessness. They were unable to prevent or terminate the traumatic experience. They had no control over what was happening to them. They were helpless. For children raised in abusive or neglectful homes, this failure to achieve a feeling of competence or efficacy often pervades their entire development. Regardless of what they do, how hard they try to please, how fast they run away, how strenuously they try not to cry—nothing stops the abuse. As a result they often give up any notion that they can affect the course of their lives in a positive way. Many children who are not physically or sexually abused are emotionally abused. Their sense of self-efficacy can be seriously undermined by disparaging comments, and by ridiculing and humiliating statements, from parents, teachers, schoolmates, and other caretakers. This absence or loss of self-efficacy can be countered with positive social encouragement, persuasion, and example. Unfortunately, helpless people often evoke rejecting and cruel responses on the part of the people they need most, those who could most influence a more positive outcome.

Decision Making

How impaired our thinking becomes depends on the magnitude of the danger and the possibility for loss. When frightened, our thinking becomes overly simplistic and we are unable to deal with a variety of categories of thought. We do not recognize all the alternatives open to us and instead tend to focus on the quickest way to escape. When severely stressed, we are unable to think clearly, to consider the long-range consequences of our behavior, to weigh all of the possible options before making a decision, to take the time to obtain all the necessary information that goes into making good decisions. As a consequence, our decisions are inflexible, oversimplied, and often very poorly constructed. At such times we minimize the effort we put into problem solving because our body has oriented us towards taking action, not towards thinking calmly about the situation. (Fish-Murray et al. 1987; Janis 1982; Janis and Mann 1977).

From an evolutionary point of view, it makes sense that when we perceive that we are in danger, we are geared to rapidly appraise a situation and take action. After all, thinking about the logical alternatives and long-range consequences of our decisions takes up valuable time that could be spent in running away from the danger. The problem, of course, is that modern life provides us with many situations that induce acute stress that are not, in fact, life-threatening situations, but our bodies and minds still respond as if they were. As a consequence, whenever we are overly stressed, we are unable to problem-solve well. The chronic experience of overwhelming arousal can lead to serious impairments in decision making over time. Thinking increasingly becomes dominated by the avoidance of stimuli that will trigger a hyperarousal response. Impulsive, violent behavior is often the result.

If escape is impossible, we will give up, and instead of searching for an escape we will turn to avoidance measures to diminish anxiety or other painful feelings. This defensive avoidance may take many forms, including distraction and dissociation, use of alcohol or drugs, dependence on someone else for decision making, or rationalizing attempts that are bound to fail and trying anyway.

Learning Under Stress—State-dependent Learning

Learning is dependent on the ability to categorize incoming material. We can categorize information and make new categories only when we are in a state of relative calm and attentiveness. High levels of stress shut down the normal categorization ability of the brain. Children who are repeatedly exposed to overwhelming stress cannot learn as well as more protected children.

Learning is also dependent on the state of consciousness we are in when the learning occurs. Fear creates a very special state of consciousness. Fear conditioning happens very rapidly in animals and humans. A single experience is sufficient, and once established, the automatic, physical response to the object of fear is relatively permanent. People can overcome their fear response, but they really do not "unlearn." Instead, higher brain centers inhibit and control the fear response but the "emotional memory" remains (Le Doux 1994). It is possible that once fear is learned, it can never be unlearned at a basic physiological level.

Whatever is learned when we are frightened gets attached to the fear "file drawer" in our minds. Whenever fear is triggered again, it is the drawer labeled "fear experiences" that is accessed, and no other file drawer can be easily accessed. When people are triggered by reminders of past trauma, they become hyperaroused, and only learning gained during past experiences of hyperarousal and danger will be available to them. If they have learned that lashing out physically at a threatening person helps to protect them, then whenever they feel threatened a sequence of automatic learned behavior will take hold, and they may lash out aggressively. If they have learned that the only way they can protect themselves is by becoming numb, they may go into a trance so that their conscious mind cannot feel the abuse. Later, when they are in another frightening situation, they may automatically enter such a trance, even in situations where they could take more effective action. In non-threatening situations, however, these same people may be quite capable of normal learning and behavior. Understanding this sequence of events can help us understand the apparently erratic behavior of so many children who the teacher knows can do better but who seem to sabotage themselves repeatedly.

This phenomenon can interfere with the efforts of others to help the victim. Most helping professionals can give examples of times they sit in the office with someone seeking advice on how to get out of or protect himself or herself from a dangerous situation. Together the therapist and the victim carefully formulate a strategy for self-protection. In the calm circumstances of such an interchange, the victim is in a state of mind that is conducive to learning. Unfortunately, once the victim returns to the threatening situation, he or she becomes quickly hyperaroused. In that very different state of consciousness, the information shared in the previous meeting with the therapist is not available. Under conditions of fear, the victim cannot think clearly and instead reverts to the behavior that he or she has learned in previous states of danger. Once calm is restored, the victim may never return to visit the therapist because of the shame of having failed.

Once an organism has had experiences with helplessness and a lack of control, it has difficulty learning that it has escaped from danger, even when it has successfully done so (Seligman 1992). Something happens to the organism's normal ability to learn from its experience. Recovery is possible, but not easy. Seligman and his colleagues tried various things to get their animals remotivated. They coaxed, they bribed, they seduced them to find out that they were safe—that they could get away. But the only thing that worked was physical demonstration—they had to literally drag the animals across the barrier so that the animals could learn to terminate the shocks themselves. After anywhere from 25 to 200 draggings the animals finally caught on, although each successive dragging required less and less force as the training progressed. The results were total and long-lasting (Seligman 1992).

In humans too, learned helplessness is hard to eradicate. It may contribute to the difficulties experienced by victims of various types of abuse when they know they are in situations of danger but are unable to escape and are unable to picture life in any other way. It has been frequently noted that battered wives often have an extremely difficult time escaping from their husbands; that prolonged captivity often results in a reluctance to leave the situation; that abused children find it difficult even as adults to leave their abusive families; that prison inmates and chronically mentally ill patients often feel safe only within institutions. But dragging people out of their "cages" is a difficult task and few helping professionals have the patience to last through two hundred potential trials, nor does the health care system any longer permit such an investment of time, effort, and money.

Remembering Under Stress

There is much yet to be discovered about the complex process of human memory. All I can hope to do in this brief section is acquaint the reader with some of the ongoing investigations and hints that we have gathered thus far about how memory and traumatic memory work. We know that there are at least two different kinds of memory (Squire 1987) and we know that memory is often profoundly altered as a result of overwhelming stress. The exact mechanisms, however, are still under active investigation.

The memory we think of as "normal" memory is called declarative or explicit memory. This memory system is grounded in our use of language. Our brain automatically categorizes every new experience. We begin creating these categories at birth and continue making new categories of information until we die. These categories comprise a system of mental schemata that are verbally encoded and become integrated into the already existing knowledge base. Most of this activity occurs in the part of the brain known as the hippocampus. This language-based system is a relatively time-consuming mechanism which does not lend itself to emergency situations in which immediate response is necessary. Thinking takes time. Additionally, the declarative memory system is open to change and distortion, both by previous experience, by new information, and by the state of arousal that the person is in at the time of recall.

But throughout every day we are drawing upon another kind of memory that does not require words, or even thoughts. This system is known by various terms including nondeclarative, implicit, or procedural memory (Southwick et al. 1994; Squire 1987; Van der Kolk 1994, 1996c). This is the memory of habits, skills, conditioned emotional responses, and conditioned sensorimotor responses. This is the memory we automatically draw upon when we go out to drive our car in the morning, or start riding a bicycle flawlessly for the first time in decades. This memory system is not language-based and appears to be controlled largely by areas of the brain separate from our normal memory, most importantly in a structure called the amygdala. The implicit memory system developed earlier in evolution than our

more recently evolved verbal, explicit memory system and may also be oper-
ational far earlier in our development than the verbal system that does not
become available until later in development when the child begins to understand speech (Le Doux 1994; Van der Kolk 1994). Children may, in fact,
have nonverbal memories long before they have memories that can be given
any kind of verbal form. These memories may then linger as vague physical
sensations, emotions, and sensory images and not as verbal messages.

The implicit memory system functions much faster than our verbally
based memory system and has been called a "quick and dirty reaction
mechanism" (Le Doux 1994). It is the amygdala that appears to attach emotional meaning to our experience, even before we have recognized what we
are reacting to or what we are feeling and then the higher critical areas elab-
orates that experience and imbues it with meaning. This aspect of memory
is especially important in the processing of "fear conditioning" and therefore centrally involved in how we manage fear. This is important because so
many psychiatric disorders, including posttraumatic stress disorder, appear
to involve some malfunction in the brain's ability to control fear (Le Doux
1994).

Under normal conditions, both memory systems are available for opti-
mal functioning. We are able to freely access information and draw upon
biographical material. Emotional experience is attached to these memories,
but our day-to-day life is not dominated by powerfully emotionally charged
memories or intrusive experiences from the past. The past remains in the
past and is not experienced as the present. Under normal circumstances
these two memory systems work in parallel and their activities are seam-
lessly interconnected at the level of our conscious experience. We are consciously aware of the information from the hippocampal system and the
other system remains unconscious, out of our awareness but always exert-
ing a powerful influence (Le Doux 1994)

Our way of remembering things—storing new memories, and drawing
upon old memories—is dramatically changed when we are under stress.
Studies have shown that emotional memories with personal relevance tend
to be quite accurate and long-lasting in contrast with memories of meaningless events that are measured in laboratory memory experiments (Yuille
and Cutshall 1989). For the past century, many observers have noticed that
the imprint of traumatic experiences is very different from the memories of
normal events.

Bremner and his colleagues (1995) recently reviewed the differences
between "normal forgetting" and traumatic amnesia. They point out that

from an evolutionary point of view, the efficient recall of memories associated with previous danger is crucial for survival. If you are in a forest and hear a loud growl behind you, it is far better for your brain to flash up an image of a threatening beast, or just a feeling of intense fear that impels you to run, than it is for your brain to stop and ponder in words a series of alternative explanations, options, or actions. After all, we are evolved from animals who lacked verbal capacities, and yet their survival depended on remembering danger. But it is difficult to explain how the over-remembering of danger associated with PTSD is adaptive or why so many people develop under-remembering, or amnesia, in the face of danger.

People who have experienced a variety of differing traumas are noted to have a wide range of memory problems with vivid intrusive memories of a past event (flashbacks) often alternating with partial or total amnesia for the traumatic events. These intrusive experiences appear to be triggered by emotions and sensations in the present that are associated with the traumatic past and the person often has amnesia for the occurrence of the flashback as well as the original trauma (Van der Kolk and McFarlane 1996).

People under severe stress secrete neurohormones that affect the way that their memories are stored. In animals—and there is a growing body of evidence to support a similar effect in humans—high levels of glucocorticoids secreted during stress impair the functioning of the hippocampus and neuroimaging techniques indicate that changes in the very structure of the hippocampus may be secondary to prolonged stress (Bremner et al 1995; Van der Kolk 1996c). This may partially or totally disable the ability of the brain to verbally categorize incoming information. At the same time, during states of high fear, the amygdala is extremely active and interferes with hippocampal functioning (Van der Kolk 1996c). The result is a partial or complete loss of the ability to assign words to incoming experience, the biological equivalent of "speechless terror" (Van der Kolk 1994, 1996c, Van der Kolk and Fisler 1995). Dependent upon words, our capacity to logically think through a problem is diminished or entirely shut down and our minds shift to a mode of consciousness that is characterized by visual, auditory, kinesthetic images, and physical sensations as well as strong feelings.

Evidence also exists that the massive secretion of neurohormones at the time of the trauma may deeply imprint the traumatic memory (Van der Kolk 1994, 1996c). The neuroscientist Le Doux (1992) has termed this "emotional memory." In studying the influence of fear in particular, he has shown that emotional memory appears to be permanent and quite difficult, if not impossible, to eliminate although it can be suppressed by higher centers in the brain (Le Doux 1992; 1994). This "engraving" of trauma has been noted by many researchers studying various survivor groups (Van der Kolk 1994; Van der Kolk and Van der Hart 1991).

But these memory effects do not happen to everyone who is exposed to overwhelming stress indicating that there must be much individual variation in the way the mind and body responds to trauma. Nor do we have a complete way of accounting for the fact that people who suffer from PTSD often have both intrusive recollections *and* amnesias. The evolving model of trauma-related memory indicates that there is a complex interaction between the event, the individual, and the context of the event. Some people are more reactive to external events than others and appear to be that way from birth. Some people more readily develop associations to different stimuli than others. Some people tend to ruminate more than others. Others are comparatively more distractible than other people. All of these factors, and probably others, may influence how memory is processed at the time of the trauma and subsequently (Yehuda 1996).

There may also be significant differences between acute and chronic stress exposure. Whereas acute stress triggers an increased level of steroids (i.e. cortisol), chronic stress produces decreased steroid levels, decreased responsiveness due to a new acute stress, and other changes that may help to explain the very complex and interactive nature of memory problems after trauma (Yehuda et al. 1995).

Traumatic memory often poses the greatest problems for people who have suffered repeated or severe traumatic experience. The intrusive symptoms of post-traumatic stress disorder—the nightmares, and the sensory, emotional, and physical flashbacks—all appear to be a result of disordered memory functioning. But traumatic experience has also been noted for the predominance of amnesia in the clinical picture as well. For the last century clinicians and researchers have been reporting the presence of traumatic amnesia in many different survivor groups (Bremner et al. 1995). This alternation between hyperamnesia and amnesia is one of the most problematic aspects of stress disorders.

On the one hand, the traumatic memories are vivid and intrusive. These memories do not fade, nor do they seem to be altered by ordinary experiences. They are state-dependent—they tend to intrude into consciousness when they are triggered by a state that resembles the state experienced at the time of the original traumatic event. Flashbacks are likely to occur when people are upset, stressed, frightened, or aroused or when triggered by any association to the traumatic event (Van der Kolk 1994, 1996c). In a study by Van der Kolk and Fisler (1995), all subjects, regardless of the age at which the trauma occurred, reported that their initial memory was not in the form of a narrative, but was instead a somatosensory or emotional flashback experience. Seventy-five percent of the subjects with childhood trauma had external confirmation of the traumatic experience.

Sleep may be seriously disturbed by vivid and horrifying nightmares that replay the events of the traumatic experience until the victim wakes up screaming in terror. Combat veterans have been known to assault their spouses during a nightmare, mistaking the body in bed next to them as the enemy in their dream. Some nightmares are the replay of the actual traumatic event and some are disguised representations of the trauma, hidden behind frightening symbols. Some nightmares decrease in frequency over time and just seem to fade away until triggered by a new stress. Others appear to become incorporated into other thematic experiences of life, often of earlier trauma or symbolized conflicts (Lansky and Bley 1995).

There is now some data available from positron emission tomography that provides more information about these intrusive phenomenon. Traumatic memories "happen" principally in the emotional areas of the brain's right hemisphere, and are accompanied by an increase in activity in the visual areas of the brain, signifying that people with PTSD actually "see" their flashbacks, while there is a decrease in the area of the brain in charge of the translation of emotional states into language (Rauch et al. 1996; Van der Kolk in press; Van der Kolk and Fisler 1995). This is experienced by the person as a total or partial reliving of the traumatic experience. It can be a sensory fragment of the trauma or the entire traumatic sequence running like a virtual reality movie. In such a state the traumatized person has difficulties distinguishing reality from flashback. The sensory experience is often quite vivid, feeding a vicious cycle of autonomic arousal that increases the sense of reality of the flashback even more.

When people experience intrusive flashbacks as visual, olfactory, affective, auditory, or kinesthetic sensations, although we term this "traumatic memory" it bears little if any relationship to the normal process of remembering. Remembering in our normal terms is based on language while traumatic recall is nonlinguistic. Gradually, as people begin to sort out these intrusive images, they begin to form a narrative as a means of explaining their experience. Once such an experience enters the narrative sphere it may be open to many of the distortions and changes related to "normal" memory processing, the distortions so highlighted by the false memory advocates. This is one of the difficulties in the public discourse about true memory and "false memory." Linguistic difficulties have helped to muddy this entire issue. The same words—"memory," "forgetting," and "remembering"—are used to describe two entirely different phenomena which appear to have different neuroanatomical and neurophysiological bases, as well as entirely different clinical presentations[3].

Amnesias are another significantly disturbing aspect of stress disorders. Amnesia develops as a result of the mechanism known as "dissociation." To understand dissociation we need to understand something about the way we order reality.

Ordering Reality Under Stress

We are a naming, categorizing, ordering species. We do it automatically, unconsciously, and constantly. We are compelled by the structure and function of our brain to make sense, to make meaning out of every experience. This demand had been termed the "cognitive imperative" (Laughlin, McManus, and, D'Aquili 1979). All new information must be mentally organized into a category that we have been establishing since birth. These categories are based on words and requires that our brain—particularly our dominant, verbal hemisphere, is working properly. When anything interferes with this categorization process we experience unpleasant feelings. One of the words for this is "cognitive dissonance." In experimental situations, when people receive anesthesia on the dominant side of the brain alone, thus preventing this normal organization of experience, they feel guilt and unworthiness, worries about the future, and a sense of loss of mastery over the environment. Overwhelming trauma appears to interfere with this organizing capacity as well. When this happens, our minds will not let us rest (d'Aquili and Laughlin 1979). The unresolvable nature of the conflict continues to arouse bad feelings and this draws our attention to the contradictory information until the mind has managed to put the confusing information into a more comfortable mental "box."

Conditions of high stress may impair the capacity to order reality normally due to the profound effects of stress hormones on the verbal capacities of the brain. When the stressed individual appraises the dangerous situation and finds it inescapable then he or she is quite likely to avoid reality, often by reordering and redefining reality entirely (Janis and Mann 1977, Schumaker 1995).

A certain amount of denial and avoidance of reality is healthy. Were we to focus constantly on our mortality we could easily become nonfunctional. Fear of dying would prevent us from living. Similarly, in the presence of life threat, avoidance of reality is a very good—often lifesaving—idea. To some extent we understand this phenomenon in its acute form. The lay term for it is "shock," the clinical term is "dissociation." After a one-time, consensually validated traumatic experience such as an earthquake, people are likely to be understanding of someone in "shock." Over the next few hours, days, or weeks the environment will provide many opportunities and cues providing the affected person with opportunities to gradually get back in touch with what has really happened and begin to integrate the experience with the overwhelming emotions.

Problems arise, however, when the trauma does not stop, or when it is too severe for anyone to deal with, or when it is a secret trauma that no one else is allowed to know about. In cases like these the gap between everyday reality and traumatic reality can continue to increase. The individual cannot deal with the traumatic experience because it continues to pose some kind of life threat and the culture cannot or will not help the person come to terms with the experience. The person is unable to establish a coherent and consistent sense of identity because the traumatized self is directly in conflict with the normal self. He or she is unable to establish a comprehensive and flexible meaning system or philosophy of life because they harbor too many internal contradictions. Under these circumstances dissociation becomes a way of life and the disintegration of the person continues.

Dissociation

The brain mechanism that allows us to define individual reality to accommodate to unsettling events, while remaining aware of another reality, is called *dissociation*. Dissociation is a part of normal human functioning and occurs under normal circumstances. When you leave the house in the morning, become deeply involved in thinking about your plans for the day and find yourself in the parking lot at work, oblivious to the details of the actual drive to work, you have been in a dissociative, or trance state. A hidden and automatic part of you has taken over the driving function, stopped at the appropriate moments, avoided accidents, and guaranteed that you arrive at your desired destination.

Dissociation is a highly evolved mechanism, allowing us increased efficiency by being able to accomplish two tasks at once. One task is in consciousness, one is happening outside of conscious awareness. But there is still a form of knowing about even what was outside of consciousness, termed a "hidden observer" (Hilgard 1986). Speculation is growing that this dual-self phenomenon may have a structural basis in the existence of two separate cerebral hemispheres that intercommunicate under normal circumstances but that each assimilate information in very different ways (Joseph 1992). Whatever the brain basis for the differences between the conscious and unconscious aspects of our mind turns out to be, it has become clear that we do not have one unified "self" but instead are "a unity and a multiplicity at once" (Beahrs 1983). It is disconcerting to recognize that we have very different and often contradictory aspects of what we think of as "me," aspects that often react and behave in ways that make us uncomfortable or ashamed. We like to believe that we are always in charge of ourselves, always in control of what we are doing, saying, thinking, feeling, and remembering. As a result, we try to avoid any recognition that we have a split nature, preferring to believe in the largely nonexistent unity of consciousness (Tinnin 1990).

As we grow up, many adults constrict their ability to lose themselves in play. But children move between various aspects of reality quite fluidly. This capacity for dissociation is natural and provides children with the opportunity to rehearse new behaviors through play that can be incorporated later as a useful piece of reality. Children often have imaginary playmates and each playmate represents a dissociated part of themselves that they can utilize as a way of mastering unpleasant feeling states while they learn how to integrate those feelings into a coherent sense of self. The good boy, Tommie, can have an imaginary bad boy, Fred, who manages the child's hostile feelings towards his parents. With healthy parental responses, the child gradually learns to tolerate both loving and hostile feelings as part of his experience of himself.

Dissociation is a particularly useful mechanism during times of high stress. When we are put in situations of danger, we become hyperaroused. Such high states of arousal can be associated with severe cognitive disorganization. Additionally, these same states of arousal are intimately connected with physiological states of high response as well, such as rapid heart rate and increased blood pressure. Past a certain point such physiological hyperarousal can be associated with death (Selye 1982). Long-standing accounts have been recorded of both children and adults being literally "scared to death" (DeMause 1982). The mind has the capacity to defend against the disorganizing, possibly life-threatening outcome of this emotional arousal—a built-in "safety valve." That capacity is dissociation.

People dissociate in different ways. Fainting is an extreme form of simply stopping consciousness. But we can also split off memories from consciousness through "amnesia." We can maintain awareness of what is going on around us but feel no disturbing emotions about it—emotional numbing. We can lose our sense of identity entirely and spontaneously create a new one and begin a new life, a condition known as "fugue." We can set aside our tortured emotions and thoughts and put the entire conflict into a physical symptom such as blindness or paralysis, a symptom picture known as "conversion disorder." We can dissociate ourselves from our value systems and our conscience, which may be what allows otherwise relatively normal people to commit unconscionable acts under acute stress.

When stress is severe, prolonged, and/or repeated, dissociation can become a preferential way of dealing with stress, particularly if the stress originates in childhood or captivity. Political prisoners and victims of torture become expert at teaching themselves to get away from reality (Herman 1992). When this occurs the person may develop very separate bodies of experience, memory, knowledge, and feeling to deal with different stressful situations. It becomes possible then, for the person who has established this tendency to enter these different states of consciousness automatically whenever the particular need arises. Under circumstances of repeated stress, the defensive capacity of dissociation is highly adaptive. But what happens when the stress is reduced and things return to normal? Do we just return to normal life, unchanged by what has happened? Does this ingenious ability have a down side, a negative aspect?

By separating thoughts from feelings, feelings from memory, or thoughts from memory, the body protects itself from being overwhelmed. The person is then able to think without being overwhelmed by terror or despair. People can get things back to normal if they have "forgotten" the events, or at least have "forgotten" the disturbing emotions of the events. If people remain totally isolated from any stimuli that remind them of the events, they may be able to wall off the traumatic events and push them out of consciousness for a lifetime. However, only rarely does a person experience a severe stress that is so isolated and unique that there are no further associations to the event. This is partly because stressful events generally occur in the context of routine daily life and partly because of the associational nature of our brains, which can form astonishingly complex networks of associations between any idea and image.

Car accidents occur on highways, in vehicles that are unavoidable if someone in the United States is to live a semblance of a normal life. Children are abused in bedrooms and bathrooms and kitchens that are equipped with mass produced furnishings that might be encountered anywhere. The stump of a finger lost in an industrial accident is a constant reminder of all of the circumstances of that accident. In order to keep those events—or parts of those events—out of consciousness the person must expend a great deal of psychic energy, which is then unavailable for full and integrated functioning. So why, then, do we often struggle so hard not to know, not to remember, to remain dissociated? That depends to some extent on the particular stress. Common to all stress however, is its tendency to evoke the same response to danger even if the stress no longer presents a danger but is now only a memory of former events. An example of how this works may be helpful.

A Cast for a Broken Heart

Paul has a heart attack while eating out at a restaurant with his wife, Mary. He receives CPR from an emergency medical team. The experience is particularly traumatic because he does not lose consciousness immediately but instead experiences the pain and terror of imminent death. He recovers from the heart attack, grateful for another chance at life, grateful to the people who helped him in the crisis. A successful person who values self-control, Paul immediately "forgets" the terror of the experience and presents to the world a model of self-sufficient post-cardiac survival. All of his emotional and physical energy at this point, needs to be focused on survival and rehabilitation. Consequently, emotional recovery, if it is even recognized as important, is delayed.

Not long after release from the hospital, however, he begins to experience some mild anxiety at indeterminate times—indeterminate only because he does not know what to look for. In fact the anxiety occurs when he sits across from a table with his wife, when he goes to a restaurant, whenever an emergency vehicle drives by or he hears sirens, whenever he sees someone with the vivid blue eyes of the EMT who gave him CPR, whenever he smells the aroma of fried onions, which permeated the restaurant. Each individual will develop their own associations to the trauma or to aspects of the trauma, and these associations that can be visual, tactile, auditory, olfactory, or ideational.

Paul makes no association between his anxiety and his heart attack. He attributes his anxiety to stress at work. The outcome of this particular scenario is as varied as the individuals who experience it. One man might begin drinking excessively to calm the anxiety, another might become addicted to tranquilizers, another might focus the problem on discomfort with his wife and end up divorced, another might vent his frustration by hitting his children, another might develop a depressive disorder; and yet another might develop a peptic ulcer.

If he does recognize that the onset of his symptoms seems to be coincident with his heart attack, or if a well-intended friend tries to tell him so, he will meet with great internal resistance. Because the original dissociation of mental contents occurred under conditions of serious danger, attempts to re-enter those conditions, even if only in imagination, are met with the same danger signals that were associated with the original circumstances.

As a result of those danger signals which he experiences as feelings of acute discomfort and fear as well as physiological arousal—increased heart rate, increased sweating, increased respiration—Paul refuses to think about the past, avoids any associations to the past, and finds any distraction he can to elude the supposed danger. We must remember, however, that at this point there is no actual threat; the only threat present is that which comes from his own memory and the attendant associated thoughts, feelings, and bodily responses. These associations have now taken on a quasi-life of their own because of the mechanism of dissociation.

This is how a formerly highly adaptive capacity turns into a habitual problem. Paul's original dissociation is useful in that it protects him from further harm that could have occurred as the result of his own overwhelming emotional state. Because he is not emotionally paralyzed throughout the time of crisis, he is able to actively participate in his own recovery and enhance the chances of his own survival. However, after the emergency is over and the threat is removed, the continued use of this defense becomes highly maladaptive.

Dissociation is an internal "cast" that the brain places around "broken" emotions to protect the break from further harm, analogous to a plaster cast on a broken leg. There is wisdom in the concept of a "broken heart." As in the leg held too long in the cast after the bone has knit together, the continued use of this dissociative cast will produce an atrophy of the emotional "muscles" that we all need to adequately propel ourselves through life in an integrated fashion.

Like the leg in the cast, the emotions that are bound up and immobilized are unavailable for normal use, thus significantly restricting the range of emotional depth and breadth. When a leg is broken, muscles in the other leg often become hypertrophied or enlarged, throwing the usually well-balanced system out of alignment. With broken emotions, a similar experience occurs because other emotions fill in for the dissociated feelings.

In Paul's case, he has dissociated the emotional experience of fear. Now, whenever a fearful stimulus is registered, he will not be able to utilize his normal fear emotion because it is immobilized in the cast. Instead, he may experience rage whenever fear should be there. Or he may have a drink or smoke a joint or a cigarette whenever something—or somebody—gets near his injury. Or he may deny the fear totally and place himself repeatedly in situations that are dangerous and should normally evoke fear as a warning that he is inadequately protected. He may refuse to follow his doctor's orders about exercise, diet, activity level, medication, or quitting smoking because any variation in his habits will remind him of his heart attack, and that will evoke the underlying fear, which is walled-off and unavailable in its emotional dissociative cast.

There appears to be some requirement for full integrity, or whole function, on the part of living systems. Although we can stay alive under circumstances of minimal nutrition, light, oxygen, water, our growth will be stunted and often full consciousness, including the capacity for learning, will be severely compromised. Evolution has provided us with excellent survival strategies that do not necessitate the realization of our full potential. The most basic functions of life will be preserved even if the higher functions are impaired or destroyed, evidenced by the many accident and stroke victims incapable of complex cerebral function, but still able to breathe and maintain other bodily functions.

It is quite possible, therefore, for human beings to function in dissociative states, to have highly fragmented personality functioning as a result, and still maintain life. It is the higher, more integrated functions that are impaired. The more complex and specialized the organism, the more vulnerable it is to the negative results of disorganization or impairment in function of any of its parts. The more complex the system, the greater the need for integration and communication.

Dissociation in Childhood

Formerly well-adjusted adults usually fare better than children who have been traumatized. They at least have some memory, some idea of what normal is or was. The situation is quite different for children. The ease with which children are able to use dissociation makes it likely that they will dissociate under conditions of stress as a preferred defense to protect themselves from becoming emotionally overwhelmed (James 1994). Given the powerlessness and defenselessness of children, dissociation is often the only thing they can do to protect themselves.

Children who are traumatized do not have developed coping skills, a developed sense of self, or a developed sense of their self in relation to others. Their system of mental schemata, of how they make sense of the world, is still forming. As a consequence, all of the responses to trauma are amplified because they interfere with the processes of normal development. Many children lack a concept of what is normal or healthy because traumatic experience has become their normative childhood experience. Raised in abusive, violent, neglectful homes, they have never learned how to think in a careful, quiet, and deliberate way. They have not learned how to have mutual, compassionate, and satisfying relationships. They have not learned how to listen carefully to the messages of their body and their senses. Their sense of self has been determined by the experiences they have had with caretaking adults, and the trauma they have experienced has taught then that they are bad, worthless, ineffective, a nuisance, or worse.

Less understood has been what happens to children's growing sense of identity when they are exposed to repeated and overwhelming stress. In these cases, their identity does not solidify around a solid core (James 1989; Putnam 1990). Instead it remains fragmented, and the fragments are separated from and inaccessible to each other. The most extreme cases were formerly called "multiple personality disorder," and are now called "dissociative identity disorder." Each separated fragment is constituted by an array of associated memories, feelings, and behaviors that remain largely unintegrated from each other.

The end result of chronic dissociation in childhood may be a serious inability to understand or contend with concensual reality. Most childhood abuse is hidden and denied. On the surface, some nonviolent forms of sexual abuse may not even appear to be traumatic. It is not necessarily the pain or terror that is the most traumatic aspect of a childhood experience but the betrayal that is so damaging (Freyd 1996). Children are helplessly dependent on their caregivers. In order to survive, they must trust those on whom they depend. When those caregivers turn out to be untrustworthy, children must deny this reality. Often this betrayal is denied or minimized by the perpetrator as well as by other family members and other members of the child's community. This means that the experience of individual reality becomes increasingly divergent from cultural reality. The individual symptoms are related to the child's or adult's attempt to individually make sense of a distorted reality (Schumaker 1995). The child, in such a situation, must make a choice. Deny your own individual reality and fit into the culture, or defy the cultural beliefs and end up alone and eccentric or even "crazy." It is an impossible choice.

Long-term Effects of Chronic Dissociation

We are beginning to understand that chronic dissociation has serious long-term consequences for healthy human functioning. As we move up the evolutionary ladder from reptiles to mammals and then to humans, there is a dramatic increase in brain integration and intercommunication between different areas of the brain. The increasing capability of computers is a result of their increasing integration and networking of bodies of information. Dissociation reduces the capacity for integration. It is "designed" to be an emergency and temporary measure to deal with specific threatening environmental circumstances. When the emergency situation has ceased to be a crisis, we are supposed to integrate the split-off mental contents back into our full range of consciousness and allow ourselves to learn from the cognitive and emotional experience. Unfortunately, what needs to happen often does not happen for various biological and cultural reasons, and as a result dissociated mental contents may continue to pose a significant impairment in the capacity for integrated function in the individual, and perhaps in the society at large. Let us speculate about the reasons why this system that starts out being so protective ends up being so destructive.

The accurate perception of our emotional states is vital to our survival. People who do not experience pain repeatedly injure themselves. People who are unable to feel anger repeatedly are victimized, while those who are chronically angry may victimize others. People who cannot feel love, compassion, or tenderness have severely impaired relationships with others in their social group. People who do not experience fear lack the capacity to protect themselves. However, these emotional states must function in an integrated way with the higher mental states of reason, moral choice, and self-control if the person is to survive adequately in a civilized world. The more complex the culture, the more necessary is a high level of integration.

As this process of dissociation continues over time, we gradually may shut-off more and more of our normal functioning (Herman 1992; Schetky 1990; Southwick et al. 1993). We will dampen down any emotional experience that could lead back to it. We will withdraw from relationships that could trigger memories. We will curtail sensory and physical experiences that could remind us of the trauma. We will avoid engaging in situations that could lead to remembering the trauma. At the same time, we will be compelled, completely outside of our awareness, to reenact the traumatic experience through our behavior. This increases the likelihood that instead of managing to avoid repeated trauma, we are likely to become traumatized again.

If dissociation continues, our sense of who we are, how we fit into the world, how we relate to other people, and what the point of it all is can become significantly limited in scope. As this occurs, we are likely to become increasingly depressed. These *avoidance* symptoms, along with the *intrusive* symptoms, such as flashbacks and nightmares, comprise the two interacting and escalating aspects of post-traumatic stress syndrome. As these alternating symptoms come to dominate traumatized people's lives, they feel more and more alienated from everything that gives human life meaning—themselves, other people, a sense of direction and purpose, a sense of community. It is not surprising, then, that slow self-destruction through addictions, or fast self-destruction through suicide, is often the final outcome of these syndromes. For other people, rage at others comes to dominate the picture. These are the ones who end up becoming significant threats to the well-being of the rest of us.

The person who has dissociated memories, thoughts, and feelings cannot utilize those mental contents in an integrated fashion. In this way, his or her long-term adaptation to the environment, and therefore survival, is compromised by the continued dissociation of emotional experience. It is relatively easy to see this mechanism in action with our cardiac patient. The dissociated mental contents may prevent him from taking proper medical advice that directly affects his health. This danger to long-term adaptation, however, can be more subtle when the adaptation under discussion is adaptation of a family or of a whole species.

People who chronically dissociate are caught in a recursive loop that informs them that they must continue to fight for their lives, long after the threat to life is over. This is why advice such as "pull yourself together" or "just get over it" or "put the past behind you" is so ineffective. They cannot control how their bodies automatically respond. They cannot command that their memories be properly restored, categorized, and stowed. They are trapped in a past that they experience as the present.

THE EMOTIONAL RESPONSE TO DANGER

Basic Affect Theory

"Affect" is the word given to the basic biological component of emotional experience. According to Tomkins, who built on Darwin's work, we are born with nine different affects—seven of which he named with two words to indicate the mild and the intense presentation of the affect: interest-excitement, enjoyment-joy, surprise-startle, distress-anguish, fear-terror, shame-humiliation, and anger-rage. The other two affects refer initially to the hunger drive and he called them dissmell (our reaction to offensive smells) and disgust (our reaction to unpleasant tastes). Each of these affects is associated with typical facial and bodily expressions that are innate and can be seen on human infants throughout the world (Nathanson 1992). Current research also indicates that each affect may evoke a separate and distinct pattern of autonomic nervous system activity and physiological response (Lazarus 1991). Additionally, each affect is linked with specific patterns of intonation, vocal quality, rhythm, pausing, and posture (Hatfield et al. 1994).

Role of Emotions

Since the affect system is innate and connected to every organ system of the body, we must assume that the experience of affect has a far-reaching survival value. Nature does not waste time evolving complex systems without vital purpose. Yet science has devoted little time or energy to researching the causes and effects of affect states. Emotions are one of those aspects of human existence that are so fundamental, so vital, and so pervasive that we fail to even think about them. We tend to notice them only when they are causing problems for us—when they are disorganizing thought, interfering with communication, or propelling negative actions. At the same time, we appear to crave emotional experiences, as witnessed by our preoccupation with emotion-evoking movies, television, books, and experiences. Depressed people often lose the capacity to experience emotions and frequently comment that a life without feeling is not worth living. So, what are emotions there for? Why did nature evolve such a complicated and troubling system? Darwin pointed out that each emotion readied the organism to act in ways that give it an increased ability to survive and that the non-verbal expression of emotion is universal and independent of cultural training (Nathanson 1992).

Cognitive Role of Emotions

According to Tomkins, affect draws our attention to something, determines what information reaches our consciousness, and motivates our behavior (Nathanson 1992). Emotions can be seen as a "sensitive mental radar" alerting us to the significance of things that happen to us externally or within our bodies (Harber and Pennebaker 1992). This has important survival value because without affect, we would be unable to pick out important information from the myriad forms of experience and objects that are constantly surrounding us. It is important that we feel fear in the presence of something that looks like a snake and pleasure when we look at water. We are biologically programmed to experience pleasure in doing things that are potentially good for us—eating, sleeping, exercising, having sex, socializing with other people, dancing, drawing, singing, playing, pretending—and distress in doing things that are potentially dangerous for us—hunger, fatigue, immobility, lack of sexual behavior, isolation from others, restriction of creative activities, detailed and repetitive tasks.

Emotions also play an important role in ordering our environment. Because we have such a powerful need to categorize and arrange information in our minds (the cognitive imperative), and because our memory is dependent on such categorization, we cannot rest as long as something remains confusing or conflictual. It is affect that keeps us aware of the discrepancy, and the affective arousal does not stop until the conflict has been resolved by our minds. There are, however, conflicts in life that cannot be resolved. If we cannot resolve the conflict, then we must find a way to turn off the emotion. That is when we dissociate.

Social Role of Emotion

Although we are born with all the basic affects, our emotional life is not simply an internal experience, even at birth. The fact that every affect is registered in a distinct and different way, on the face and in bodily expression from the time we are born, indicates that affect plays a vital social and communicative role for affect. Affect is the connecting bridge between the individual internal world and the social external world from birth to death. Recent work on early child development shows that the infant and its mother comprise a complex caregiver system (Solomon and George 1996). The main currency of exchange at this stage of development is emotional information. The infant comes into the world as a *broadcaster* of emotional information and the infant's primary caretakers are the *receivers* of this information through a process known as *affective resonance* (Nathanson 1992) or *emotional contagion* (Hatfield et al. 1994).

Emotional Contagion

Research shows how profoundly influenced we are by other people's affect states, from birth on, how rapidly our interpersonal affective responses occur, and how dynamically our physiology responds to others' affect states (Hatfield et al. 1994). This information is conveyed not through language but through nonverbal communication that makes this system available to us even in the early stages of development. Infants only have nonverbal means of communication available to them. Babies signal their distress by crying and mothers respond to this signal by administering care to the distressed babies. Such information exchange is vital if infants are to survive. But this emotional information exchange, or emotional resonance, does not stop in childhood. We are a supremely social species, and our survival has been dependent on our individual ability to mobilize the group. An individual scout, spotting danger, is able to convey this sense of imminent threat to the group through emotionally charged tone of voice, gesture, and facial expression. The necessity for such a response preceded the development of language and is well-organized, sophisticated, and easily transmitted.

We continue to resonate to each other's emotional experience throughout our lives. How many times have we said to a intimate partner, "It's not what you said that hurt me, it's the *way* you said it." The nonverbal components of speech (called "prosody") develop in parallel with language and are controlled by the nondominant hemisphere of the brain, the same hemisphere that appears to be activated during traumatic recall. But we are usually far less aware of the way we are saying things than what we are saying, although we are exceptionally skilled at perceiving those aspects of language, even outside of consciousness, and at responding to the nonverbal communication even more strongly than we do the verbal content.

We "catch" each other's emotions all the time. The more our attention is riveted on someone else, the more interrelated we are with someone else, the more we are able to read their nonverbal expressions, the better they are at expressing their feelings nonverbally, and the more stressful the situation, the more likely we are to catch other people's emotional experience. This describes many situations of highly charged group danger in which panic rapidly rises, or in which people appear to "hysterically" catch the symptoms of each other (Hatfield et al. 1994). In such a state of danger, people will be in an altered state of consciousness, able to distort reality, easily susceptible to the contagious effect of emotion, and open to the suggestion of someone else. For similar reasons, people can have an enormous positive influence on a highly aroused individual. If they can maintain clarity and calmness, this too can be contagious, thus reducing the other person's level of arousal both emotionally and physiologically. We actually have an enormous, underestimated, and often neglected role to play in other people's emotional lives.

Emotional Arousal

Emotional reactions are also an important part of the flight-or-fight response. The dominant affects that are aroused are fear and anger. Anger prepares the person to fight an enemy and mobilizes our innate tendency toward xenophobia, or fear of the stranger. Fear prepares us to flee the situation and mobilizes our protective defenses. Too much emotion however can be self-defeating. Too much fear results in paralysis, panic, an inability to mobilize defenses. Too much anger can cloud the capacity for thought and also impair defense. Shame which is triggered when we experience ourselves as weak, incapable, inadequate, or helpless, is cognitively disorganizing, a phenomenon Nathanson (1992) has called "cognitive shock." An overload of emotion can itself kill. Dissociation can help us avoid these self-defeating maneuvers in times of danger.

It is not just actual dangerous events that trigger powerful emotional reactions and dramatic changes in the body. People can voluntarily and involuntarily stimulate their bodies to evoke the stress response even when the source of danger is imaginary or symbolic. If you concentrate on remembering a past stressful event you may notice that your heart is beating fast, your palms are sweaty, and you feel frightened. The same stress response explains how we can sit in a movie theater and be terrified or enraged by events that are purely imaginary and not part of the reality that is occurring to us at all. The movie screens of our minds present us nightly shows in our dreams, and occasionally these dreams are so real or frightening that we wake up in stark terror or rage. Fear conditioning is important as well, because as mentioned above, once we have become conditioned to a fearful stimulus we will always be afraid when that stimulus is presented. Our higher-order functions may attempt, with more or less success, to suppress the fear response, but it will be there under the surface, nonetheless.

Interference With Thought

Under normal conditions, emotions serve as "sensitive mental radar" alerting us to the significance of things around us. When people have been traumatized they no longer can predictably count on their emotions to provide the proper evaluative information. After all, powerful negative emotions can, post-traumatically, be associated with such apparently nontoxic objects as a clock on the wall, or a color of a room, or an otherwise useful kitchen object. This means that people who have been traumatized can no longer trust what they feel. Activities that should evoke pleasure may instead evoke terror, rage, or despair. People who have been sexually abused as children often find normal sexual arousal and enjoyment impossible because of the flood of noxious emotions. Likewise, activities that should be avoided may instead by sought out. People who have been traumatized often seek out high-risk and dangerous situations.

The cognitive consequence of all this is confusion. The normal ordering process of the brain is disrupted if the traumatic distortion occurs in adulthood. But it may never develop properly if the traumatic distortion begins in childhood. This confusion can disrupt learning, problem solving, decision making and all other higher order functions.

Expression and Inhibition of Emotion

The conclusion we can draw from all this is that feeling a wide ranges of emotions is normal, that experiencing very intense emotions under stress is also normal but can interfere with thinking, and that we need each other to help us modulate overpowering emotions. A growing body of research indicates that healthy human beings need to confide their thoughts and feelings about troubling events to other people and—perhaps most importantly—to themselves. Inhibiting the expression of emotion has negative consequences for both mental and physical health, and expressing emotions, particularly about traumatic events, is health-producing. Some theorists have even gone so far as to propose that self-disclosure of upsetting experiences is a basic human motive (Pennebaker 1989). The theory, which has growing research support, is that the inhibition of feelings requires physiological work that over time becomes a cumulative stressor and is associated with increases in stress-related diseases.

Unfortunately for the victim of trauma, one of the long observed results of traumatic experience is the loss of the ability to identify specific emotions and put those emotions into words that can then be shared. This phenomenon has been called "alexythmia" (Krystal 1978). The person who demonstrates alexythmia often finds other forms of expression through psychosomatic diseases or violence. The development of this problem is particularly evident in populations of abused children and may have a neuroanatomical and neurophysiological basis (Cichetti and White 1990, Van der Kolk 1996). The person who is alexythmic cannot make use of the health-promoting effects of disclosure. Instead, he or she can become locked in a cycle of isolation, traumatic re-experiencing, and traumatic reenactment.

Numbing and Loss of Modulation

The emotional effects of repeated or prolonged traumatic experience are profound. The loss of the ability to modulate internal states means that people become very labile, with rapidly shifting, easily triggered, and powerful negative emotions that are beyond their control. This loss of the ability to control one's emotional states reinforces the already established learned helplessness. Alexythmia prevents the health-promoting effects of talking about feelings with other people. The resulting internal states are so noxious that people will do whatever they can to decrease their emotional exposure. They will shut down as much as possible. This leads to emotional numbing often accompanied by a profound depression and apathy.

But no attempts at numbing are totally foolproof. As a result, emotional outbursts are not uncommon. Typically, the traumatized person has a great deal of trouble managing anger appropriately. Long periods of passivity reaching to masochism may be interrupted by bouts of uncontrollable rage in which the person may do physical harm to himself or herself or others. Accompanying this is a loss of the experience of pleasure termed "anhedonia," the loss of the ability to laugh, to cry, to experience joy, or to accept comfort from others.

Psychosomatic and Stress-related Disorders

People who are traumatized must learn to inhibit their emotional experience, partly because emotional arousal is so disruptive of normal functioning, partly because other people are unwilling to deal with people who are emotionally upset. Such inhibition appears to be intimately related to stress-related illnesses. Short-term inhibition causes increased arousal of the autonomic nervous system and long-term inhibition is a low-level and cumulative stressor. This association has held true with cancer, coronary ailments, and breast cancer as well as other illnesses (Harber and Pennebaker 1992). Inhibition is also associated with impairments in assimilating information. Certainly medical research has established that overwhelming life experiences can result in an increase in physical and psychological health problems (Holmes and Rahe 1967). The literature reviewing the relationship between trauma and health consistently demonstrates an association between catastrophic stress, adverse health reports, medical utilization, morbidity, and mortality among survivors. The findings are so significant that Friedman and Schnurr (1995) have commented, "We believe that PTSD is distinctive among psychiatric disorders in terms of its potential to promote poor health because of both the physiological and psychological abnormalities associated with this disorder." Likewise, expressing powerful emotional experiences has been found to decrease psychosomatic symptoms, but victims of trauma must contend with the reality that emotional expression is frequently culturally discouraged (Harber and Pennebaker 1992).

Impaired Social Role of Emotions

Emotions have important signal value between people. We express our emotions to each other in a variety of nonverbal ways. People who have been traumatized have extreme difficulties with emotional control. As a result they unwittingly give signals to others that are quite disturbing. Sometimes they signal too much emotion, inappropriate to the given situation. In other circumstances they signal too little, unintentionally maintaining an external mask of blankness that is confusing to the observer. Often, however, this confusion on the part of the other is not conscious. Most of what we register about each other's emotional states occurs at a level below consciousness although it profoundly effects the way we interact with each other. Because this communication experience is nonconscious, it is not usually open to spontaneous exchange between people, an exchange that could lead at least to the possibility of explanation and understanding on both people's parts.

Instead, the signals given off by the traumatized person have a strong tendency to evoke unconscious distancing and rejecting responses on the part of the other. Researchers have studied listeners' responses to victims' disclosure. What they found is very disturbing, but understandable. Listeners "don't want to hear it." They tend to disrupt trauma stories by switching the topic of conversation away from the trauma, by attempting to press their own perspective of the trauma upon the victims, or by simply avoiding contact with the victims altogether. Researchers propose that listeners have a hard time listening because the stories of the victims' traumas threaten the listeners assumptive world views about justice. As a consequence they tend to exaggerate the victims' personal responsibility, often ending up blaming the victims for a traumatic experience that they could not avoid (Coates et al. 1979; Harber and Pennbaker 1992).

Given what we know about emotional contagion, such reactions on the part of listeners become relatively easy to understand. Confronted with a traumatized person who has little if any control over negative affect, the listener is quite likely to become empathically upset as well, with all the physiological disturbances that accompany emotional arousal. Ultimately, victims recognize that people are pulling away from them or avoiding them, and they consequently begin to inhibit their own emotional expression and avoid discussion of the trauma. This goes in exactly the opposite direction of what they need to do (Harber and Pennebaker 1992). The result: "Victims may be trapped in a complicated dilemma, in which they can maximize their social acceptance only at the expense of their personal adjustment" (Coates et al. 1979).

For these reasons, our culture has strongly supported the continuing maintenance of emotional inhibition, suppression, dissociation. After traumatic experience, the traditional folk wisdom says, "just forget about it dear, put it out of your mind." All of us have been reared with repeated admonitions to control our emotions and keep our feelings to ourselves. Emotional control is seen as a requirement of adult behavior. Unfortunately, after trauma emotional control is difficult to attain without the suppression of emotion that turns into repression and amnesia for the feelings themselves.

THE SOCIAL RESPONSE TO DANGER

Need for Social Connectedness

Human social life originates with the evolution of parental care and the mother-infant bond. The behavior between mother and infant, and later between father and infant, is the foundation stone for adult bonding, friendliness, and love—all of which are at the heart of social organization (Eibl-Eibesfeldt 1989). Unfortunately, all mammals, including humans, demonstrate ambivalence about other people. As powerfully wired as we are for social contact, so too are we wired for "xenophobia," the fear of strangers. This fear begins during the second half of the first year of life, and although it is modifiable by culture it is never totally absent from human social relationships. This inherent conflict is probably what propelled our evolution into relatively small social groups; we needed social bonds, and yet we had to minimize our fear-arousing contact with strangers. Thus, the perfect solution is a fixed group of familiar people (Eibl-Eibesfeldt 1989). Modern urban life, of course, poses serious problems in this regard.

There is a social response to danger as well. When danger is signaled, people who are attached to each other feel compelled to draw together. This makes a great deal of sense from an evolutionary perspective because human safety is so dependent on the protection of the group. This behavior originates in the infant-mother bond and proximity-seeking behavior on the part of both of the pair is innate. This increased attachment behavior in the face of danger or threat and in the service of survival has been noted in all social species. As children, our only safety is to be found in the protection of others and therefore, whenever fear is aroused we seek protection from others, even when we are adults. Under such circumstances we also become more obedient and open to suggestion (Eibl-Eibesfeldt 1989; Schumaker 1995).

In situations of danger, our sense of stranger anxiety also increases, and our bonding to an in-group escalates along with our perception of threat from an out-group. When we are frightened we want to be with people we trust, and we want to touch them as well. Tactile communication is extremely important among primates and humans and has a calming, positive effect (Eibl-Eisbesfeldt 1989). Coming together as a group in times of danger has many obvious benefits. Defense is easier if we are not alone. We can pool our resources and information and better prepare for the danger. We can read each other's level of emotional expression and gauge our own level of arousal accordingly. We can use others to help us modulate our own level of arousal if it is becoming dangerously high. If we are in an avoidant state that could have destructive consequences, other people can help us confront the situation without being overwhelmed by it, thus increasing our own level of potential competence.

This biologically based behavioral sequence is obvious in any kind of disaster and is probably the reason why in these situations people's "stranger

anxiety" is so diminished and why people draw together and are more helpful to each other than under other, more normal circumstances. It is also
part of the reason why secret danger is so damaging. The person who must
keep silent about a dangerous situation cannot utilize these innate human
responses to help modulate anxiety and arousal.

Trauma-bonding

When danger is especially severe, repeated, or prolonged it often is not
shared. In fact, in many of these cases, the people who are closest are the
same people who are the perpetrators of the traumatic acts. This is most evident in cases of child abuse, where the primary caretakers are the sources of
the trauma for the child. This is an extremely problematic situation. The
result is increased attachment to the abusing person, a phenomenon known
as "trauma-bonding." As a result, highly untrustworthy and destructive relationships come to be considered normative (Dutton and Painter 1981;
Herman 1992; James 1994; Van der Kolk 1989). The natural, innate protective mechanism of turning to people to whom you are attached for safety is
turned on its head. Your persecutors become the same ones you turn to for
relief. If these same persecutors also provide intermittent nurturance in the
form of food, shelter, relief from pain, or even affection, then the situation is
even more confused, both cognitively and at a basic biological adaptive level.

This is a part of the complicated picture for battered spouses, abused
children, prisoners and victims of torture, and any other situation in which
the abuse is prolonged and repeated (Herman 1992). Their conscious mind
says that their perpetrators are a source of danger, while something deeper
and far less conscious directs them to stay near to the person to whom they
are attached. This is yet another form of confusion and cognitive dissonance for which the traumatized person finds only pseudosolutions. If a
woman is being beaten by her husband, her mind will signal danger. But her
husband is her primary attachment figure, and. therefore, seemingly para-
doxically, the beating may well enhance attachment to him *because* of the
danger he has aroused, and she may feel even more frightened to leave him
than to stay with him.

Social Skills

People who have been traumatized since childhood often are severely incapacitated in their ability to get along with other people. In the first place,
the normative aspects of trauma-bonding will mean that they will tend to
be attracted to abusive relationships in which they may take the role of the
victim, the abuser, or alternate between the two. Because these are estab-

lished norms for relationships, people may feel an unverbalized sense of security and freedom from anxiety only when they are in such a relationship. After all, they know about the parameters of abusive relationships. They know what to expect, they know what comes next, the relationship is trustworthy to the extent it is predictable. Because of this ability to predict the outcome of any interaction, they can exert some control, at least over their own protective defenses and feel less helpless. It is nonabusive relationships that are anxiety producing, confusing, unpredictable, and frightening. The feeling of vulnerability that may be aroused in a nonabusive relationship may not be endurable. This is a particularly powerful influence if the entire family is characterized by abusive relationships. The group normative aspects of this kind of a situation further reinforce the behavior.

Children who grow up in such situations demonstrate an impaired capacity to trust other people, and may even feel more trusting in abusive relationships than nurturing ones. To the extent that they have experienced a lack of emotional resonance from their primary caretakers, they may be unable to experience resonance with the pain of others. They will therefore treat others with the same callous disregard that they have experienced themselves. This has become the standard within their families, the standard for survival.

As a result, victims of repeated trauma often have profound difficulties with any kind of social relationship. Intimacy poses problems because healthy intimacy cannot be established in a relationship based on fear, anger, and danger. They may have a very difficult time getting along in a group of people, tending instead to attempt to unwittingly replicate the problems within their families of origin. Their sense of self and identity may have become so compromised that it will be quite difficult for them to exercise a sense of social responsibility or commitment to a larger social purpose. Their healing may be delayed or prevented because healing is so dependent on sharing and integration with others. They may not be able to turn to others for emotional support, confession, or guidance.

Their wariness of kind behavior on the part of others leads to subtle and overt but unconscious attempts to get other people to behave in ways with which they are more familiar. This cueing plays an important role in traumatic reenactment. The response on the part of others is predictable— "They don't really want help; they are impossible, they are resistant." In this way, victims of childhood abuse end up replicating their situations throughout a lifetime. The lack of empathy they have experienced is duplicated by the surrounding environment. This is complicated by the fact that other people do not really want to know what has happened to the victims. One of the common results is the scapegoat phenomenon.

Scapegoating

A recent survey found that 54 percent of people questioned feel that people get the suffering they deserve (Wuthnow 1991). The scapegoat is one of our oldest cultural motifs. A scapegoat is a person made to bear blame that should fall on others. In ancient Jewish ritual the scapegoat was a goat on whose head the high priest symbolically laid the sins of the people on Yom Kippur, and which was then allowed to escape into the wilderness. We have a long tradition of using people as scapegoats—as "poison containers" (DeMause 1982)—for our own unacceptable feelings and our own unresolved traumatic experiences. If we can get someone else to act out those feelings we can often avoid feeling them ourselves. In more primitive days, human sacrifice was the preferred and ritualized form of scapegoating. One person or a group of people would be designated to be the sacrifice to whatever deity required it, and the sacrificial victim, often a child, would be ritually killed. As Patrick Tierney has pointed out, "Our own society has child sacrifice written on our twin foundation stones—the attempted sacrifice of Isaac, son of Abraham, on Mount Moriah, and the sacrifice of Jesus, Son of God, on Mount Calvary" (Tierney 1989).

Rather than seeing scapegoating as the inevitable consequence of "Homo necans, man the killer" (Tierney 1989), it may be more useful to view scapegoating as a result of repeated traumatic experience involving the entire social group. As we know, people who are repeatedly traumatized learn to be helpless and are unable to defend themselves. They easily become targets for those in the social group who have been traumatized and have identified with their perpetrators. One of the reactions to helplessness is to become preoccupied with the use and abuse of power. These people become bullies who target the scapegoats for more abuse and in doing so reenact their own traumatic experience—only this time as the perpetrator. The rest of us stand by, preferring to silently or overtly align ourselves with the powerful perpetrator rather than the helpless victim— the "bystander effect" (Staub 1989). As an increasing number of people in the culture begin responding this way, there is an increased tolerance for antisocial acts.

THE BEHAVIORAL RESPONSE TO DANGER

The obvious behavioral response to danger is to get away from it, to stop it, to protect oneself or others from harm. The entire fight-or-flight response directs the individual to make a behavioral response. But, in any situation of danger, the actions that we take are multidetermined. The signals from our body combine with past memories of danger, immediate choices in the situation, long-standing habits of behavior, and the influence of others around us. To some extent, whether we fight, or freeze, or flee is determined by habits. Because fear conditioning is so potent, even one experience with danger can result in the development of habits that may or may not be effective under circumstances that are different from the original danger.

Habits

We are creatures of habit. Much of what we do each day is based on habits. Life would be unendurable if every day, in every way, all was brand-new. This tendency to form habits easily, to repeat behaviors and thought patterns that have guaranteed survival constitute a way that we order our existence and make sense of the world. We are conservative creatures—Nature's way of trying to protect us from making too many fatal mistakes—and we tend to look to the past for solutions to today's problems. The more powerfully life-saving the reason for the habit formation, the more anxiety we experience if we try to alter that habit. Habits become dissociated from our usual consciousness—that is what makes them habits and therefore automatic. Any attempt to alter them or eradicate them will lead us to re-experience the initial fear that created the need for the habit. The strength of the fear will determine the strength of the habit. As a consequence, we rarely change habits unless we are forced to by some change in our environment, a change that evokes greater fear than the original fear or need that created the habit.

Relational Behavior

The behavior of other people has a great deal to do with our behavioral responses to situations of danger. This relational aspect of dangerous situations has been studied by the military most intensively. It is well-recognized that people tend to come together seeking aid and comfort. This finding has been borne out in field studies of infantry platoons, air crews, and disaster control teams as well as through social psychological experiments with college students (Janis 1972). This heightened need for affiliation leads to greater dependency on the group and an enhanced tendency to conform to group norms.

In their seminal work on World War II, Grinker and Spiegel noted that, "The impersonal threat of injury from the enemy, affecting all alike, produces a high degree of cohesion so that personal attachments throughout the unit become intensified. Friendships are easily made by those who might never have been compatible at home, and are cemented under fire. Out of the mutually shared hardships and dangers are born an altruism and generosity that transcend ordinary individual selfish interest" (1945).

As one might expect, however, this positive relational response to danger has a great deal to do with many other factors that are inherent in each individual situation. In situations where social structures have been radically and rapidly destroyed, relationships can entirely break down, even in the face of great danger (Turnbull 1972). When the danger is chronic and difficult to identify, particularly when those causing the danger fail in their ability to resolve the difficulties, as in the case of industrial and technological disasters, relational behavior can be severely damaged so that individual victims become alienated and psychologically impaired, suspicious, paranoid, hypervigilant, and unable to screen out signs of potential danger (Erikson 1994; Kroll-Smith and Couch 1993). In situations of poor leadership, overcrowding, extremes of temperature and noise, deprivation of food, shelter, or other necessities, relational behavior can become alienated, paranoid, and violent (Forsyth 1990).

Creative Expression

Creative expression is the voice of our nonverbal self. Integration of creative inspiration with the verbal self produces works or experiences of art that can be shared with others. There is good reason to believe that all forms of creative expression—painting, sculpture, music, dance, drama, storytelling, writing, poetry—evolved in parallel with language and that the exercise of these abilities is absolutely necessary for the attainment and maintenance of human health (Bloom 1996; Dissanayake 1992). Healthy human beings express themselves creatively in a myriad of ways and they actively participate in the creative endeavors of others.

But what of the role of creative expression in the human response to danger? The basis of creativity is our mimetic ability. Through mimesis we reenact or represent an event or relationship. This mimetic level of representation predates language and underlies all culture, human communication, and the arts. This preverbal communication system is quite apparent in animal species that have ritualized, nonverbal ways of communicating signs of danger to others of their kind. For humans, group mimesis became the basis for ritual, our earliest attempts at controlling nature—both outside of us and within us. Rituals help us order reality and prepare for a safe or safer future as well as help us manage aggression (Driver 1991; Schumaker 1995). Rituals also help us manage emotions. And ritual is accompanied by the rudiments of behavior that eventuate in what we consider art. Musical rhythms synchronize specific physiological rhythms and activate different emotional states (Lex 1979). This is presumably the origin of military marches, designed to stimulate the soldier in preparation for danger. Tribal cultures traditionally prepared for war through costuming, dancing, music, and reenactment of tribal myths. We must conclude that one motive force behind the evolution of the arts was a proactive and uniquely human response to danger.

Humor and Play

Healthy human beings enjoy laughing, playing, and having a good time. They experience humor as a form of personal and shared intimacy between people. On a physiological level, laughter strengthens the respiratory system, increases the amount of oxygen in the bloodstream, increases the heart rate, and accelerates breathing and circulation while relaxing muscles (Williams 1986). There are also indications that laughter releases endorphins which act as painkillers and generally increase the sense of well-being (Åstedt-Kurki and Liukkonen 1994). Evidence exists that laughter improves health in various disease states (Cousins 1976). Epinephrine, which is secreted whenever we are stressed and aroused, increases laughter (Hatfield et al. 1994). In situations of danger, humor can enhance group cohesion, diminish paralyzing anxiety, release tension, help reduce stress, and diminish hostility.

Fixation to Trauma

To early workers such as Freud and Janet, it became obvious that traumatic experience had the effect of halting development. Traumatized individuals become attached to the trauma. They are unable to make sense out their experience. As a result, they develop difficulties in integrating new experience (Van der Kolk and Van der Hart 1989). This internal fixation and fragmentation makes integration of the personality impossible. When the traumatic experience occurs in childhood, before the personality has fully developed, the person may develop severe personality problems, such as multiple personality disorder.

Another form of this problem can be seen in people who are said to have a "borderline personality disorder," in which their sense of self is divided into a "good self" and a "bad self," and their external world likewise becomes divided into "good" and "bad," along with all the people in their lives. These people are unable to function in a mature and integrated way, particularly within the context of their intimate relationships and their view of themselves. We know now that a very high percentage of these adults were seriously abused as children (Herman 1992; Herman et al. 1989; Perry et al. 1990).

Many perpetrators of criminal violence have had serious childhood traumatic experiences. This population is less well-studied because they do not show up with a high degree of frequency in psychiatric centers, nor do they tend to be compliant with treatment or research. However, workers treating prisoners and familiar with the effects of childhood trauma are beginning to publish information about their findings. James Gilligan, M.D., after spending much of his professional career working with violent offenders, before becoming Director of the Center for the Study of Violence at Harvard Medical School, has stated, "The violent criminals I have known have been objects of violence from early childhood." (1996). In such cases, their early experiences have done such damage to them that they have become detached from other human beings and are incapable of empathy, often on a permanent basis. Because they are severely impaired in their capacity to form attachment bonds, they are unable to attach to other people, or to a civilized system of laws and beliefs. They are unable to love and care for life other than their own, and even their capacity to love and respect themselves is severely impaired or missing on all levels other than that of pure survival. It is very possible—and by clinical experience probable—that the damage done to many of these children in early childhood is irreversible by any means presently known to psychiatric science.

Adults who are traumatized also become fixated on the trauma, and it is from these adult experiences that we have derived a great deal of information about the trauma response. In the history of the study of traumatic experience, the initial emphasis was on the inability of the individual to cope with the traumatic experience (Peterson, Prout, and Schwarz 1991). The traumatized person was seen as simply not strong enough to cope with the trauma. The problem remained focused within the person, not on what had happened to the person. Now we understand that this fixation can occur to virtually anyone if the circumstances are "wrong" enough.

Self-destructive Behavior and Traumatic Addiction

One of the more puzzling aspects of human psychopathology has always been the tendency of disturbed people to harm themselves in any number of ways. Psychiatry has focused on those whose self-harm ends up largely focused on their own bodies. The penal system and the political system have largely taken jurisdiction for those whose self-harm ends up hurting other people. Because our reaction to the latter is largely one of punishment, we know relatively little about what makes them do the things they do, or what could prevent it. For those who harm themselves the picture is becoming somewhat clearer as we understand more about the long-term effects of severe trauma.

Endorphins and Stress—Addiction to Trauma

The endorphins our bodies produce are not just painkillers. They reduce anxiety, rage, depression, and fear. They are vital to attachment behavior from birth to death. They increase when social support increases; they decrease when social support is withdrawn. Lack of early care in animals effectively reduces endorphins and may do so in people as well. Not surprisingly, given their powerful analgesic and calming effects, large amounts of endorphins are released as an integral part of the fight-or-flight response (Bremner et al. 1993; Van der Kolk 1996b; Van der Kolk and Greenberg 1987). After all, if we are running from an enemy and sprain an ankle, it is far better if we are unable to feel the pain until we have reached safety.

But what happens to the normal endorphin response when people are exposed to chronic and repeated stress, when their bodies are repeatedly exposed to these powerful agents? Stress-induced analgesia has been described in animals following exposure to inescapable shock. In severely stressed animals, signs of opiate withdrawal can be triggered by stopping the stress or by giving the animal a drug that counteracts the effects of the endorphins (Van der Kolk 1996b). One theory is that some chronically stressed people may become addicted to their own circulating endorphins because of overexposure and impaired regulation of the endorphins as a result of chronic stress. Whenever the stress is relieved, they feel worse, not better. They go into an opiate withdrawal syndrome that is similar to heroin withdrawal. They feel anxious, irritable, depressed, and miserable (Van der Kolk et al. 1985; Van der Kolk and Greenberg 1987). In order to feel better they must do something to get their endorphin level back up, and that means doing something stressful. What they end up doing is determined by what works, their own experience and inclinations.

Stress-addicted children are often those children in the classroom who cannot tolerate a calm atmosphere but must keep antagonizing everyone else until the stress level is high enough for them to achieve some degree of internal equilibrium again. Violence is exciting and stressful, and repeated violent acting out, gang behavior, fighting, bullying, and many forms of criminal activity have the additional side effect of producing high levels of stress in people who have grown addicted to such risk-taking behavior. People who self-mutilate, who literally cut and burn their arms, legs, and torso have always puzzled psychiatrists because this self-mutilation did not seem to be aimed at suicide. People who self-mutilate report a rising sense of internal tension that is relieved when they cut themselves. Self-mutilators may generally be people who as children were abused, often sexually abused and have learned that hurting the body will evoke a calming response because of endorphin release. They have not been able to find comfort from other people and instead must rely on their own methods, even if that means self-harm. Many people appear to seek out high-risk jobs or forms of recreation and talk about the "high" they feel, even at risking their lives. An important element of these behaviors is *control*. All of these examples are ones in which people have the opportunity to overcome and defeat helplessness by taking control. No one else is hurting them, risking their lives, threatening them—they are playing with life and death themselves; they are in charge.

Traumatic Reenactment

It was Sigmund Freud who drew attention to what he called "the repetition compulsion," the all-too-human tendency to repeat the past. He connected it to traumatic experience and pointed out that through their actions people unconsciously repeat the past (Van der Kolk and Ducey 1989).

It has become clear that the very nature of the trauma response determines this repetitious behavior leading to the use of a more descriptive term, "traumatic reenactment" (Van der Kolk 1989). The memories of the traumatic experience are dissociated, nonverbal, and unintegrated. Over and over, people find themselves in situations that recapitulate earlier trauma and lack any awareness of how it happened much less how to prevent it from happening the next time. The lack of awareness is due to the dissociative blockade that places the behavior out of the context of verbal and conscious control. Since words are not available to sufficiently explain the experience, thinking cannot really occur. Under these circumstances, people will usually come up with explanations for their strange and mysterious behavior, because the rational part of their mind is struggling to make sense of the situation. But without access to the dissociated material, the rational mind flounders helplessly, interpreting behavior in a simplistic, often stupid way, while the person helplessly reexposes himself or herself to further trauma.

This lack of control over the repetition of trauma, combined with an insistent, albeit unconscious need to repeat the traumatic scenario is called a compulsion. A compulsion, by definition, is impossible to resist—the person is compelled to do what he may even consciously know is wrong to do. The power that motors this behavior is the energy that derives from the dissociated mental contents pressing for expression. When we are able to see it coming, we can stop acting and begin thinking about, and ultimately feeling and integrating the split of mental contents. This may be the most important function of psychotherapy.

People have a strong compulsion to repeat traumatic experiences, sometimes overtly but more frequently in a disguised, often highly symbolized, way. These reenactments which consist of the repeated establishment of the traumatic scenario that then gets relived over and over can come to dominate a person's entire life. In this way, Shakespeare's observation that the world is a stage is particularly apt. Each of us experiences the early drama of our own life, and then, for the rest of our years, we reconstruct the pattern over and over, using different people, places, and things, to play the same old roles, usually with the same old endings.

We must assume that as human beings, we are meant to function at our maximum level of integration and that any barrier to this integration will produce some innate compensatory mechanism that allows us to overcome it. Splitting traumatic memories and feelings off into nonverbal images and sensations is life-saving in the short-term, but prevents full integration in the long-term. For healing to occur, we must give our overwhelming experiences words. In "Macbeth," Shakespeare told us "Give sorrow words; the grief that does not speak whispers the o'er fraught heart and bids it break." Both Janet and Freud claimed that the crucial factor that determines the repetition of trauma is the presence of mute, unsymbolized and unintegrated experiences (Van der Kolk and Ducey 1989). Freud wrote that in order for feelings to be experienced (for affects to become conscious), words had to be linked to them. It was the linkage with word representations that allowed the affect to cross the repression barrier and become conscious (Sashin 1993).

But we cannot find the words by ourselves. That is the whole point— traumatized people are cut off from language, deprived of the power of words, trapped in timeless, speechless terror. But they do speak. They speak the language that existed before we had words or language, the language of action. Mimesis is defined as "the ability to produce conscious, self-initiated, representational acts that are intentional but not linguistic" (Donald 1991). Through mimesis we reenact or represent an event or relationship. This is a form of self-expression and social communication that precedes the development of language and is evident in primates. It is the level of communication that underlies all modern cultures and forms the most basic medium of human communication and is central to all the arts (Donald 1991).

Mimesis is the basis of ritual behavior and the arts and in many ways is the basis of the human condition (Driver 1991).

Reenactment behavior is repetitive and ritualized. It is so because it is usually not seen or heard for what it is—a signal to the social group. We are a social species. Once trauma has occurred and our consciousness has been split into fragments, there is nothing internally that will put "Humpty-Dumpty" back together again. The evolved mechanism for healing is not fundamentally biological—it is social. In their apparently crazy behavior, traumatized people are desperately trying to get the attention of their social group. Psychiatric patients have always been accused of "trying to get attention." It is true. They *are* trying to get attention. But that is because getting attention is precisely what evolution has programmed them to do. The problem does not lie with the body of the traumatized person. We have seen how their body has responded to danger in exactly the appropriate way. The problem lies with the corporate body, the social body, that refuses to play the role it is duty-bound to play. It is not the traumatized person who is basically sick. It is those people who fail to understand our oldest, bonded, interconnected language. Let's look at two examples of traumatic reenactment. The first describes an individual, the second describes three generations of reenactment behavior.

Until Death Do Us Part

Connie came to see me for the first time when she was already well on the road to recovery from a lifelong history of trauma. She had had years of treatment, much of which had been very successful, and now wanted guidance in how to live a more normal life, how to have healthier relationships. The hard work was already accomplished. But the story Connie told was an instructive one.

Connie had been reared in a middle-class home in the suburbs of New York. Her mother and father were respected members of the community. Connie had an older brother. To anyone outside the home, their family looked like every other normal American family.

But what no one saw was the tortured relationship between mother and daughter. Connie's mother had been raised by parents who were religious fundamentalists of German background. Connie did not know what kind of childhood her mother had except that her mother said that her father and mother had been very "strict" and refused to talk further. Whatever the reality behind the scenes, Connie's mother had some strange ideas about child rearing. After her husband went to work, Connie's mother performed a daily morning ritual that extended as far back as Connie could remember.

Her mother would wake her up, take her into the bathroom, beat her, and then give her enemas, which were supposed to "clean all the bad out of me." Secretly, and behind closed doors, this torture went on almost until adolescence.

Connie dealt with this situation in the way so many abused children do—she dissociated. Children often create imaginary friends as part of their play. Children who suffer often use their imaginary friend as a source of comfort. And children whose suffering is prolonged, repeated, and inescapable often turn their imaginary friend into a separate personality of their own who then conveniently learns to handle the pain and suffering, thus protecting the child from being overwhelmed by the experience.

Connie used this defense quite effectively. Every morning, her alter personality, Sarah, would emerge to handle the scene with her mother. Sarah was a stoic who never cried or showed any emotion as her mother was involved in her compulsive destructive behavior. When her mother released Connie, Sarah would go back "inside," and Connie would go to school, apparently happy-go-lucky and free from care. Connie had no memory of the events that had gone on in the morning and could therefore be free to do her schoolwork, play with her friends, and live an apparently normal childhood existence. Sad and stoical Sarah did her job dutifully for many years.

Adolescence is a difficult time for children who have been abused because adolescence is the time when it becomes necessary to synthesize all the childhood identities into one integrated sense of self in order to prepare for the stages of normal adult development. For Connie, such a synthesis was impossible. Although the physical abuse had stopped by this time, if not the emotional abuse, Connie remained seriously split inside, preventing her from developing a healthy adult self.

People who are internally split as a result of abuse learn only one way to protect themselves from other people—and that is by splitting, by using their alter personality to handle abuse, rather than stopping it. Children are supposed to be protected by their parents until they are old enough to protect themselves. But people who have produced a dissociated and protective alter personality cannot really grow up. Inside they remain children, able only to use dissociation when danger comes from outside. Like other victims of trauma, victims of childhood abuse are compelled to repeat trauma. The power of this unconscious force in determining behavior is awesome. In late adolescence, Connie met Frank. Blinded to Frank's negative side, Connie looked to him as her savior, her ticket out of her disturbed home. They married, and not long thereafter Frank began physically and sexually abusing her.

During the day, Connie went out and worked, rising in position and status in the advertising business. Her secret life at night was a source of ongoing pain and shame. She continued to dissociate as she had in her childhood when the beating began. Only years later did she recall being tied to the bed repeatedly, raped, and sodomized. Over the course of the years, Connie gave birth to four children. To cope with the stress of a high-pressure job, four children, and an abusive husband, Connie began taking tranquilizers. Uppers and downers became her way of staying alive, of maintaining an unsteady balance. The split in her personality and the drug abuse prevented her from ever being fully aware of her situation and so the past just kept repeating itself. The children were witnesses to a highly dysfunctional and loveless marriage, and although Connie did not know this until many years later, her husband sexually and physically abused the children as well. Connie could not protect herself or her children.

This disturbed situation would have remained the same had not Frank's behavior deteriorated even further. His drinking increased and one night he drew a gun on Connie, and pointed it at her head with his finger on the trigger. Connie likely would have been another murder statistic had he not passed out at that moment in a drunken stupor. It was at this point that something finally clicked inside for Connie. The dissociative split that allowed this abuse to continue was created initially to serve a protective function. When Connie saw and finally believed that her life was almost lost as a result of being unable to protect herself, the contradiction seemed to bring about some kind of insight. The next day she took the children, found a shelter, started court proceedings, and with the help of the court, assumed a new identity that enabled her to move out of the state and create a new life for herself.

But in her new job and new life, she still had the substance abuse to deal with, four traumatized children to support, and she was still divided into two personalities. She sought treatment, was hospitalized and detoxified from the medications, and then spent years in therapy integrating her two personalities along with all the memories and repressed emotions from the terrible years of her past. Connie's story is a good example of the cost of child abuse and the power of traumatic reenactment. Clearly, her mother had been raised in circumstances that are shrouded in mystery. But we can be certain that her mother's bizarre conduct came out of the need to repeat horrors of her own family past. According to some authorities on the history of childhood, the idea of children needing enemas to purge them of "bad humors" and "inner demons" was a common practice of the late seventeenth and early eighteenth centuries (DeMause 1982). Victims of abuse do not always become perpetrators directly themselves. Connie's mother did, and if we knew more of the details of her life we could probably understand how it happened. But Connie chose not to act against her own children. Damage occurred just the same, however, because Connie was drawn to a man who was disturbed, and in doing so she illustrates one of the primary disturbances among those who are abused: the inability to self protect.

People who are abused as children are often unable to protect themselves or others from abuse in adequate ways. Connie's compulsion to repeat trauma attracted her to Frank, a man who was violent, incapable of empathy, and highly disturbed. For her, abusive relationships had become more normative than loving ones. Because of the tendency of abuse victims to experience increased attachment to abusers, Connie became increasingly attached to Frank as a result of the abuse, much as she had to her abusing mother, and even produced four children within the context of that attachment. In doing so she produced four new victims for Frank and spread the "disease" to another generation.

Connie found some healthy and not-so-healthy ways to cope. She poured her energy into her job. Her capacity to dissociate and maintain that dissociative split enabled her to do so. But as her defenses began to break down, she required more and more drugs to help her maintain her position. As a result, she developed yet another problem—addiction. Her inability to protect her own children from the abuse left her feeling guilty, remorseful, and ashamed, and this additional impairment in her self-concept made recovery even more difficult. The longer this situation went on, the more difficult it became to do anything to correct it. This is typical of a deteriorating, abusive, and traumatic situation. Trauma produces reenactment and more trauma as the victim follows a downward spiraling life course.

It is ironic that an attempted murder caused a reversal in Connie's fortunes. Faced with the life-and-death decision of whether to stay and die or take a leap into the unknown and leave, something inside Connie, a deep instinct for survival, gave her the energy to make the decision to change, and from that point on there was no turning back. Connie had the strength to leave her batterer, but her healing would have been impossible without the support, encouragement, limits, guidance, and push she got from other people—her co-workers, her therapists, her support group in Alcoholics Anonymous, and her friends. They were willing to hear what her behavior meant, willing to support her while they pushed her to redirect her traumatic reenactment scenario to a happier ending.

Multigenerational Transmission of Traumatic Reenactment

Our lives are reenactments not only of our own buried traumatic experiences, but also contain our family history. To the extent that our family history has been traumatic, the family traumatic reenactment then compounds and magnifies the individual traumatic reenactment. Intergenerational trauma has been best studied in research on the offspring of Holocaust survivors (Danielli 1985, Freyberg 1980, Kestenberg 1980, Sigal and Weinfeld 1989). and can be summed up in one sentence: "The children of survivors show symptoms which would be expected if they actually lived through the Holocaust" (Herzog 1982). Lenore Terr (1990) quoted a survivor and psychoanalyst as saying, "My thirty-five year-old son told me recently that he has had nightmares in which the Gestapo come up his stairs. You realize what this means? My son was born and raised in America. But he dreams my nightmare, MY life."

War experience has also shown to be problematic for the next generation. It has been noted repeatedly that many of the symptoms of PTSD have a severe, ongoing, and disruptive effect on marital and family life (Figley and Sprenkle 1978; Matsakis 1988; Rosenheck 1986). One study of eighty-six children of Vietnam War veterans with PTSD showed that children with a violent father were significantly more likely to have more behavior problems, poorer school performance, and less social competence than children with a nonviolent father. Within this high-risk group, a lower level of family functioning, father's past combat experience, and current violent behavior were all significantly associated with the behavior problems of the children (Harkness 1993).

The intergenerational transmission of child maltreatment is also being studied. There is extensive evidence to show that parents who were maltreated are more likely than nonmaltreated parents, to abuse their own children. About one-third of parents who were abused as children continue a pattern of seriously inept, neglectful or abusive parenting. One-third do not. Another third remain vulnerable to the effects of social stress and are more likely to become abusive under such influences (Oliver 1993). This generational transmission happens in a number of ways. A growing body of evidence demonstrates that one mechanism is through the attachment relationship. Mothers who have been rejected by their mothers tend to be rejecting of their own infants (Main and Goldwyn 1984). In a large study of the intergenerational transmission of corporal punishment, social learning, passed from one generation to the next appeared to be the most important factor (Muller et al. 1995) although the effect of establishing a family norm which then gets passed on from one generation to the next also may play a role (Jacobs and Campbell 1965). Other research focuses on the damage that child abuse does to the brain which interferes with normal parenting of the next generation (Teicher et al. 1993).

Breaking the cycle of abuse is more likely to happen if parents have current social support, particularly a supportive spouse, if they have had a positive relationship with a significant adult during childhood, and if they have had therapy as an adolescent or an adult which allows them to remember, talk about, express anger over, their abuse while holding their abuser, not themselves, acountable for it (Cicchetti and Lynch 1995)

The "Sins" of the Fathers to the Third Generation

Sam is a World War II veteran who returns from extremely traumatic and life-threatening experiences in a Japanese prisoner-of-war camp. In the camp he was subjected to humiliation, torture, and prolonged deprivation of basic needs, and he felt an overwhelming helplessness. After his return he never talks about his experiences and is encouraged by well-meaning people to put the past behind him. He returns to civilian life, gets a job, marries, has children, becomes successful at work. To the world he appears to have no deficit as a result of his experiences.

What the world does not see—or refuses to see—are the emotional deficits Sam carries with him. He cannot really get close to anyone, even his wife, Alice. Feelings of tenderness make him feel terribly vulnerable and helpless, which evokes memories of his captivity. His wife knows that he loves her. Their relationship predates the war, a time filled with happy memories. But she constantly feels abandoned and betrayed because he is unable to offer her comfort when she most needs it. Their sexual relationship has become quite compromised as a result of his emotional unavailability and her chronic anger. His infrequent but violent nightmares which neither of them discuss, have led them to occupy separate beds, though they still share a bedroom. Yet she senses within him some terrible pain and vulnerability, and she often becomes as protective of him as she is with her children.

He knows what he should do as a father and attends ball games and school plays dutifully, but does not allow himself to get close to his children. His son, Ed, has asked him about his war experiences and short of telling him that he was a POW, he avoids discussion and his son senses immediately that the subject is taboo. When his son has particularly angered him, Sam has been known to fly into an uncontrollable rage, demonstrating an anger totally out of proportion to his son's misdemeanor of the moment and resulting in some physical violence. Everyone in the family knows about these rages, but they are so discontinuous with Sam's normally controlled behavior that no one talks about what happens. The next morning, everyone pretends nothing went wrong and after a while they actually do manage to forget the incident—until the next time that Sam flies into a rage.

The family manages to survive these internal problems and deficits relatively well, at least by external appearances. They live in a lovely home and have a comfortable standard of living. Ed and his sister, Sarah, attend good schools, and their academic performance is excellent. Ed grows up, goes to college, joins ROTC because that is what seems natural to do. Sarah grows up and goes to college as well. At this point in time, a family snapshot would show what appears to be a healthy, happy family with two successful children and a marriage that has lasted.

If we could see below the surface of this snapshot, we would see a son who always longed for closeness with his distant but respectable father, a boy who has learned that men never show tenderness or fear and sometimes lose control and vent their anger on those less powerful than them. Ed has learned to shut off his feelings of fear, vulnerability, and need for intimacy, using his father as his role model. He has learned that it is best not to talk about uncomfortable feelings or situations, even if they are in the distant past. He assumes that this is the way men are supposed to be. Once, in his early adolescence, he got embroiled in a fight with a much younger boy and probably would have seriously injured the boy if other children had not been pulled him off. Ever since then he has feared his own anger and tends to be too passive and too compliant, particularly with people in authority.

Sarah, has also always yearned for closeness with her father and is mystified by what she perceives as men's emotional coldness and propensity for rage, yet somehow all the young men she dates behave the same way. When confronted by her mother about her poor choices in men, she becomes quite protective of the boy and she and her mother end up fighting. She has concerns about her own sexual feelings which she shares with no one, and is very confused about the role of sexuality in a relationship. She has never seen much open expression of affection between her parents, knows they sleep in separate beds, and has sensed some kind of related tension between them but doesn't understand what it is about. She is determined to live her life differently from her mother, whom she perceives as angry and disappointed with her life. Her mother out of loyalty to her husband, cannot say anything to Sarah, but she is badly frightened about the boys Sarah brings home. They seem so much like Sam, and though she loves him, she does not want Sarah to end up like her.

War breaks out while Ed is in college, and he signs on to go to Vietnam. Sam is overwhelmed by emotion when he gets the phone call from his son. Fleetingly he has thoughts about helping him run to Canada or calling a senator he knows and pulling some strings, but a voice inside him tells him that is not right. Instead, he pushes the fear aside, a well-practiced habit by this time, and encourages his son to do what he thinks best. His mother stands by, helplessly crying, enraged that her only son is to be sent to war. She knows that war has done enough to her and her family, yet she cannot say these things, dare not even think them, for to do so would be to somehow betray her husband and all he suffered for, and she has spent her life protecting him. So Ed dons his Army uniform and marches off to Southeast Asia, carrying, he thinks, his parents' blessings.

Vietnam is a hell that no middle-class American boy can even imagine. The goals of the war are unclear, leadership seems to be in disarray, the living conditions of the soldiers in the field are abominable, the enemy is a guerrilla enemy who can strike at any time. The only safety is the safety of one's brothers-in-arms, and Ed bonds firmly with his comrades. Men who allow themselves to experience fear, sorrow, or vulnerability frequently become easy targets for the enemy. Ed has been well-trained by his father in dissociating these feelings and he becomes like his father, a good soldier, respected by the other men and fierce in combat.

Ed becomes particularly close to his commanding officer who reminds him of his father, but who is tender with his men after battle, protective of them under fire. One day, while out on patrol, the platoon comes across sniper fire in a small village. Ed follows standard procedure to deal with the situation until a shot hits the officer. Ed finds himself in a blind fury, shooting every civilian—even the children—in his line of fire, incensed by their diminutive stature and Oriental eyes. Only later, back at the base, does he realize what he has done. His shame and guilt bury the experience far out of consciousness, never to be discussed again. Nor does he even consciously register that not only does he have his own reasons for killing Orientals, but buried within him is his father's desire for vengeance as well.

Meantime, Sarah becomes seriously involved with a man at school. He pushes her to have sex, and despite her reservations, she acquiesces. She becomes pregnant, and they marry, thus somewhat attenuating her parents' disgrace. Later she recognizes that she has married a man even more withdrawn than her father, but also more in need of her psychological protection. Although their sexual life is unfulfilling, he is a good provider.

Ed returns from Vietnam, finishes college, gets married, and begins a family. Sam and Alice are proud grandparents. Problems arise, of course, but are just considered part of everyday life. So everyone is astonished when Ed's teenage son and Sarah's teenage daughter begin having serious problems. Ed's son starts shoplifting at thirteen, is truant at fourteen, begins using drugs at fifteen, and is a high school drop-out at sixteen. He is, and always has been, an emotional and sensitive child and he began having conflicts with his father as soon as he reached adolescence and began to question authority. Sarah's daughter has already been hospitalized after a suicide gesture, is now on antidepressants and continues to declare that life is not worth living, even though she is beautiful, talented, and a gifted student.

No one in the family can make sense of this situation. The kids' parents blame the schools, their friends, drugs, and television. The grandparents stand by helplessly, willing to provide assistance but clueless about how to do that. Our cultural refusal to accept the biblical wisdom about the "sins" of the parents being passed on to the third and fourth generation is apparent to an outside, trained observer, but is hidden—dissociated—from the members of the family. Because the problem is never properly identified there can be no adequate solution.

Children learn as much in their families by what is *not* said than by what is. Ed never consciously noticed that his father became distressed and enraged whenever a show came on TV that showed Oriental-looking people. Nor did he notice that his own body registered this fear and anger coming from his father. Ed certainly never knew that his own deep sense of rage at his father for being so withdrawn, and shame at himself for having participated in atrocities, was conveyed wordlessly to his own son, preventing his son from establishing a clear and healthy identity in his own adolescence.

Alice never talked to Sarah about her sexual frustration or rage at her husband Sam, yet Sarah knew deep inside all about it and repeated her mother's life in her own, lacking any conscious control to stop it. And Sarah certainly never meant to convey to her own daughter the sense of hopelessness about ever having her own needs met. And yet her daughter sensed it, without words, and assumed the same applied to her.

What happens is that the traumatic affect gets passed on to each successive generation unattached to a verbalized memory experience that could help the next generation make sense of the feeling and place it in its proper context. The intent initially is not malicious, but protective. And yet we have totally underestimated the power of emotion and emotional inhibition. Emotion gets conveyed to the people we are close to in an inevitable and uncontrolled way if we do not take responsibility for it and talk about what we feel. By ignoring traumatic affect and memory we do *not* make it disappear; we just create a psychic abscess that infects the rest of the person *and* subsequent generations.

By the time the traumatic affect has reached the third generation, and even worse, the fourth generation, the affect is passed on automatically without any cognitive framework that would help the child make sense of what he or she feels. These feelings are passed on through the nonverbal intricacies of basic attachment behavior between parents and children. The children then assume that there is something fundamentally wrong with them, or that this relationship behavior is the norm, rather than being able to understand that because they have been *less* traumatized than their parents, they are more sensitive and tuned-in to their parents' unexpressed and unresolved emotional states than their parents are. When this occurs, we say that the children are "too sensitive" and label them as disturbed, bad, lazy, or sick, and look for every explanation for their problematic behavior other than the obvious one—the unresolved, unverbalized, and unhealed legacy of pain in their family of origin.

The parents, grandparents, and great-grandparents, if any of them are still alive, have a vested interest in blaming the children for the problem because any other route would lead to the past, back to the original trauma and the original pain, which was originally walled-off in the interests of *survival.* Once the survival programming is in place, defying this programming and opening up old wounds becomes very difficult—yet this is the only way that the children and the entire family can heal.

In this situation, and most others like it, whom do we blame for the problem? In the present, the grandchildren suffer from a familial emotional dissociation that has become highly maladaptive for adequate function. And yet, as the example of Sam and Alice and their family illustrates, the adaptation that each successive generation makes comes from protectiveness and the need to survive. Trace back almost any American family history, and you will find repeated experiences of overwhelming traumatic experience that have produced impairment in the capacity for healthy and loving parenting. Each traumatized generation has done its best to guarantee minimum survival.

The intergenerational problems begin when the emergency measures that have been activated to protect family survival operate long past the time when they are necessary. Separated from their original purposes, these emergency measures become family styles of interacting, family belief systems that rapidly become impermeable to change. And even if we can name the sin and its perpetrator, no one commits shameful behavior outside of a social system that encourages and supports that behavior. In this case, Sam and Ed were patriots, who were taught that going to war when your country demands it is the right thing to do if you are a man, but they were also taught from early childhood that killing is a mortal sin. Alice and Sarah grew up in a social system that encourages women to support men's patriotism and to surrender control of their lives to men's desires, while taking care of their men who are wounded inside. When the children of the third generation become old enough to question and challenge—through their maladaptive behavior—all of these internal contradictions, not only do their parents and grandparents not want to hear the meaning in their message, but the entire society denies their perceptions and labels them as sick.

CONSEQUENCES OF THE RESPONSE TO DANGER—MAKING MEANING

If the human response to danger is effective, the individual and the group survive without sustaining any major or long-lasting damage. Healthy human beings function as an integrated whole. Danger produces a suspension of those integrated functions as each aspect of our physical, mental, and social self organizes for its special function in times of alarm. There appears to be no built-in biologically derived mechanism or instructions for integrating dissociated material. Integration does not appear to usually occur naturally or spontaneously, probably because of the contradictory need to continue to self-protect against the powerful and frightening feelings aroused at the time of the danger.

The social group apparently has the obligation to provide a mechanism for conscious integration after any kind of dissociative experience. If alarm is followed by a restoration of calm, and no serious damage or loss has occurred, then the person returns to baseline. The danger has been successfully mastered, and the normal pace of life is resumed. The person reviews his or her response, the social group spontaneously reviews the situation, and members share their experiences. In this self-and-other exchange, fragments of sensory experience and memory are integrated into a meaning scheme and stored for future reference. When done properly, the social group provides various, often ritualized, ways for the victim to put their experience into words using language.

This may be one of the main functions for which language and writing evolved. Any learning that has been gained will be put into a narrative form to be remembered and transmitted to others and to the next generation.

The translation of remembered images, feelings, smells, sounds, and bodily experiences into words through celebratory and ceremonial rituals and works of art provides a way for us to organize the memories. This reordering and integration of information allows us to fit it all into schema that permits us to integrate the experience into a meaningful, and therefore controllable, explanation of the world that incorporates the recently experienced danger. Physiological calm is restored through alleviation of the dangerous provocation and through communal sharing of emotions and perceptions. Fright is turned into humor and pride. For a while, social contact is enhanced, people are drawn to each other and feel a heightened sense of safety with each other. But what happens to the meaning system when the response to danger goes wrong, when the trauma does not end, or is pervasive, or repetitive, or secret, or when the social group does not respond in ways that are healing?

Destroying the Assumptive World

People who suffer profound trauma may no longer feel that they are alive. Instead, they feel like zombies, the walking dead wandering in the wilderness. Trauma sets people outside the bounds of the normal human community. We are able to get out of bed and leave our house in the morning because we make basic and unconscious assumptions that the world is safe, meaningful, and we can function adequately well in it. We rarely if ever think about these underlying assumptions because they *are* underlying premises that are just taken for granted in a consensual way. Trauma shatters the assumptions upon which each of us bases our sense of safety and freedom in the world. The victim may perceive the world as no longer meaningful, or benevolent, and perceive themselves as worthless, helpless, and hopeless (Janoff-Bulman 1992).

Loss of Benevolence

When people are traumatized, these assumptions are at best challenged, and at worst demolished. When we experience the trauma, the world can no longer be seen as a benevolent place. The more rejecting the social response is to the trauma, the more this lack of benevolence is exaggerated. The world becomes less benevolent when a woman is raped, then even less benevolent when the judicial authorities blame her for the rape, and even less benevolent when her husband accuses her of inviting the rape. Children raised in homes filled with malice may never even get to fully develop the concept of a benevolent world before their tender assumptions are shattered. These may be the people who end up in our maximum security prisons.

Loss of Justice

Most people base their sense of safety in the world on a sense of meaning that they have derived individually from their own experience and from the social milieu of which they are a part—their gender, their family, their community, their ethnic group, their racial group, their religious community, their national group. Man is the meaning-making animal. All of our cultural achievements are directed at making sense of the world we live in and of each other.

Children do not need to be taught about "fairness"—it seems to be built-in (Callahan 1991; Wilson 1993; Wright 1994). One of the fundamental ways in which we make sense of the world is through this native sense of justice. We assume that the world is just and that we are rewarded for right behavior and punished for wrong behavior. The corollary of this belief system is that if bad things happen to us, it is because we are bad in some way and are being punished. Somehow it is our fault.

Loss of Order

Because we need the world to be meaningful, the traumatized person has to fit the trauma into some kind of schema that makes sense. But most trauma does not make sense. It is meaningless, unfair, and tragic. Overwhelming traumatic experience challenges our assumptions about the nature of reality. Traumatized people often do not have a moment that is not contaminated by the trauma. It is so real that they can taste it, smell it, see it, hear it, feel it. But for even their most intimate companions, the trauma has no reality, and they want to distance themselves from whatever reality is conveyed through the emotions of the victim. Because much of what we define as real is defined that way through our cultural framework, the victim of trauma is set outside of this safe space, one foot in the world of others, another foot in the traumatic reality.

Loss of Meaning

Traumatic experiences destroy the sense of meaningfulness of the world in which the victim lives. And yet trauma rarely destroys the sense of justice that resides within—at least as it applies to judging the self. As a result many victims of trauma come to believe that their self is *not* worthy, because if it was, the trauma would not have occurred. They become deeply ashamed of whatever imagined fault has caused the trauma to have befallen them and stolen from them a sense of mastery. When other people scapegoat them, it is a further confirmation of their blameworthiness. Burdened by such a sense of shame, victims often cast themselves into the wilderness, outside of the realm of human community.

Loss of Comfort from Others

Victims of trauma often become increasingly isolated from other people. They may destroy relationships that already exist, and refuse to start new relationships. They may be unable to pursue a vocation or avocation because they cannot find meaning in anything they do. They often resort to self-destructive behaviors including substance abuse, which relieve them briefly from the feeling of alienation and oppression. They are lost, alone, bereft, and unable to find comfort or solace anywhere, waiting for life to be over or taking the matter into their own hands and attempting suicide.

Loss of Faith

This loss of faith in oneself is mirrored in loss of faith in the capacity of others to provide help or comfort, as well as the loss of faith in a benevolent higher power to whom one can turn. Without an ability to alter one's reality positively through the use of other people or a group setting, the person often becomes overwhelmed by what has become his or her reality, unable to perform the self-deception that appears necessary for health (Schumaker 1995). Without a fundamental ground of meaning or a shared meaning system it is often difficult to create, honor, and maintain a consistent set of ethical rules. And people who have learned to be helpless do not demonstrate an ability to mobilize for social action (Bandura 1982).

TRAUMA-ORGANIZED BEHAVIOR

The lives of these people I used as examples, Connie, Sam, Alice, and their children and grandchildren, all demonstrate that our lives can become completely organized around trauma. Trauma can become the central organizing principle for human thought, feelings, behavior, and meaning.

If children are exposed to danger repeatedly, their bodies become unusually sensitive, so that even minor threats trigger this entire sequence of physical, emotional, and cognitive responses. They can do nothing to control this reaction; it is a biological, built-in response, a protective device that goes wrong only if we are exposed to too much danger and too little protection in childhood or as adults. As we have seen, if trauma occurs in adult life, the same sequence of events occurs but is far less likely to skew normal development because the brain and character traits of the adult are already established. For children, every aspect of the self will be distorted and bent in the direction of the traumatic exposure. Through the overwhelming power of traumatic addiction, traumatic reenactment, and emotional contagion, they and their entire social support system will unwittingly become a "trauma-organized" system (Bentovim 1992). Although evidence for this effect in childhood is abundant, there is also evidence that prolonged and repeated exposure to trauma, even in adult life, can warp character as well. (Southwick, Yehuda, and Giller 1993; Tichener 1986; Van der Kolk 1996a).

If traumatic experience is so damaging, and human history has been so traumatic, how have we survived and thrived? The key to the answer to such a question resides in attachment—our attachments to each other and to our social group that follow us from cradle to grave. Attachment theory is the next thing we must understand before we can construct a more generalized understanding of how to go about helping people heal from traumatic experience.

two

Attachment
Constructing the Social

Post-traumatic stress disorder is a social disease. Its effects spread across and down the generations. The key to eliminating post-traumatic stress disorder is preventing trauma. The key to treating post-traumatic stress disorder is other people. Now that we have seen what happens to people who are traumatized, how the normal adaptation to danger turns into disorder, we must begin to develop some premises for how to reverse that order. To do that, we have to have a better idea of the powerful effect human beings have on each other. The social aspects of being a human being are as innately wired as our need to eat, drink, and sleep and every bit as important to our survival. As Felicity de Zulueta notes in her book on trauma, attachment, and violence, "We matter deeply to one another for our very well-being. It is not just that we need each other to *satisfy* our hunger or our sexual needs as Freud saw it; it is not only that we need to feel good with one another to feel good about ourselves. What is becoming clearer is that our social interactions play an important role in the everyday regulation of our internal *biological* systems throughout our lives, such an important role that we cannot do without significant 'others' and remain in health" (de Zulueta 1993).

ATTACHMENT AND SEPARATION

Although people have long been aware of the importance of the mother-child bond, it was Dr. John Bowlby in England who spurred the current interest in studying the vital importance of early relationships in all subsequent human endeavors. Bowlby said, "Attachment behavior is held to characterize human beings from the cradle to the grave" (Bowlby 1979) and that assertion has stood as a clarion call to study the mechanisms and dynamics of attachment behavior.

The reasons for attachment behavior seem pretty clear. Increasing mammalian intelligence was accompanied by the rapid growth of large heads to accommodate those bigger brains. But large heads have difficulty getting through narrow birth canals, and with each increase in intelligence, the offspring is born in a less developed state. Mammalian development necessitated a new evolutioary adaptation—parental care (Eibl-Eibesfeldt 1989). The human infant is the most dependent mammal born and has the longest period of dependency. Parenting, for the human species, requires a larger investment of time and energy than in any other species. Nature had to devise effective mechanisms that would keep child and parent attached to each other for the years necessary to protect human offspring.

Response to Separation

John Bowlby is the person most responsible for pointing out the importance of attachment in human growth and development. In his book *Attachment* (1982) he points out that although mothers and poets have been alive for a long time to the distress caused by separating a child from its mother, science has only begun to study these effects. Not until World War II were careful scientific observations made of children and infants separated from their mothers (Spitz 1945).

Since then, confirmations of these observations have come from many different sources, on children from many different backgrounds, of different ages, and under various circumstances. All of the data confirm the fact that children experience extreme distress when separated from their primary caregivers. And it is not just children who respond poorly to separation (Schore 1994). Numerous studies have demonstrated a strong connection between separation, loss, and depressive illness in adults (Reite and Boccia 1994). A strong connection also exists between separation, loss, and various medical disorders, probably because of the combined effect of a generalized dysregulation of the autonomic system physiology and alterations in immune function, both of which accompany loss (Reite and Boccia 1994).

Protest, Despair, Death, or Detachment

All mammals are dependent on their caregivers. Given this fact, mammals had to evolve a means for achieving and maintaining closeness between the baby and its mother. These behaviors are called attachment behaviors. All mammalian species emit a "separation cry" when the baby animal is separated from its mother, a cry of distress that elicits predictable responses in the caregiver or, in sub-primate species, any caregiver. In primates and humans over a certain age, not just any caregiver will do. Primates and humans become attached to a specific caregiver and the separation cry sounds whenever they are separated from that caregiver. Human communication begins with this separation cry and evolves into speech, and for the rest of our lives, speech becomes a way we maintain and secure attachments.

These observations describe the response of children ages fifteen to thirty months. Until about six to nine months, the child may allow another caretaker to substitute for mother. Stranger anxiety begins by the ninth month and is accompanied by the child's specific preference for its own mother. The child's initial response to separation from its mother is protest, which lasts from hours to weeks. During this time the child is obviously distressed and does whatever is within its power to find its mother. There is also a pronounced physiological response with many different signs of hyperarousal (Van der Kolk 1987a, 1987b). Usually the child will reject all attempts at being comforted by another caretaker. The child will cry loudly, look eagerly for any signs of the mother's return, shake the bed, throw his or her body around.

If his mother does not return, the protest stage is succeeded by the stage of despair and the child begins to behave in a way that appears to represent a sense of hopelessness. The crying decreases in intensity, physical activity slows down, the child becomes withdrawn and uninterested in the surroundings. This can be mistaken for a decrease in distress instead of being recognized for what it is—a deep and inutterable sense of grief. Research has shown that the deeper the affectionate bonds and the more satisfactory the relationship between mother and child are before the separation, the greater the child's upset during the separation.

Some children actually die from failure to thrive (Spitz 1945; Benoit, Zeanah, and Barton 1989) or succumb to various diseases, referred to by the poets as "dying of a broken heart." This phase is characterized by retarded activity, reduced food and water intake, and collapse, indicating a basic neurobiological failure, even in the presence of sources of physical maintenance (Kraemer 1985). If the child survives, after some time has elapsed, he or she will appear to be recovering. The child begins to show more interest in the surroundings, accepts care and food from others, and becomes more sociable. The child may appear normal in many ways until the mother returns to the scene. Then it is possible to see that this stage is not recovery but detachment. The child shows none of the expected joy over reunion. Instead the child turns away from her, as though she is a stranger.

If the child repeatedly loses caretakers to whom he or she has become attached, the child may eventually act as if neither mothering nor contact with other humans matters very much. He will become increasingly self-centered and preoccupied with material things such as food and toys, instead of people. If the mother reappears, the child will be interested in the presents she brings, but not in her. Although the child may appear superficially normal socially, he or she is likely to have difficulty sustaining intimate relationships (Jones 1983).

LESSONS FROM OUR ANCESTORS—PRIMATE RESEARCH

Looking at the behavior of our primate cousins helps us to develop some ideas about how human attachment behavior evolved and how much of human behavior is innate rather than learned. A massive amount of research has been performed over the last several decades on studies of primate behavior and attachment (Harlow and Mears 1974; Kraemer 1985; Suomi and Ripp 1983).

Protest, Despair, and Dysfunction: Harlow's Monkeys

Harry Harlow began studying monkey behavior a few decades ago (Harlow 1962; Van der Kolk 1987a, 1987b). He took baby monkeys away from their mothers and isolated them alone in cages with various forms of what the experimenters called "evil mothers"—dummies made only of wire mesh, dummies covered with a cloth-covered frame, dummies that shook when the baby monkey clung to them—all formed to substitute for the warm, responsive, biological mother. These babies came to be known as the "motherless monkeys." "Eventually we realized that we had a laboratory full of neurotic monkeys" (Harlow 1962). Since then, Harlow's monkey research findings have been confirmed and extended. This research has been shown to be consistent with that of researchers who have studied early infant separation experiences in humans and indicates the enormous damage that occurs when infant attachment bonds are damaged. Let us look at these specific primate studies in a little more detail.

Baby monkeys who are separated from their mothers in the first year of life and raised instead with "surrogate wire or cloth mothers" become highly disturbed adolescent and adult monkeys. They are very socially withdrawn, unpredictably aggressive, and aggressive against themselves. They do not know how to engage in normal monkey behavior, are unable to mate properly, and do not know normal monkey social cues. If the female monkeys are artificially inseminated or manage to get pregnant naturally, they often mutilate and kill their babies. These animals are unpredictably aggressive, and engage in self-destructive behaviors. They also develop more tumors than normal monkeys and are more prone to various infections (Mason 1968; Van der Kolk 1987a,b)

The degree of impairment depends on the amount of time spent in isolation (Kraemer 1985). Monkeys isolated for the first three months of life, if subsequently placed in a nurturing environment, seem to recover. If monkeys are separated from their mothers after three or six months of social experience, they are not as severely debilitated, but they do show persistent abnormal social and sexual behavior. Monkeys isolated during the second six months of life show inordinately high levels of aggression when put back in with other monkeys. Monkeys who are isolated for the first twelve months are severely disturbed. These monkeys show a devastating loss of social competence and can not respond normally to social cues (de Zulueta 1993). If isolated monkeys are reunited with their mothers and peers quickly the effects of the isolation can be reversed, although males are more affected by the effects of isolation than females. Interesting for human developmental research as well is that isolates have been found to be ineffective in perceiving and sending facial expressions and they do not respond appropriately to the facial expressions of other monkeys (Kraemer 1985).

Some of the damaging effects can be attenuated if the monkeys are housed with their peers, even if separated from their mothers. When the monkeys have been raised with their peers, then separation from their peers will produce the same protest/despairing response as separation from mother. Repeated separations will diminish the protest response but the despair response persists (Van der Kolk 1987b).

Motherless Monkeys Grown Up

If the adult "motherless monkeys" are put in social groups composed of normal three-month-old monkey peers, monkeys raised normally with their mothers, the motherless monkeys are initially extremely maladjusted and very aggressive. But after time has passed they are able to learn new behaviors in parallel with their normal younger monkey peers. The younger monkey "therapists" are suitable teachers because they have not yet developed the normal aggression towards strangers that is seen at seven months of age. They tend instead to cling to the disturbed monkeys, thus providing them with the warmth, contact, and play that the disturbed animals had never received. The motherless monkeys calm down and begin to look more and more like the normal monkeys. The researchers who noted this effect coined the term "monkey therapists" to allude to the therapeutic effect the normal monkeys have on the disturbed monkeys (Suomi and Harlow 1972; Suomi, Harlow, and Novak 1974).

But even so, problems arise for the motherless monkeys when they are socially stressed. When they become physiologically aroused they tend to become either socially withdrawn or overly aggressive compared to normal monkeys and fail to obey normal monkey social cues. Their sexual behavior often continues to be disturbed as well (Anderson and Mason 1978). They also show responses to other circumstances that differ from normal monkeys. When motherless monkeys who have been normalized by monkey peers are given amphetamines, they become acutely violent and kill their peers. Normal monkeys do not respond in this manner (Kraemer 1985). The response of motherless monkeys to alcohol also differs from their normal monkey peers. If the motherless monkeys are given alcohol, they drink much more than normal monkeys. The previously separated monkeys drink more alcohol than their normal peers both during and after separation (Van der Kolk 1987b).

Researchers have also studied the effects of social deprivation on the second generation (Ruppenthal et al. 1976; Suomi and Ripp 1983). Female monkeys who are separated early in life from their own mothers, particularly for prolonged periods, are severely impaired in their ability to provide adequate mothering for their offspring. They are prone to mutilate and kill their babies; the younger the mother, the greater the likelihood of abuse. Motherless monkeys are three times more likely to provide adequate care for their female offspring than their male offspring and their male offspring are four times more likely to be abused. Motherless monkey mothering improves with practice. If the motherless monkeys are allowed to be abusive with their firstborn, their mothering improves with each subsequent child as long as they were not separated from their firstborn, a finding that is common in human clinical work, in which the eldest child is often the most severely abused. These studies consistently show that primate infants subjected to abuse and deprivation have significantly more difficulty as adults, particularly the males, dealing with aggression than their normal peers. The females learn to suppress their aggression but remain distrustful of sexual contact while the males continue to be violent (Harlow 1974).

MOM AND DAD AS BRAIN MODULATORS

The human infant comes into the world totally helpless, with a brain that is still actively developing. Most of the development of axons, dendrites, and synaptic connections that underlie all behavior takes place *after*, not before, birth, and therefore it takes place in the context of interaction with primary caretakers. The maturation of the prefrontal cortex, the part of the brain that truly distinguishes us from other species, occurs after birth. This brain development occurs during "critical" or sensitive periods. Critical periods are periods of intense growth during which the brain is particularly susceptible to environmental conditions that can lead to developmental arrest if they are not within the proper range (Schore 1994). This concept also implies that if the proper stimulus is not applied during this critical period, the development will never occur.

The Immature Brain

The neonate's brain is able to handle a smaller amount of the information per unit of time as that of the adult, and the brain circuits function more slowly while the cerebral metabolic rate is very low compared to the adult (Schore 1994). As a result, the child needs the mother to be the external regulator of his or her own internal biochemistry. Even many genetic programs are dependent on transactions with the infant's environment, and maternal behavior is thought to be significant in mediating genetic influences. The mother also is a hidden regulator of the infant's endocrine and nervous systems (Schore 1994).

How does this happen? How can someone outside control another being's body inside? Apparently through affect, through the emotional contagion that we discussed earlier. In studies of emotional contagion we know that human beings automatically and rapidly mimic each other's nonverbal expressions, both facial, vocal, and postural. In doing so, we spontaneously evoke a similar emotional state in ourselves as in the person we have mimicked. This emotional state is, of course, accompanied by the level of physiological arousal typical of the particular affects elicited (Hatfield et al. 1994). The emotional, nonverbal transactions between the child and mother appear to regulate internal neurochemical changes (Schore 1994).

The Face Shows All

The face is our "affect screen." Each affect has a distinctive facial and postural appearance (Nathanson 1992). The neonate preferentially attends to the human face at birth and prefers the mother's face by two to seven weeks. The baby's facial recognition abilities for different people and different emotional expressions develops rapidly, so that by seven months the baby can even begin to categorize certain facial changes expressing emotion. Over the course of the first year of life, the mother induces changes in emotional state in her infant, and in doing so directly influences the infant's learning of how, how much, and whether to feel (Schore 1994).

Evidence also attests to a synchrony among activity, behavior, and speech rhythms between human mothers and infants, as well as complex patterns of social interactions. Brazelton concluded that "[t]his interdependency of rhythms seemed to be at the root of their 'attachment' as well as communication" (Reite and Boccia 1994). We apparently have discovered an essential biosocial bridge; the link between the internal physiological world of the infant and the internal physiological world of the mother, that paves the way for all later relationships.

Affect States and Brain Development

These changes in affect state are so vital because of the effect that these states have on brain development. The arousal of specific levels of affect, at specific critical times, triggers the release of specific neurohormones in the brain that determine actual brain development (Schore 1994). The level of arousal will determine brain effects such as regional blood flow, the vascular delivery of vital nutrients, and the regional metabolism which determines the actual growth of brain cells.

Additionally, the mother-infant relationship changes over time, and these changes result in reorganization of brain structures. The heightened levels of positive emotion and play behavior that occur between infant and mother at the end of the first year are particularly important in regulating the development of the prefrontal cortex. This is at least partly due to the stimulation of opioid production in the brain and these substances help to regulate the development of neurons in key centers of the brain (Schore 1994).

In the second year, the mother's role shifts from pure caregiver and joy-promoter to agent of socialization—the "no" phase. In this period, the mother-infant interactions are more stressful, and these changes induce maturation in the cortical system that self-regulates emotional states. The basic regulation of affect between the young child and the mother will determine whether the child is able to regulate shame; dysregulation may lead to various forms of psychopathology, including depression. Since rage reactions are related to separation responses, the development of affect regulation between infant and mother, when successful, leads to the transformation of unmodulated rage into healthy aggression and the development of autonomy (Schore 1994).

The Beginnings of Moral Development

At eighteen months, children normally first exhibit moral prosocial behavior in the form of comforting, which means regulating the negative affect of a distressed other. This response is dependent on having had the proper affect regulatory experiences with mother which helped develop the appropriate frontal lobe circuits in the brain that subserve moral development.

Gendered Caregiving and Receiving

At this time, the father becomes an important emotional resource for the baby, and he plays an increasing role in arousal modulation and stimulation, thus also influencing cortical development. (Schore 1994). Most of the developmental research has focused on the role of the biological mother as the primary caretaker, in part because this work has its roots in animal research in which the biological mother *is* the primary caretaker. But what about father caregiving in humans? Some researchers, combining what we know about animals and humans, suggest that caregiving behavior is built into both males and females but that male caregiving is less readily evoked than female. If a human male has sufficient exposure to a young child, he will become a caregiver (Ainsworth 1991).

The Beginnings of Autoregulation

By the middle of the second year of life, a child who has had a healthy developmental experience can access mature areas in the frontal lobes and the limbic systems of the brain that autoregulate the child's autonomic nervous system and endocrine systems (Schore 1994). It is possible to see that many things can go wrong in this early learning experience, and research is just now being performed. For now, it is important to recognize that the modulation of important brain biochemicals is dependent on interaction with another person from birth onward. Lack of proper modulation from parenting figures results in a physiological hyperarousal for the infant or child that is emotionally noxious, physically dangerous, and cognitively stupefying. We are beginning to understand that this basic biochemical vulnerability does not stop in childhood, that adults remain vulnerable to massive swings in biochemical states as well. So let us now look at what we know about disrupted attachments in childhood and how they affect adult development.

DISRUPTED ATTACHMENTS

We have seen the devastating effect of disrupted attachment on young primates. It should come as no surprise that we see a similar pattern of maladaptation among children who have disrupted attachments. Because children are dependent on their caretakers for safety and the fulfillment of their basic needs, any traumatic situation may disrupt the child's primary attachments and sense of basic trust. This disruption is particularly profound when the source of the trauma *is* the primary caretaker.

Disorganized Attachment

Mary Ainsworth and her colleagues have taken advantage of normal stranger anxiety to discover the different ways in which children attach to their caregivers (Ainsworth et al. 1978). The typical patterns of normal attachment are well-organized and consistent over time with that particular caregiver although the pattern may be quite different with a different caretaker. Longitudinal research has begun to show that these patterns of attachment are predictive of a child's behavior in school, at home, and in social situations at least to the tenth year. A child's attachment style is also consistent with parenting characteristics and parental attachment style (Berman and Sperling 1994).

The most recently identified attachment style has been called the disorganized/disoriented attachment (Main and Hesse 1990). This style is characterized by a lack of coherent strategy of relating to the caregiver. The behavior of these children is inconsistent and contradictory without the usual sequencing of behavior and with the addition of quite unusual behaviors such as freezing and hand flapping. These children appear to be caught in dilemma—their attachment figure is also the source of fear. They respond to this conflict with mental, emotional, and behavioral disorganization and confusion. This style of attachment has been found to be highly correlated with parents who have unresolved traumatic loss in their own backgrounds. The parent's state of continuing fear and the behavioral components of this fear state frighten the child (Main and Hesse 1990).

Intergenerational Transmission

This last disturbed attachment relationship paves the way for what we call "trauma-bonding" and is probably how the multigenerational transmission of traumatic experience actually happens. Considerable evidence suggests that an individual's relationship history is an important variable determining parental behavior (Zeanah and Zeanah 1989). In other words, we tend to raise our children similarly to the way we were raised. This does not mean that maltreated children inevitably maltreat their children in the same way. Only a relatively small percentage do. But what can be repeated, down through the generations, are attachment styles that become organizing themes of relationships (Zeanah and Zeanah 1989).

ATTACHMENT IN ADULTS: THE CONTINUING NEED FOR SOCIAL SUPPORT

Adult attachment has been defined as "the stable tendency of an individual to make substantial efforts to seek and maintain proximity to and contact with one or a few specific individuals who provide the subjective potential for physical and/or psychological safety and security" (Berman and Sperling 1994). The bonds of adult attachments appear to have their roots in the childhood attachment bond. This does not mean an absolute one-to-one correlation. It simply means that early attachment experiences set the tone, they are likely to determine the kinds of partners with whom new attachments are formed most easily and the developmental course of new attachments (Weiss 1991).

Thus, over the long haul, attachment styles appear to organize emotional and behavioral responses (Bowlby 1978; Grossman and Grossman 1982; Main et al. 1985; Sroufe 1989; Sroufe and Walters 1977; Stern 1985). Bowlby's theory was that they do this through the creation of an "internal working model" that guides us to recreate the original attachments throughout a lifetime, a sort of cookie-cutter pattern into which we jam anything that doesn't quite fit the mold. Then, in the form of a self-fulfilling prophecy, the more we make new relationships replicate the old, the more we become convinced that our relational models and assumptions are correct. The result: If we are lucky, have loving parents, establish secure relationships with them throughout childhood and adolescence, then that is what we repeat. But what if we are not so lucky? What if we experience a traumatic loss or traumatic betrayal of parental care? What role do other people continue to play in our lives, for better or for worse? Let's take a look at what we know about the elusive quality called "social support."

The whole idea of social support dates back to at least the last century when, in 1897, the sociologist Durkheim wrote one of the first books to show a marked increase in concern for the physical and mental health of modern society. In his classic study on suicide he discussed the way suicidal behavior evolves out of diminished social connections to family, friends, and community. According to Durkheim, when an individual does not feel that he is a part of a group, when he recognizes no higher purpose or meaning, and has few social supports, suicidal behavior becomes more likely (Durkheim 1951). His conclusion was that the social conditions that underlie the rising suicide rate and other forms of social pathology "result not from a regular evolution but from a morbid disturbance which, while able to uproot the institutions of the past, has put nothing in their place" (Bellah 1973).

Social support theory provides a direct line of connection between childhood attachment, adult attachment, and social connectedness. Caplan described support systems as an enduring pattern of social ties that play a major role in maintaining the psychological and physical integrity of the individual (Caplan 1974; Greenblatt et al. 1982). This sense of being cared about is possible because of the human capacity for emotional resonance and empathy.

Other important work has related the effects of social support on physical health, particularly as it is related to stress. Support provided by key people and groups in a person's life are seen as playing a significant role in cushioning or "buffering" the individual against both physical and psychological consequences of stress (Cassel 1976; Vaux 1988). At the same time, many forms of stress also cause major disruptions in social ties which then exacerbate the stress, creating a vicious downward spiral. Certainly, as a result of the research that is being done in the field of post-traumatic stress we are beginning to understand how social support, to the extent that it helps people deal more effectively with stress, can lower the amount of hyperarousal, thereby changing the internal biochemistry of the stressed person and in so doing, positively affect the immune system (Pilisuk and Parks 1986). In study after study, social isolation increases the risk of developing coronary disease and other life-threatening illnesses, and among people who already have coronary disease, people who are socially isolated have a two- to five-fold higher death rate than those observed in nonisolated patients (Williams 1995).

As we learn more about emotional contagion and the ways in which we directly affect each other's physiological states, we can begin to develop an understanding of *how* and *why* other people can have such a profound effect on us. Certainly, other people's capacity for creating negative effects, as witnessed by the extraordinarily high incidence of interpersonal trauma, is only too evident. We need to be spending at least as much time and energy trying to figure out how to maximize the positive influence we can exert in each other's lives, in many different kinds of ways. The social support literature is diverse, complicated, and even in some ways conflicted, but nonetheless it does go to show that there are numerous ways of defining social support. We need different things from different people at different times in our lives. But we never cease to need something from other people.

In treating victims of trauma, my colleagues and I have focused our attention on the neglected aspect of psychological treatment—the social context. It is time now to look in more detail at *The Sanctuary* and how a trauma-based paradigm changed us, the way we treat our patients, and even the way that we now view the world.

three

Remembering the Social in Psychiatry
Deviance

Deviance refers to "any behavior or attribute for which an individual is regarded as objectionable in a particular social system ... anything that violates prevailing norms" (Glaser 1971). There are many different kinds of deviants. People who are criminals and people who are mentally ill are considered to be deviants. The line between who is deviant and who is not changes dramatically over time and place. But always, a community tends to show its most degrading side when it attempts to deal with those whom it has labeled deviant. Historically and sometimes today, we lock them up, run them out of town, humiliate them, torture them, deprive them of basic human rights, even kill them. Once we have decided that a person or a group is deviant, we build up a complex and convoluted system of legal tenets and ethical justifications to demonstrate that grave differences exist between the way we, as a social group, treat deviants and the way they treat us. One of the most obvious differences of course, is power. Whoever has the most power determines who is deviant and what should be done about their deviance.

It is important that we as a society become better equipped to deal with deviant people for several reasons. The first is that people who are judged to act in deviant ways pose many of the problems that give pause for great concern to the rest of us; and second, there appear to be more and more deviant people. Almost thirty years ago, Laing pointed out that a child born in the United Kingdom was ten times more likely to be admitted to a mental hospital than to a university: "This is an indication that we are driving our children mad more effectively than we are genuinely educating them" (Laing 1967). Today, five out of six people will be victims of violent crimes at least once in their lifetimes (National Victim Center 1993). These crimes will be committed by men and women who will be defined as deviants once they enter our ballooning prison system. According to the Justice Department, from 1980 to 1992 the American state and federal prison population soared nearly 150 percent, from 139 to 344 jailed for every 100,000 of total population—the Western world's highest ratio (Starer 1995).

Psychiatry is the profession that is socially assigned to deal with a certain class of deviants—the mentally ill. As a major social institution and therefore supporter of the status quo, the psychiatric profession has always had an underlying conflict, forever arguing over the etiologic foundation of the disorders that come under its purview. Those inclining toward biological predisposition have always been in conflict with those who place a stronger emphasis on social and environmental factors as the sources of psychiatric dysfunction. But, the voice arguing for social and political factors has always been a quieter voice, and has rarely been heard for very long. Many of these voices have been largely silenced, available now only in libraries or antiquarian bookshops, though their message is more relevant now than it has ever been. The purpose of this chapter is to remember, to hear again some of the voices of the past conveying a wisdom that is timeless, vital, and yet repeatedly ignored.

A BRIEF HISTORY

There have been at least three major historical paradigms to deal with deviance: deviance as sin; deviance as crime; and deviance as sickness (Conrad and Schneider 1980). The dichotomy of madness as moral trauma and madness as disease goes back at least to the Greeks. This essential conflict over the roots of mental illness was never resolved by the Greeks, and has never been resolved since (Porter 1987). However, modern psychiatry begins at the historical period, when deviance in all its forms began to be seen as sickness, rather than sin or criminality. This period coincides with the Enlightenment, when ideas of Reason, Liberty, Democracy, Equality, and the Rights of Man filled the air and changed the entire political landscape.

Throughout the Middle Ages, the mad were often executed as witches, thrown into prisons, or banished and sent to roam outside of their towns. Some towns would charter entire ships—"Ships of Fools"—to take the insane to distant and uninhabited places and abandon them (Foucault 1965; Kittrie 1971). As society became increasingly structured and compartmentalized from the late seventeenth through the nineteenth centuries, there was a greater need to insist that people follow established norms, so as not to upset the social order. The result of this was what Foucault called "the Great Confinement," during which period all kinds of institutions prolifer- ated to take care of problem children, criminals, the poor, and the mad (Foucault 1965). In Paris alone, about one percent of the population was locked up within a few years. Foucault and others have attributed this enor- mous social change to forces related to the economics of capitalism, indus- trialization, and a market economy. In these institutions, resources were scarce, the problems of management were enormous, and order was achieved through mechanical and physical restraint. No real differentia- tion was made between the violent and the nonviolent, and nothing that could be called "treatment" was available.

Pinel in France, Chiarugi and Pisani in Italy, Langerman in Germany, and many practitioners influenced by the Moors in Spain, were all men of the Enlightenment who believed mental illness was the result of a combi- nation of heredity and life experiences. Treatment was to be relational, based on the physician's understanding of human motivation and his abil- ity to develop the patient's trust. The mentally ill were not animals, as the prevailing notions would have it, but wounded souls who needed the com- fort of others, occupation, sound health measures, respect, and benevo- lence (Alexander and Selesnick 1966).

A group of English Quakers led by William Tuke, opened the York Retreat in 1796 as a direct response to the brutal treatment and death of one of their Quaker colleagues at an asylum. The new asylum was to be "a place in which the unhappy might obtain a refuge—a quiet haven in which the shattered bark might find the means of reparation or of safety" (Busfield 1986). The form of treatment they advocated came to be called Moral Treatment, the precursor of the therapeutic milieu, and of The Sanctuary.

MORAL TREATMENT

In 1813, Samuel Tuke, grandson of William, published a book titled *Description of the Retreat, an institution near York for insane persons of the Society of Friends*. In his book, he gave an account of "moral treatment." Physical coercion and restraint were deplored and were replaced with rela- tionships with attendants who were carefully selected to offer inmates guid- ance and treat them humanely. Patients were to be treated with respect, as adults, not as children, and were to be urged in the direction of self- restraint and self-control (Busfield 1986). The violent were separated from the nonviolent. Environmental factors were seen as playing an important role in the etiology of the mental problems. Attention to the social milieu largely replaced physical methods of treatment.

The mad were not seen as animals, but as suffering humans who had gone astray and who could be led back to the right path through kindness, compassion, and rational conversation. Moral treatment was a profoundly social form of treatment. The experience of madness was to be corrected by placing people in humane and caring social environments that emphasized social interaction and the cultivation of latent faculties and healing processes. Moral treatment had far-ranging effects on the face of institutionalization in Europe and in America. The book that Samuel Tuke wrote about the York Retreat spurred the investigation and reform of madhouses throughout the Continent (Macalpine and Hunter 1993).

Moral treatment spread rapidly to the United States. Benjamin Rush, considered the founder of American psychiatry, believed that disease, political institutions, and economic organization were so interrelated that any general social change produced accompanying changes in health. For him, proper political stimuli and a stable and ordered society were required for health. "Mental health implied a society which would provide the proper stimuli and necessary conditions for well-being" (Rosen 1959).

As a result of the influence of the Tukes, Pinel, and others, the asylum movement grew rapidly, and soon every population center in America had a beautifully constructed asylum created to provide the mentally ill with the most modern forms of social treatment in a safe and humane environment. By 1844, American proponents of moral treatment had amassed an impressive body of evidence to support their belief that mental illnesses were treatable and that asylum treatment could restore patients to health. By 1837, Eli Todd at the Hartford Retreat had cured 91.3 percent of his recent cases, and Woodward at Worcester had discharged more than 82 percent as recovered. They proposed that the mentally ill had as much chance for recovery as a person who was ill with any other acute disease of equal severity (McGovern 1985).

But moral treatment required the intensive involvement of many staff members with small groups of patients, and this kind of treatment was more expensive than domiciliary care. As the asylums became available, they were seen as the last resort for many different kinds of problem populations—the senile, syphilitics suffering from the tertiary stage of the disease, the mentally retarded, alcoholics, opium addicts, impoverished immigrants, and other patients suffering from chronic disorders for which little treatment existed. The resultant increase in the chronic population reduced the rates of cures, making it harder for the asylums to justify the increasing level of funding required from state legislatures (McGovern 1985).

Meanwhile, the sheer numbers of patients demanding care resulted in the massive growth of mental institutions, thus defeating the original premises of moral treatment. Hospitals designed to accommodate small patient populations were faced with demands for admissions of anyone considered deviant or unmanageable. As the management of these unwieldy institutions became more and more bureaucratized, the care became more impersonal, controlling, neglectful, and harsh. The funding of asylums became a political hot potato. Legislatures grew increasingly unwilling to fund the asylums. Charismatic and inspired asylum directors gave way to men with the political savvy to attempt political bargaining with state legislatures but who did not necessarily understand the initial goals of Moral Treatment (Dwyer 1987; McGovern 1985; Rothman 1980). Administrations became increasingly corrupt, until by 1891, Burdett, an English physician surveying American institutions, depicted "overcrowding, deteriorated physical facilities, extensive use of physical restraint and manipulation, and only occasionally a hospital with a therapeutic orientation" (Almond 1974). These asylums were the huge and impersonal institutions that we have been busy disassembling for over twenty years.

The relationship between the social and the individual has been and remains a raging academic debate. How much is nature? How much is nurture? What is the etiology of mental illness? If it is illness, like any other biological disorders, then why bother with social forms of treatment. If it is not illness, then what is it? Moral weakness? Evil spirits? Bad character? Philosophers, too, have long been wrestling with our relationship to the larger social context.

THE SOCIAL PHILOSOPHERS

By the end of the nineteenth century, while Freud and his followers were developing a complex theory of individual development and pathology, other thinkers were focusing on the massive social disruptions of the Industrial Revolution. In doing so, they were compelled to look at the connection between individual maladjustment and social forces.

Emil Durkheim, considered the founder of scientific sociology, tried to understand the unconscious sources of social existence as Freud was trying to understand the unconscious sources of personal existence. For Durkheim, society is the source of morality, personality, and life itself at the human level. It is something on which we all depend, whether or not we know it. Durkheim saw modern societies as being sick, and a sign of the sickness was not only the rising suicide rate but also the appearance of what he termed "pessimistic philosophies." George Mead, another social philosopher of the late nineteenth century, saw human group life as an essential condition for the emergence of consciousness. He described the dialectical relationship between the individual and society, pointing out the development of individuality and the development of social institutions are both part of human evolutionary experience. Individuals change and are changed by social institutions (Mead 1934). Another sociologist, Charles Cooley declared in 1909 that human nature cannot exist separately in an individual but is, in fact a "group-nature," a "social mind," and that wherever there is an individual aspect of human function there must also be a social fact (Cooley 1967). In 1920, McDougall asserted that "We can only understand the life of individuals and the life of societies, if we consider them always in relation to one another . . . each man is an individual only in an incomplete sense" (1920).

John Dewey, one of America's most influential philosophers, saw the individual as so embedded in the social milieu, that mind is capable of operating only by the continual stimulus of the social group. Social living is the origin of the self (Campbell 1995). Alfred North Whitehead noted that philosophy has been haunted by a misconception throughout the centuries, the notion of independent existence: "There is no such mode of existence. Every entity is only to be understood in terms of the way it is interwoven with the rest of the universe" (Douglas 1986).

PSYCHIATRY AND THE SOCIAL

Although Freud was fully aware that the development of human personality must be seen in terms of the influence of the prevailing social standards and values to which the person is subjected (Alexander and Selesnick 1966), other psychiatric workers focused more on the interpersonal dimensions of human experience. William Alanson White, an influential early twentieth-century psychiatrist observed "society, while it is composed of individuals, reflects its degree of development in each individual psyche, so that man and society occupy relations of mutual interdependence, each profoundly affecting the other" (White 1919).

Trigant Burrow helped found the American Psychoanalytic Association in 1911 and became its president in 1926. His work has been largely ignored because he took a radical turn away from individual psychoanalysis and toward a study of the group. In his papers and books from 1914 on, he developed the idea that the neurotic elements that Freud had identified in individual patients were embodied in the entire society. He gathered around him a group of colleagues, family members, and patients and they formed the nucleus of a group of investigators that remained together in an experimental community for more than thirty years. In this group setting, called the Lifwynn Foundation as of 1927, they spent their time observing interrelational processes through their own interactions, using themselves as the laboratory agents. Burrow regarded conflict, alienation, crime and war as major public health problems that could be solved through science (Burrow 1984). "Man is not an individual," he said. "His mentation is not individualistic. He is part of a societal continuum that is the outgrowth of a primary or racial continuum" (1926). Later he warned, "My researches clearly indicate to me . . . that with the enhancement of individualism the balance in favor of group survival has been placed in serious jeopardy. Today the very existence of the species is threatened because the antagonisms characterizing man have been largely divorced from his biological needs and actualities" (1953).

Early in his career Alfred Adler worked with underprivileged laborers and was struck by the deplorable conditions under which they worked and how these conditions contributed to their physical and mental problems. At least in part as a result of these experiences he had a well-developed social consciousness. In his later writings, he stressed that mental health could be judged by the degree to which a person could direct himself to his work, love his fellow man, and fulfill his social and communal obligations. In his book *Social Interest,* he stated, "The growing irresistible evolutionary advance of social feeling warrants us in assuming that the existence of humanity is inseparably bound up with 'goodness'" (Alexander and Selesnick 1966).

Adolph Meyer had a vital impact on American psychiatry. He was influenced early in his career by Clifford Beers, a reformer who had himself received horrendous treatment in mental hospitals and devoted his life to reforming them. He was also influenced by his wife, Mary Brooks Meyer. Around 1904, Mrs. Meyer began visiting the families of her husband's patients to learn more about their background and in doing so she became the "first American social worker." He said of these visits, "We thus obtained help in a broader social understanding of our problem and a reaching out to the sources of sickness, the family and the community." Meyer believed that the individual must be understood as a complete whole, a unique entity, and could best be understood by searching for all forces that react upon him and that affect his interaction with the social milieu (Alexander and Selesnick 1966).

Harry Stack Sullivan considered mental illness as related to disturbed relationships between people, seeing the basic conflict as located between the individual and his interpersonal environment. During the years between World War I and World War II, he played a key role in altering the traditional focus of psychiatry from the individual to the interpersonal. "Personality," he wrote in 1938, "is made manifest in interpersonal situations, and not otherwise." His work paved the way for the socially oriented therapies that were to dominate post war psychiatry (Grob 1991). Karen Horney's theories placed human development firmly in a cultural context, and she believed the neurotic person was one who had experienced injurious cultural influences in childhood (Portnoy 1974).

Developing his ideas in the first half of this century, Moreno, the originator of psychodrama, said, "Mankind is a social and organic unity." He termed his area of interest "sociatry" and saw its aim as the healing of normal society. "Sociatry treats the pathological syndromes of normal society, of interrelated individuals and of interrelated groups. It is based upon two hypotheses: 1) The whole of human society develops in accord with definite laws; 2) A truly therapeutic procedure cannot have less an objective than the whole of mankind" (Moreno 1953).

SOCIAL PSYCHIATRY

Social psychiatry is concerned with the relationships between mental disorder and sociocultural processes
—Alexander Leighton 1960, *An Introduction to Social Psychiatry*

As early as 1922, Dr. E. E. Southard of Harvard Medical School, taught his students about "social psychiatry," which he termed "an art now in the course of development by which the psychiatrist deals with social problems" and as "that part of the knowledge of psychiatry which has a bearing upon social problems" (Southard and Jarrett 1922). As a result of the massive disruptions of World War II, American and British psychiatry took on a decidedly social and political complexion. Maxwell Jones referred to this as the "general tendency to change which was apparent in many spheres during war-time" (Jones 1953). The First World War had shaken psychiatry and medicine as a whole, because of the considerable incidence of battle neurosis, or "shell shock."[1] Experience in that war led to the development of special hospitals and clinics for servicemen and then for civilians, at least in Great Britain (Rees 1945). But it was World War II that brought about major changes in the psychiatric system and ideology.

As a result of World War II, military psychiatrists came to some important conclusions: that neuropsychiatric problems were more serious than had been previously recognized, that environmental stress was a major contributor to mental maladjustment, and that purposeful human interventions could alter psychological outcomes. Their experience with the number of men rejected from military duty because of mental health problems led them to conclude that mental illness was a more serious problem then had been recognized. Fourteen percent of men ages eighteen to thirty-five were disqualified from service because of neuropsychiatric disorders (Menninger 1945). It also became vividly apparent that a continuum existed between mental health and mental illness that was related to the degree of stress a person was forced to endure. A year after the end of the war, J. W. Appel and G. W. Beebe concluded that combat exposure for 200 to 240 days would break anyone and that psychiatric casualties were as inevitable as gunshot and shrapnel wounds (Herman 1992). Early treatment in noninstitutionalized settings appeared to confirm the need for a different way of viewing hospitalization (Grob 1991).

These psychiatrists had seen that treating servicemen in the context of their social relationships was essential. With enough supportive forms of psychotherapy, combined with rest, sleep, and food, severely stressed combatants were able to rapidly return to the front. And it was not the specific treatments that mattered. "Successful treatment seemed to depend less upon specific procedures or specific drugs than upon general principles— promptness in providing rest and firm emotional support in a setting in which the bonds of comradeship with one's outfit were not wholly disrupted and in which competent psychiatric reassurance was fortified, symbolically and physiologically, by hot food and clean clothes and by evidences of firm military support and command of the situation" (Grob 1991). They had also seen that the effects of overwhelming stress, were in fact, treatable. William C. Menninger believed that the war demonstrated the significance of group cohesion, leadership, and motivation. He believed it was vital to determine the "more serious community-based sources of emotional stress" if effective strategies were to be developed to treat that stress (Grob 1991).

When they left the service these psychiatrists applied the same notions to civilian care and began to emphasize treatment in a family and community setting, rather than within the state hospital systems exclusively. New epidemiological work focused on the general population rather than the institutionalized mentally ill. These studies supported the wartime experience that cultural factors that caused significant stress played a central role in mental health and mental illness. William Menninger said that every institution in American society had to to evaluate its program "in terms of the contribution to individual and group mental health" and that it was vital to determine "the more serious community-caused sources of emotional stress." These observations led to a dramatic increase in social activism and an optimism that was typical of the times. Prominent psychiatric leaders called upon the mental health professions to deal with "ignorance, superstition, unhealthy cultural patterns, and the rigidities and anxieties of parents, as well as with social conditions which foster the development of neuroses and maladjustments" (Grob 1991).

Social psychiatry developed out of the work of these and other pioneers. Rennie wrote, "Social psychiatry is etiological in its aim, but its point of attack is the whole social framework of contemporary living." The goals of social psychiatry were broad: "To include all social, biological, educational, and philosophical considerations which may come to empower psychiatry in its striving towards a society which functions with greater equilibrium and with fewer psychological casualties "(Jones 1968b). The horrific events of the First and Second World Wars had convinced many people that the individual could not be treated as separate from the society and that the society contributed greatly to mental disorders.

The principles of social psychiatry were summarized in six postulates:

1. Human behavior can only be understood in the context of the total social and other energies (including living and inert physical matter) of this universe.
2. A person should always be a subject and never an object of an interpersonal transaction.
3. There is meaningful interrelationship, a relativity, between the behaviors of one individual and all social and mythological institutions and groups.
4. Social problems, including individual, institutional and group deviant behaviors, cannot be solved without collaboration between all the institutions and disciplines of human knowledge, influence, and action.
5. Values of compassion, caring, and consideration for all human beings are essential to the operations of social psychiatry.
6. Human behavior acquires purpose and meaning in reference to and by virtue of adherence to these postulates (Carleton and Mahlendorf 1979).

Adherents of social psychiatry tried to place the patient and his or her symptoms within a total sociopolitical context. "The mentally ill person is seen as a member of an oppressed group, a group deprived of adequate social solutions to the problem of individual growth and development" (Ullman 1969). Other clinicians and theorists began to view each patient's symptoms as an adaptive response to dysfunctional systems, most importantly the patient's family. In 1969, one of the original family therapists, Don Jackson, said, "The important point here is that the behavior which is usually seen as symptomatic in terms of the individual can be seen as adaptive, even appropriate, in terms of the vital system within which the individual operates." Recognition grew that deviant behavior was not just irrational, insane, animalistic, and inexplicable, but could be understood in a relational context. "Deviant behavior can be seen as a form of communication, but to elicit and understand what lies behind such behavior is a difficult and painful process" (Jones 1968b).

Around the same time, increasing numbers of critiques were published about the overall health—or lack thereof—of the entire society as well as an attempted redefinition of the role of the therapist in dealing with this sick society. From 1914 on, Trigant Burrow was convinced that sometime in the course of social evolution our primary unity was inadvertently distorted, and that subsequently we substituted an arbitrary standard called "normality." He believed that this maladaptation had become so extensively systematized that a social neurosis exists throughout the species (Burrow 1984).

In 1936, Lawrence K. Frank wrote: "Today we have so many deviations and maladjustments that the term 'normal' has lost almost all significance. Indeed, we see efforts being made to erect many of the previously considered abnormalities into cultural patterns for general social adoption.... The disintegration of our traditional cultures, with the decay of those ideas, conceptions, and beliefs upon which our social individual lives were organized, brings us face to face with the problem of treating society, since individual therapy or punishment no longer has any value beyond mere alleviation of our symptoms" (Sanford 1966).

The tumultuous 1960s, provided an opportunity for the reevaluation of psychiatry's traditional role. The fundamental health of society was questioned. Given two world wars, slavery, genocide, racial discrimination, discrimination against and abuse of women, child abuse, and gross economic inequality, could our society be construed as healthy in any way? If someone whom we designate as mentally ill actually sees the contradictions and hypocrisy more clearly than we, can that person be truly considered mentally ill or are our definitions distorted by our own misperceptions? Should we be helping them "adjust" to a sick society, or should we be doing something to make the society less sick?

In 1963 Eric Fromm wrote a book titled *The Sane Society*, in which he echoed and extended the thinking of Durkheim and presented a cogent argument for the essential sickness of what we call normal society. In *Path-*

ways to Madness, written in 1965, Jules Henry wrote, "Under the proposition that 'he was doomed by his upbringing' we acquit all the institutions in our culture except the family of complicity in the destruction of the individual."

Strident criticisms began after the war and continued through the 1970s of what had become mainstream psychiatry, particularly in the profession's apparent willingness to support the status quo, even to the detriment of patients. Thomas J. Scheff wrote in *Labeling Madness*, "What I am suggesting is that researchers in the field of mental illness . . . are helping to further confound the moral issues by giving laymen the impression, however subtly or unintentionally, that there is absolute scientific justification for the prevailing American world view. . . . It is our responsibility as scholars and students of human behavior to make visible the hidden moral values in psychiatry and mental health, so that they can be made the subject of research and open public discussion" (1975).

Dr. Eugene Brody, M.D., in a 1973 book titled *The Lost Ones*, described the results of a study looking at the relationship between social forces and mental illness in Rio de Janeiro. He concluded: "Psychiatric symptoms and attitudes cannot be understood without reference to the social context in which they occur. . . . The major dilemma for mental health professionals lies in the fact that primary prevention of mental handicaps and the assurance of overall community health is total. It involves the whole social system and is thus beyond his power as well as his expertise. . . . There is no reason to believe that most mental health professionals have the interests or capacities which would allow them to become expert or to develop the political power necessary for effective action regarding most of these issues" (1973).

Out of these critiques, and the growing social activism of the 1960s, some psychiatric workers began more seriously addressing the issue of prevention. "Preventative psychiatry" as defined by Caplan was both theoretical and practical—a public health approach. The traditional focus of psychiatry is on treating illnesses that are already well-established, or in simpler terms, fixing someone who is already broken. Caplan and his colleagues became interested in discovering ways to prevent mental illness from occurring in the first place—primary prevention, and to reduce the spreading damage of mental illness once it had already started—secondary prevention. Tertiary prevention would reduce the amount of impairment that would result from already existing mental disorder (Caplan 1964). This focus on prevention led inevitably toward a movement to correct the environment forces that were so obviously contributing to mental and social illness.

Jerome Frank wrote in 1976 that "anyone who takes the goal of prevention seriously is bound to recognize that it involves social reform. We go on trying to fix up damaged adults in one-to-one relationships when a more proper professional function would be to spend a considerable portion of our energies trying to fix up a society in ways that will increase the strength and stability of the family, thereby affecting positively the mental health of generations to come ... for prevention people like ourselves would be needed as teachers, researchers and especially, as radical social activists, proselytizing for changes in our society to make it more supportive, less dehumanized."

GENERAL SYSTEMS THEORY AND FEMINIST CRITIQUES

Another important scientific and philosophical conceptual framework that emerged about the same time also influenced psychiatry: general systems theory (Von Bertalanffy 1967 1974). The concept grew up out of quantum physics and cybernetics but profoundly influenced the ecological movement as well. The main premise was that every individual component of any system influences and is influenced by every other component. General systems theory provided a theoretical underpinning for some of the observations that were central to the lessons of WWII. Psychiatry came to recognize that individuals could be understood and helped only in the context of understanding their family system, their cultural framework for constructing reality, and the larger systems within which they live and work—school, workplace, friendship patterns—as well as the network of connections that comprise each individual's personal and cultural history (Gray 1969).

Feminism provided another important influence in the overall intellectual environment. Throughout this time, feminist thinkers were attempting to define an alternative, feminist style of thinking, relating, and defining the world. In doing so they offered critiques of the dominant male view of every important area of life, including the practice of psychiatry. This critique actually had its inception much earlier in the work of women such as E. P. W. Packard, who was committed to an asylum by her husband because of her religious views. She was completely released only when members of her community assisted her in obtaining a court hearing which resulted in her release. She devoted the remainder of her life to successful reform regarding the rights of women in several different states (Packard 1882).

Phyllis Chesler's *Women and Madness* was published in 1972. In it she exposed the social and political underpinnings of psychiatric diagnostic criteria and treatment as it was directed at women, demonstrating that only men could be mentally healthy because it is male behavioral norms that establish the definitions of normality. She discussed how women's reality-based experiences of rape, sexual abuse, and physical abuse were denied, minimized, or blamed on the victim (Chesler 1972). Ehrenreich and English extended this critique to include all of medicine (Ehrenreich and English 1978). Building on the work of workers such as Karen Horney, later writers—Jean Baker Miller, Nancy Chodorow, Judith Lewis Herman, and others—opened up a powerful corrective to the predominantly male voices of traditional psychoanalysis and psychodynamic psychotherapy (Chodorow 1978; Herman 1981; Miller 1973 1976).

THE THERAPEUTIC MILIEU

The events of the first half of the twentieth century shook many fundamental systems of meaning, particularly the relationship between the individual and the community. Psychiatrists who showed a willingness to confront these issues at home, after the war, called themselves social psychiatrists. They were often to be found working in milieu settings that were quite different from the traditional psychotherapeutic setting and the traditional psychiatric hospital. Psychoanalytic psychotherapy and all its offshoots were grounded in an approach to the patient that focused almost exclusively on the individual. The relational aspects of therapy were implicit in the relationship between therapist and patient, but the main source of problem and motivation for change was seen as being intrapsychic—within the individual. The social and political contexts were not relevant and were largely disregarded. Sarason observed in 1981, that "the theories generated by these studies [psychological research studies] have been, for all practical purposes, asocial. That is to say, it is as though society does not exist for the psychologist. Society is a vague, amorphous background that can be disregarded in one's efforts to fathom the laws of behavior."

The therapeutic community—or milieu—concept was one attempt to apply the tenets of social psychiatry and systems theory to the institutional treatment of various kinds of deviance. The hospital was seen as being a microcosm of the larger society, an experimental laboratory for social change (Tucker and Maxmen 1973).

One of the most interesting aspects of this development was the widespread use of group forms of therapies. Faced with the need for intensive treatment of combatants during the war with limited resources, military psychiatrists developed group forms of treatment that had been extremely helpful in treating battle-fatigued soldiers. In England, J. R. Rees, who was the director of the Tavistock Clinic, was appointed consultant psychiatrist to the army in 1938. In this capacity, he and his team were led to consider the far-ranging implications and problems of psychiatric work in wartime. Their focus shifted from the individual to the larger problems of group relations (Bion 1991; Foulkes 1964; Foulkes and Prince 1969; Manning 1989; Rees 1945).

Meanwhile, the British army set up a treatment unit at Northfield Hospital under the leadership of Tom Main, who originated the concept of the "therapeutic community." In a paper published in 1946, Main wrote, "The fact must be faced that radical individual psychotherapy is not a practicable proposition for the huge numbers of patients confronting the psychiatric world today.... The Northfield Experiment is an attempt to use a hospital not as an organization run by doctors in the interests of their own greater technical efficiency, but as a community with the immediate aim of full participation of all its members in its daily life and the eventual aim of the resocialization of the neurotic individual for life in ordinary society" (Main 1989).

During the same era in the United States, Harry Wilmer, a psychiatrist stationed at the Oakland Naval Hospital, used his own experience as a patient in a tuberculosis sanitarium at the beginning of World War II to create a program based on group therapy for returning veterans. His experience was similar to that of his British colleagues. He refused to use any control other than social control, and the staff were taught to establish the firm expectation that the patients could and would control themselves. This required the staff to learn ways of managing difficult patients without using the usual forms of external control—seclusion, restraint, and punishment. The result was that many patients who had been hostile, belligerent, and assaultive in other settings were treated in the therapeutic milieu without resorting to violence. "I never found it necessary to isolate even one of the 939 patients with whom we dealt, despite the fact that almost every type of acute psychiatric disorder was represented in the group. This result was achieved largely because the staff, no longer free to use methods of control that brutalize both themselves and their patients, had to find new ways of dealing with patients. They found the new ways more effective and infinitely pleasanter than the old" (Wilmer 1958).

It was Maxwell Jones who most enthusiastically developed the concepts of the therapeutic community both in Britain and in the United States and attempted to spread those concepts to institutions outside of the formal psychiatric system. Another army psychiatrist, Jones first developed a program during the war to treat soldiers suffering from "effort syndrome," a psychosomatic disorder that was related to combat fatigue. The approach was focused on education in a group setting which led to the development of a "group atmosphere." Treatment was no longer confined to a therapeutic hour but became a continuous process operating throughout the waking life of the patient. To accomplish this, Jones had to reorder the hospital society and flatten the traditional hierarchical pyramid of authority to promote more interaction between patients, nurses, and doctors. Even before Moreno's techniques about the use of dramatic techniques as a form of treatment had become well known, Jones was using drama as an effective technique of social therapy (Jones 1953). The patient would write, direct, and act in his or her own personal play with the help of the entire community, as part of an intensive therapeutic experience.

After the war, Jones developed a program for ex-prisoners of war and continued experimenting with the use of discussion groups, educational films, psychodrama, and discussions of community life. The results of the work impressed the government enough to ensure the development of a postwar program at Belmont Hospital to treat the chronically unemployed neurotic. Patients who were admitted were those considered unsuitable for either psychotherapy or physical methods of treatment such as electroshock, but excluded psychotic patients. He described the treatment population as "[i]nadequate and aggressive psychopaths, schizoid personalities, early schizophrenics, various drug addictions, sexual perversions, and the chronic forms of psychoneuroses. Our patients represent the 'failures' in society; they come largely from broken homes and are unemployed; inevitably they have developed antisocial attitudes in an attempt to defend themselves from what appears to them as a hostile environment; as often as not their marriages are in ruins and there is little or no attempt to keep up any of the more usual standards of behavior in their home life" (1953). These were not the worried well, but severely dysfunctional, nonpsychotic patients. These same kind of patients today may wind up in the mental health system but are just as likely to constitute a large proportion of our growing prison population.

Jones and his colleagues performed follow-up studies and six months after leaving the hospital, two-thirds of the patients they traced had made a fair adjustment or better. Just over one-half had worked the full time since leaving. Patients generally stayed in the hospital for two to four months, but some patients stayed up to a year, while others stayed a much shorter time than two months. Jones based his work on the idea of "social learning." The term "social learning" describes the little understood process of change which may result from the interpersonal interaction, when some conflict or crisis is analyzed in a group situation, using whatever psychodynamic skills are available. . . . Learning of this kind is complicated and painful: old learned patterns, adequate in previous situations, must be unlearned because they stand in the way of acquiring new and more adequate patterns of behavior" (Jones 1968b). To his way of thinking and working, every social interaction or crisis presented a "living-learning situation," which provided the grist for the therapeutic mill and the opportunity for changing and learning how to change.

Under the influence of Jones, Main, Wilmer, and others (Caudill 1958; Rapoport 1960), combined with the publications of critiques of the existing mental health system (Greenblatt et al. 1957, Stanton and Schwartz 1954) and the sociopolitical influences that permeated the psychiatric world, the concept of the therapeutic community and its attenuated form—the therapeutic milieu—caught on in Britain and the United States and dominated the field of inpatient psychiatry throughout the 1960s, presenting a potent challenge to the traditional organization and modus operandi of state hospitals (Grob 1991).

The most striking characteristic of the therapeutic milieu was that the community itself—and all the individuals who constituted it—were the most powerful influence on treatment. Unlike many other settings, many of the values that formed the underpinnings for every milieu were clearly articulated—egalitarianism, permissiveness, honesty, openness, trust (Almond 1974; Leeman 1986; Leeman and Audio 1978; Rapoport 1960).

All therapeutic communities rested on several assumptions: patients should be responsible for much of their own treatment; the running of the unit should be more democratic than authoritarian; patients were capable of helping each other; treatment was to be voluntary whenever possible, and restraint kept to a minimum; psychological methods of treatment were seen as preferable to physical methods of control. Psychotherapy, individual therapy, and various forms of group therapy were used routinely and were usually psychoanalytically informed (Almond 1974; Cumming and Cumming 1962; Wilmer 1981).

By 1969, Abroms was describing milieu therapy as a "treatment context rather than a specific technique ... a metatherapy." Tucker and Maxmen described the treatment milieu as a "laboratory wherein the patient may safely experiment with newly acquired adaptive skills." The aim of a modified therapeutic community was to "promote a corrective emotional experience, enhance personal understanding, and maximize healthy ego growth" (1973).

The therapeutic milieu concepts, as advocated by Jones and others, were powerful influences on many of us who trained in psychiatry during the 1970s. The tenets of the therapeutic community provided the foundation for our first attempts at creating a new community.

CREATING A LIVING-LEARNING ENVIRONMENT

When my colleagues and I began our professional careers our training was clear. We were the experts and the well people; the patients were sick, ill, disturbed, maladjusted. We were to help them get well, become less disturbed, make a better adjustment. Unfortunately, just how we were supposed to accomplish all this was not so clear. None of the explanatory systems available to psychiatry seemed to adequately encompass our patients' reality. In my training program I had been exposed to most of the major schools of thought. But there was no integration. The psychoanalysts focused on the patient's intrapsychic world and frequently viewed medications as a poor substitute for good analysis. The biological psychiatrists derided the importance of psychotherapy and magnified the importance of drugs. The behaviorists chimed in that insight was not necessary, that behavioral forms of treatment could cure most neurotic problems as well. Years spent watching analysts fight with behaviorists and biologists, all of them sounding like medieval priests arguing over angels on the heads of pins, left me firmly convinced that none of the groups knew what it was talking about *and* that they all did to some degree.

All of them were partially correct, but none saw the whole picture. Early in my career, as a psychiatric aide, I thought this was my own ignorance; later, with training and experience, I learned that it was an accurate assessment of the state of knowledge. I learned that the psychiatric diagnoses did not really *mean* anything. They were labels, descriptions of behavior, not explanations for pathology. They didn't say anything about "Why?" but only "What?" Labeling behavior was in the academic air, however, highly valued by the profession and proof of psychiatric ability. As a result, we would often act as though we had actually achieved something by agreeing on a label when we had only managed to organize our own thinking in an arbitrary way, failing to grasp the totality of the being before us.

If we decided someone was a schizophrenic that meant, in our shorthand, that the prognosis for cure was poor and that the best thing to do was to start the patient on medication quickly. If we decided someone was the new hot category, "a borderline," that meant that the patient was probably a female, would cause a great deal of trouble, would be astonishingly manipulative and would probably not respond very well to treatment. If someone fell into the category of being "a hysteric," that meant that the patient was either a female or a gay male who should be carefully kept at a distance by male staff members because she or he would probably try in some way to seduce them. If someone was "a sociopath," that meant that the patient was a male and probably should be in prison, not on a psychiatric unit, and that you could not trust a thing they said and should discharge them as soon as possible.

Drugs, of course, were big. There were all different kinds of drugs—drugs for too much depression, drugs for too much elation, drugs for too many hallucinations or paranoid thoughts, drugs for too much anxiety. And the drugs did help—sometimes they even saved lives. They just did not help enough. Drugs seemed largely unable to help improve self-esteem. They often failed to stop stubbornly persistent symptoms such as self-mutilation, self-starvation, bingeing, purging, murderous impulses, chronic suicidal behavior, lying, stealing, manipulation, and addictions. They also often failed to do anything to improve disturbed family functioning, oppressive work situations, abusive marriages, or troubled children. Nor did they address questions of meaning, existential dilemmas, or soul-searching riddles.

Talking also was big. Based on a particular theory that we were supposed to have learned in our training, we were expected to know what to listen for, what to say, what not to say, and what information to obtain. The theory was supposed to provide you with a way of thinking about and understanding other human beings, and out of this comprehensible and systematic body of thought you could derive successful interventions. If you had been trained as a Freudian, certain kinds of information were valued more than others. If you were a behaviorist or a cognitive therapist, or any of a number of other "ists," then certain information was admitted and other information could be ignored. However, if you had failed to be converted to any particular school of thought, then you were likely to spend a great deal of time perplexed by the enormity of the problems with which you were confronted.

In 1980, I was offered an opportunity to gather some colleagues together and form a psychiatric unit from scratch. As our unit evolved, it took on much of our shared characters. We were all somewhat intolerant of hypocrisy and double standards, so the rules that applied to us within the system also had to apply to our patients as much as possible. Since we did not like restrictions nor were particularly comfortable with the exercise of power over others, our unit was created to be strictly voluntary and open, meaning that no patient could be kept on our unit without his or her consent and that there were no locked doors to keep people inside. None of us liked too much regimentation, fixed hierarchy, or unnecessary restrictions. So we created a unit that had a leadership structure in which roles could be fundamentally interchangeable, with a relatively horizontal hierarchical structure. We created policies and procedures and a system of rules and regulations, but we based these largely on the structure that is necessary for any large group of people to function together in a practical, efficient, and safe way. We all had a low tolerance for boredom, so our program was designed to be educational, creative, and intensive.

This same intolerance for boredom fueled a desire for diversity, so we tried to hire other staff members who shared similar values but who could make their own unique contribution by virtue of their own selfhood. For similar reasons we designed the unit to accommodate men and women of all ages. None of us had a dogmatic therapeutic orientation, so our program was eclectic and included everything from individual psychodynamic therapy to family therapy, process groups, psychodrama, art therapy, recreation, and twelve-step programs. Each of us placed a very high priority on a sense of humor, so we liked patients who also had a sense of humor, who could help create a relaxed and even funny atmosphere in the midst of the miasma of pain and suffering that was all around us.

We had all been trained in settings that had sprung from the original "therapeutic milieu" concepts, and we had adopted a belief system that reinforced the notion that the whole is greater than the sum of the parts, that there are emergent qualities of any system that cannot be explained solely by an analysis of the parts of the system. This meant that we were all responsible for creating and maintaining the system within which we wanted to work together and treat our patients. And this meant that we had to pay attention to the workings of the system by surfacing and resolving conflict on a regular basis without becoming so compulsive that we would drive ourselves crazy and lose our focus on the goal, which was to help psychiatric patients improve their level of functioning.

Clearly, we had learned a great deal. By 1985, we were proud of the environment we had created. It was a safe place for us and a benevolent place for our patients. Most of the time, they left us in better shape then when they were admitted. Sometimes the changes were remarkable. We felt good about the service we were providing and satisfied that we had created an environment within which we could grow and learn as well.

Unresponsive Problems

But, there were problems, inexplicable complications, confusing cases, disturbing conflicts. After all, we had created a human setting, not a heavenly enclave. There was always ongoing conflict with the larger medical system within which we were embedded. We were in a medical institution, and although psychiatry is a medical subspecialty, the medical model of understanding and dealing with human beings is vastly different from the psychiatric model—or at least *our* psychiatric model. The medical model puts the power into the hands of medical authority, and patients are discouraged from questioning this authority. The corollary of this is that medical providers are expected to fix what is wrong. We did not care to assume that much authority over the lives of our patients, nor were we able to make any claims that we could "fix" what ailed them. And in any system there is always competition for resources, and ours was no different.

More worrisome was the fact that we had no real way to understand what it was we were doing or why it so frequently worked, at least to some extent. We could not communicate our methods to people outside of our system because so much of what went on was based on our interconnected knowledge and understanding of each other and our respect for each individual team member's area of expertise. We had no cohesive cognitive framework for explaining how we understood what we did understand intuitively and emotionally. We had no language that could be shared outside of our own personalized code. To even explain to each other we had to use the language of metaphor and simile. The situation presented by "Joan" was very similar to that of "Alexander" who was on the unit two years ago. Or the community is doing to "Sam" what another community had done to "Oscar." But we did not have a systematic, shared, and cohesive framework to understand the biological, psychological, social, and existential dilemmas presented by our patients and experienced by us.

And there remained a troublesome and varied group of people who kept turning up, reappearing on the unit with a discouraging frequency, who did not seem to respond to what we had to offer even when it seemed as though they should. Some were patients who had symptoms that were characteristic of someone considered to be psychotic—hallucinations, delusions, any number of odd perceptual experiences, brief episodes of paranoia or other odd behavior—and yet who did not warrant the diagnosis of schizophrenia or related disorders and showed a relatively poor response to the traditional antipsychotic medicines. Often they were people who functioned quite well between these bizarre episodes, holding down responsible positions in many different professions. Then came the people—usually women—who persistently mutilated themselves, but did not actually attempt suicide. What could make a usually pain-aversive human repeatedly seek out pain? Masochism—but what exactly was that? What did it really mean?

Then there were all the people who actively sought out relationships but were terrible at maintaining them. We would, with all good intentions, be kind to them, and they would readily accept our kindness. But soon they turned into emotional vampires, demanding more and more kindness until we were drained, at which point they would turn on us with a rage that was difficult to bear. Others were addicted to all kinds of substances and behaviors, and they became overwhelmed and unable to cope if their substances were withdrawn or their behaviors curbed. We noticed the growing similarities between all kinds of addictions—legal drugs, illegal drugs, alcohol, nicotine, sex, bingeing, starving, purging, shopping, shoplifting, exercise, religion, working, money-making, even relationships. People seemed to need their addiction of choice to simply go on functioning while meanwhile the addiction was taking over their lives.

We also had the risk-takers, those confusing people who seemed to feel good only when they were putting their lives in some kind of danger. They seemed to find danger and violence exhilarating. They would often not last very long on our unit because of our low tolerance for violent acting out. They provided a contrast to another puzzling group—the chronic depressives who failed to respond dramatically to any antidepressant, who temporarily felt better when their circumstances changed, but who lapsed back again into the misery of lives often characterized by miserable marriages, miserable family lives, miserable jobs, and a miserable history. Occasionally we also puzzled over a complicated medical case, referred by one of our colleagues because he or she suspected a strong psychological component to the medical problem. Often these were people who had had numerous medical procedures and even surgical interventions for disorders that turned out to be nonexistent and who had been made worse by the complications of the medical and surgical procedures themselves.

Just as we could not really explain why what we did worked when it did, likewise we were largely unable to explain why we failed when we failed. As a result, we tended to resort with time worn, tried-and-true explanations that mainly settled on blaming the patient and his or her "resistance." Now, resistance is a real thing. When we do not want to become aware of something we already know but which is painful and conflictual, we frequently do avoid confronting our own self-knowledge and we will fight against anyone who tries to urge or push us to look. This happens to everyone in friendships, in marriages, at work, and at school, and it also happens in therapy. But we were unable to differentiate between the patients' resistance and our own lack of understanding or skill. Since we were unclear about exactly what we were doing or how to do it, we could not tell the difference between their failure and our own. And since we were the ones with the power to define failure, it was always theirs. Those who have the power are the ones who define deviance and the responses to deviance. We were not always wrong, of course, but we rarely saw the whole picture.

Readiness for Change

By 1985, we were ready for a change. We had tried our hand at practicing what we had already been taught. We knew by then that few of our former ideological beliefs about psychiatric patients seemed to help us deal with many of the problems we encountered. Looking back now, I can see that we were at that critical point that Thomas Kuhn described so well in 1970, when a shift in basic assumptions is about to happen. We had no way to really adequately order the reality we saw in our psychiatric community. We knew that the explanations that we had been taught were not sufficient. Some of them reflected a part of the reality, and others just seemed to be completely misguided. But even taken altogether, they did not show us how to be more helpful to patients. The extent to which we were helpful had much more to do with our unique personalities, styles, and intuitive understanding and compassion for human suffering as well as our sense of humor in the face of all this.

BEGINNING TO MAKE A SHIFT

The high incidence of traumatic experience in the histories of our patients hit us powerfully and suddenly. Because Dawn's clinical picture was so dramatic, she provided me with my index experience—but about the same time—every member of the treatment team had at least one patient who was their agent of change. As a result, we began asking other patients about their histories. About 80 percent recounted horrific stories of trauma of all kinds, which occurred usually but not always, in childhood. The stories were not just a result of increased suggestibility on our parts. When we reviewed past charts of patients we had been working with over time, we saw that there were many times we had carefully obtained the past history of trauma, meticulously written it down, and then casually ignored it. The history had simply played no role in our case formulation or treatment. But most of the time, we had just failed to ask the questions, assuming, perhaps, that people would volunteer such information, while also failing to recognize the incidence of violence in the home.

This is consistent with research data that came out in 1987 and 1990 but which was actually performed in 1984—long before there was a generalized increased awareness of sexual abuse or the long-term effects of trauma and about a year or two before we began noticing the same phenomena. Jacobson and colleagues interviewed 100 hospitalized psychiatric patients and asked them about physical or sexual assault. Eighty-one percent had experienced major physical and/or sexual assaults (Jacobson and Richardson

1987). Forty patients—one in six men and one in five women, reported abusive genital sexual contact as children. Forty-four percent had never revealed the abuse to anyone (Jacobson and Herald 1990). When the researchers reviewed the previous charts of these patients they found out that only 9 percent of the assault histories obtained during research interviews were mentioned on the patients' charts. Eighty-five percent of physical assaults in childhood and 90 percent of physical assaults as an adult had never been charted, and 100 percent of sexual assault in childhood or as an adult had not made it into the patients' histories, largely because they had never been asked the questions about previous assaults (Jacobson et al. 1987).

The patients who gave a history of trauma did not fall into any neat diagnostic category. In fact, they covered the spectrum of psychiatric classification. Though often still ignored by many in the psychiatric profession, this point has been made repeatedly since that time. Whether we look at depressive disorders, eating disorders, personality disorders, psychosomatic disorders, substance abuse disorders, adjustment disorders, or a number of other psychiatric and medical dysfunctions, what keeps coming up in study after study is a high incidence of previous severe and often, repeated, trauma.[2]

Since that time we have talked with many clinicians who have had similar experiences and none has described a gradual learning curve. For most people, this understanding about the role trauma plays as an etiologic factor in the evolution of both personal and social disorders comes as a shock, a sudden—and largely unwelcome—perceptual shift. This is certainly understandable. Such recognition is disordering to our working view of reality on several different levels. Although intellectually we may know that life is often cruel, unfair, and notoriously brutal to the weak, the young, and the infirm, our present social and political paradigm does not really function consistently on the basis of this assumption. We are immersed in an individualistic philosophy that holds each person accountable for his or her failures and shortcomings. This philosophical principle is centuries old and the basis for much of what we think and how we behave. We like to believe that we get what we deserve and that we live in a basically just world (Janoff-Bulman 1992; Lerner 1980).

The Hebrew concept of *teshuwa* best describes the experience that we, along with so many of our colleagues, were immersed in. The basic meaning of teshuwa is a "turn around," referring to a turning from the wrong path (Bianchi 1995). The word carries with it connotations of conversion, repentance, reconciliation, and atonement as well. It is rather astonishing now, in retrospect, to look at our own previous arrogance in applying an individualistic, reductionistic, and dichotomized belief system to people suffering from overwhelming life experiences. The self of the therapist—our philosophical and ethical stances, preconceived ideas, and ideological positions—has received little attention in the clinical or scientific literature (Shay 1995). And yet I can see now, how much our beliefs, values, ideals and prejudices determined how we viewed our patients and our conduct towards them, without any awareness on our part.

Certainly we always felt compassion for our patients' suffering. Compassion, at least, allows a little distance from the pain. Empathy is a far more dangerous personal experience. Empathy requires that we vicariously *experience* the trauma that our patients have survived. Empathy is not conscious or willed—it just happens. It is the shattering of a barrier between two human beings that is normally present under the circumstances of our present social structure. We do all kinds of things to keep our distance from other people. An important part of what we do is define reality in such a way that good things happen to good people, and bad things happen to bad people. In such a world, justice is relatively easy to delineate and if we are fortunate, we can remain safe by always being good and doing the right thing.

Listening to the stories of trauma and abuse sustained in childhood shatters our carefully constructed and sustained "just world" theories. Beatings, incest, abandonment, neglect, humiliation, rape, assault—these things did not occur to responsible and empowered adults, but to innocent and helpless children who were powerless to do anything to change their fate. And then we wonder why these same children have trouble differentiating right from wrong and developing a respect for justice and the law. Once we stepped into the shoes of the children our patients once were, we were in deep waters. From that starting point it became relatively easy to understand how they had tried to cope, how few were their resources, how they had found it necessary to make enormous sacrifices just to go on living and functioning. Step by step we could follow their desperate and often resourceful movements as they took a course necessary for immediate survival but destined to lead them into psychiatric and social disarray. Just like us, they too had bought the "just world" definition of our mutually shared reality and the consequence to them was a loss of a good self and the acquisition of badness, unworthiness, guilt, and personal responsibility for pain.

This narrowing of the distance between "us" and "them" was very disconcerting. As the psychic distance narrowed, the unwelcome realization dawned that if it could happen to them, it could happen to me! For some of us, it had, in fact, happened, and we had to deal with the surfacing of our own histories of abuse, neglect, and maltreatment. For others of us, this realization brought in its wake an uncomfortable hyperawareness that bordered, at times, on paranoia. I recall driving down a beautiful country road, looking at all the warmly lit houses, a model of domestic tranquillity and asking myself cynically, "Oh, sure, it all looks good from the outside, but I wonder what is *really* going on inside those houses?"

By now, ten years later, this phenomenon has become well-recognized under several different terms: vicarious traumatization compassion fatigue, secondary traumatic stress, secondary victimization, covictimization, and secondary survivor (Figley 1995; McCann and Pearlman 1990; Pearlman and Saakvitne 1995; Stamm 1995). It is commonly seen among the friends, relatives, and colleagues of anyone who experiences a traumatic event, and is common among therapists and other helping professionals who use a trauma model as a way of understanding psychiatric disorder. It is an example of the effects of emotional contagion and results in symptoms that are similar to, although usually less intense than, the symptoms of the trauma victim. This phenomenon helps to explain why this material has been so resisted in the medical and psychiatric professions, as well as among the public at large. The reality of trauma is frequently just too painful to bear.

The only resource that we had to help us cope with this emotional, physical, and spiritual distress was each other. We practiced in a relatively isolated setting. At the time, we knew of no other clinicians who were experiencing what we were going through. Very little academic discourse or research literature was available at the time, and what did exist lay, for the most part, outside freely available psychiatric journals. We had reached a crisis point. We had noticed for years that the psychiatric paradigm that we were taught did little to explain or help us address many of the problems that we routinely saw on our unit. And yet we had no other way to think about these problems. Then, we observed things about our patients that directly contradicted much that we had been taught and assumed to be true. In describing a similar state in his own field, Einstein said, "It was as if the ground had been pulled out from under one, with no firm foundation to be seen anywhere, upon which one could have built" (Kuhn 1970).

Then we got really lucky. I signed up for a course in psychological trauma that Harvard was offering as a continuing education course. I had never heard of the two people who were teaching the course, Judith Herman, M.D., and Bessel Van der Kolk, M.D., but it looked interesting, and besides, it was in Aruba, and I needed a vacation. I saw very little of the beach that week. Drs. Herman and Van der Kolk taught as a team, every day. They told us about the research on Vietnam veterans and what post-traumatic stress was all about. They brought us up to date on the outcome of research on the Holocaust survivors, and victims of rape, other violent crimes, and disasters. They taught us about the effects of domestic violence, political torture, child abuse, and particularly incest. They talked about the biology, and the psychology, the sociopolitical context, and even the philosophical impact of trauma on any human being. Kuhn had noted that "to reject one paradigm without simultaneously substituting another is to reject science itself (Kuhn 1970). This evolving theory about trauma was providing us with a new paradigm. Finally we had another way of thinking, of understanding our observations. We were beginning to see the outlines of this new paradigm, this new way of thinking about human experience, human tragedy, and the universal human response to that tragic experience.

When I came home from my "vacation," I convened a meeting of my entire inpatient and outpatient group. I passed on to them much of what I had learned, and I watched them, too, make the shift I had made. The soil had been prepared by their own clinical experience. The seeds had been planted by the patients. The theoretical and research base about trauma provided us with the trellis we needed to support our observations and encourage the growth of our own dialectical process of theory and practice. We began to speculate on the implications of this material. How did our inpatient unit need to change if we were to provide a better healing environment? If our patients were less "sick" than they were "injured," what kind of setting is most conducive to help people recover from injuries, even psychic ones?

To answer these questions, we called upon our newly honed empathic skills. If our patients were more like "us" than any abstract and diminished "them" we had construed in the past, then what kind of environment would be best for *us* if we were injured? In what kind of setting would we want to be sheltered and comforted? What would it take for us to feel truly *safe*? All of our previous and combined experience was evolving into a space and an idea that we called *The Sanctuary*.

four

Creating Sanctuary
Reconstructing the Social

I've never felt safe a day in my life. I don't know what it would feel like. When my father wasn't beating us, my mother was, and then I found my husband.
> —forty-five-year-old victim of domestic violence,
> seen in intensive care after severe beating

CREATING A SAFE SPACE

To begin the process of creating a sanctuary, we had to start with the idea of safety. But what exactly does safety mean? We always recognized the importance of physical safety. Our refusal to tolerate violence of any sort constituted our best defense against any breach in physical safety. But a physically safe environment, although necessary, was not sufficient. So there had to be other kinds of safety, which I have termed psychological safety, social safety, and moral safety.

Psychological Safety

Psychological safety refers to the ability to be safe with oneself, to rely on one's own ability to self-protect against any destructive impulses coming from within oneself or deriving from other people and to keep oneself out of harm's way. This ability to self-protect is one of the most shattering losses that occurs as a result of traumatic experience, particularly childhood trauma. Normally, children learn how to protect themselves on the basis of the way their caretakers take care of them. When their caregivers have respected their children's bodies, wishes, needs, and feelings, children learn these as normal behaviors and learn adequate self-care skills and attitudes. But when the caregiver is neglectful or abusive, children learn that this is the way they are supposed to treat themselves and other people. As adults, although intellectually they may know that using addictive substances, failing to get proper medical care, indulging in compulsive behaviors, deliberately inflicting self-harm, or repeatedly placing themselves in situations of danger are all bad for them, their normative childhood experience is what actually determines their adult behavior. The inability to eradicate this internal conflict leads to many kinds of further dysfunctions, including denial of the conflict, lying, rationalization, and trying to inflict those "normative" standards on other people, including their own children.

To create psychological safety, these normative aspects of self-destructive behavior need to be consciously, actively, and relentlessly challenged. So too does another aspect of post-traumatic psychological adaptation—the experienced helplessness, worthlessness, and essential badness of the self. People who have been traumatized have injuries or deficits in their sense of self-efficacy, their basic sense of ability and power in the world. They enter treatment as if bearing the mark of Cain, some nameless internal designation that has labeled them as evil and has set them apart from the rest of humanity, outside of the realm of normal human discourse. To reestablish psychological safety, they must regain, or gain for the first time, a sense of empowerment, an experienced recognition that they *can* alter their lives for the better, that they can express anger without being abused, that they can relax and enjoy themselves without punishment, that their actions can make a positive difference in their lives and in the lives of others. And they must begin the long process of reframing the traumatic experience as their own personal tragedy, largely unwarranted and undeserved, but theirs nonetheless to transform, if they wish, into personal victory and accomplishment.

Trauma robs the self of power and control, but it also steals off with speech and memory and feeling. We ordinarily experience ourselves as sensing, thinking, biographical creatures. We define who we are with labels and titles, with what we have done and where we have gone, by what we have felt, how deeply and widely our emotions stretch to encompass our experience. Trauma robs us of whole chunks of our experience and in doing so, appropriates all or part of our identity. It extorts from us any sense of normal emotion and leaves us instead with wildly swinging and often inappropriate emotional expression alternating with a numbing coldness that makes life not worth living. To achieve psychological safety, victims must regain the power of speech, a narrative of memory, and the symphony of modulated feelings that constitutes full humanness.

The overall process of achieving psychological safety is one best characterized by the concept of conscious integration. Traumatic experience is fragmenting; a healing experience must be defragmenting or integrating. Different aspects of the self must learn to live together in harmony. Memory must be recaptured and put into words so it can reenter the stream of time. Speech reconnects us to others but also reconnects us to ourselves. Memory, speech, cognition, and feeling must all be integrated into a narrative whole. Out of integration comes wholeness and out of wholeness can come meaning. Trauma creates existential dilemmas that are overwhelming and incomprehensible. We are a meaning-making animal. To achieve psychological safety, we must make sense out of what has happened to us or our reality is not bearable. Making sense out of child abuse is difficult to do.

Social Safety

Social safety describes the sense of feeling safe with other people. Though we know little about creating physical or psychological safety, we understand even less about how to create social safety. Individualism has been such a dominating force in American psychological theory and practice, that relatively little attention has been paid to understanding how environments help—or hinder—human healing and growth. Most of what we know derives from social psychiatry, the practice of the therapeutic milieu, the study of group dynamics, general systems theory, and feminist theory and practice. But the question of how to create socially safe human environments is essential if we are to do more than put a metaphorical finger in the dike. There are many more traumatized people than there will ever be individual therapists to treat them. We must begin to create naturally occurring, healing environments that provide some of the corrective experiences that are vital for recovery.

This is difficult to do for several reasons. Victims of trauma—particularly interpersonal trauma—have serious difficulties in their ability and willingness to trust other people. Experience has taught them that people are dangerous, betraying, two-faced, and duplicitous. If they have been injured as children, then they have come to expect bad treatment and are often suspicious of kindness. They will exert pressure on the other to conform to their normative expectations of abuse. The miracle is not that so many are distrustful; it is, instead, that so many are willing to try trusting again, and again, and again, despite their past experience. But for victims of trauma, interpersonal relationships continue to pose enormous challenges.

Then, for those of us who bear the responsibility for creating a socially safe setting, we are at a disadvantage to the extent that we have never actually experienced such a setting ourselves. How many of us have ever felt truly safe in a social setting, a setting in which we felt safe, cared for, trusted, free to express our deepest thoughts and feelings without censure, unafraid of being abandoned or misjudged, unfettered by the constant pressure of interpersonal competition, and yet stimulated to be thoughtful, solve problems, be creative, and be spontaneous? Our families are supposed to be the prototype experience for this kind of security and safety, but such a family setting is relatively rare. And yet it is the kind of setting that human beings need to maximize their emotional and intellectual functioning in an integrated way. Our social system is created to produce human beings who will fit into a highly industrialized, competitive, often cutthroat capitalist environment that still prepares at least half of us for mortal combat. Our social system is not designed to maximize the human potential for growth, self-exploration, mutual cooperation, nurturing of the young, artistic endeavor, or creative expression and exploration.

We were trying to create a sanctuary yet had never been in one, had never seen one, and until that time, had probably never even spent much time imagining one. The closest environment I could think of to a socially safe environment is the fictional portrayal of "Star Trek: The Next Generation." And we have a very long way to go before we reach that stage of social evolution.

So, we started by defining our values, by openly stating our belief system, our creed. John Gardner, founder of Common Cause, has said, "Families and communities are the ground-level generators and preservers of values and ethical systems. No society can remain vital or even survive without a reasonable base of shared values" (Etzioni 1993). We called our shared value base the "trauma model" and began to discuss our shared fundamental assumptions, goals, and shared practice that could help us define our position, our view of this new reality (Bloom 1994a).

SHARED ASSUMPTIONS

I've always known I was nuts. I've been raped, beaten, and humiliated since I was a little boy. Even my priest did it to me. This doesn't happen to everyone—it's got to be something wrong with me.

—thirty-five-year-old factory worker,
referred for evaluation after stalking a woman at work

1. Patients begin life with normal potentials for growth and development, given certain constitutional and genetic predispositions, and then become traumatized. "Posttraumatic stress reactions are essentially the reactions of normal people to abnormal stress" (Silver 1986).

2. When people are traumatized in early life, the effects of trauma frequently interfere with normal physical, psychological, social, and moral development.

3. Trauma has biological, psychological, social, and moral effects that spread horizontally and vertically, across and down through the generations.

4. Many symptoms and syndromes are manifestations of adaptations, originally useful as coping skills, that have now become maladaptive or less adaptive than originally intended.

5. Many victims of trauma suffer chronic post-traumatic stress disorder and may manifest any combination of the symptoms of PTSD.

6. Victims of trauma can become trapped in time, their inner experience fragmented. They are caught in the repetitive reexperiencing of the trauma, which has been dissociated and remains unintegrated into their overall functioning.

7. Dissociation and repression are core defenses against overwhelming affect and are present, to a varying extent, in all survivors of trauma.

8. Although the human capacity for fantasy elaboration and imaginative creation are well-established, memories of traumatic experiences must be assumed to have at least some basis in reality.

9. Stressful events are more seriously traumatic when there is an accompanying helplessness and lack of control.

10. Traumatic experience and disrupted attachments combine to produce defects in the regulation and modulation of affect, of emotional experience. Human beings require other human beings to respond to their emotions and to help contain feelings that are overwhelming.

11. People who are repeatedly traumatized may develop "learned helplessness" a condition that has serious biochemical implications.

12. Trauma survivors often discover that various addictive behaviors restore at least a temporary sense of control over intrusive phenomena.

13. Survivors may also become addicted to their own stress responses and as a result compulsively expose themselves to high levels of stress and further traumatization.

14. Many trauma survivors develop secondary psychiatric symptomatology and do not connect their symptoms with previous trauma. They become guilt-ridden, depressed, and exhibit low self-esteem and feelings of hopelessness and helplessness.

15. Trauma victims often have difficulty managing aggression. Many survivors identify with the aggressor and become victimizers themselves. A vicious cycle of transgenerational victimization often ensues.

16. The more severe the stressor, the greater the likelihood of post-traumatic pathology. The same is true the more prolonged the exposure to the stressor, the earlier the age, the more impaired the social support system, and the greater the degree of exposure to or involvement in previous trauma.

17. Attachment is a basic human need from cradle to grave. Enhanced attachment to abusing objects is seen in all studied species, including humans.

18. Childhood abuse often leads to disrupted attachment behavior, inability to modulate arousal and aggression toward self and others, impaired cognitive functioning, and impaired capacity to form stable relationships.

19. Although it may be a lifelong process, recovery from traumatic experience is possible. Over the course of recovery, survivors may temporarily need safe retreats within which important therapeutic goals can be formulated and treatment can be organized.

20. We are all interconnected and interdependent, for good or for ill. Safety must be constantly created and maintained by everyone in the community as a shared responsibility.

21. The whole is greater than the sum of the parts.

SHARED GOALS

> My only goal in Vietnam was to stay alive. But I died, out there, with my friends. I still wake up screaming, seeing Pete's head—no body—lying along a path. Now I just want to get it over with, I just want to get out of my body and away from this pain.
>
> —forty-eight-year-old Vietnam War veteran,
> admitted after shooting himself in the abdomen

Our shared goals were to make conscious what is unconscious, to make peace and eschew violence, to create an atmosphere of kindness, respect, mutual regard, and tolerance rather than one of hostility, fear, disrespect, shame, or intolerance. Together we would work towards alleviating the suffering and improving the level of functioning for the patients who sought our help. To enter and remain in this environment every person—patient or staff member—had to be dedicated to striving for health, wholeness, and safety.

Shared Goal Setting

We recognized that we had to share goals if we were to be successful. Helping patients to set achievable goals and restricting ourselves to goals that could potentially be met in a very short time were always challenges. Patients who have been severely traumatized begin the process of recovery with an extraordinary amount of work that they must accomplish if their lives are to truly change for the better. Over time we became more realistic about how rapidly change could occur, and what could practically be expected of each person. We had to struggle with defining these goals for each other and telling each other when we thought one of us was expecting too much, too fast. We also had to spend time helping the patients to become more realistic about their goals. Naturally, someone who was extremely depressed wanted to set a goal that they would feel good before they left the hospital, that everything would be "fixed." Our job was to help them break this goal down into manageable parts that could be attained with the few days or weeks that they would be able to stay. Our primary initial focus was aimed at helping our patients develop a plan for becoming safe with themselves.

As managed care companies became more involved in treatment decisions, this became increasingly difficult. These companies expected people to be in and out of the hospital in a matter of days, so their goals were often such behavioral goals as, "patient is no longer suicidal," so that the patient could be sent home. The problem was that suicidal patients often became rapidly less suicidal as soon as they entered the safe structure of the unit. We were perfectly aware, however, that the likelihood remained high that the suicidal ideation would resume if they were released with no other changes having been accomplished. Goal setting was difficult enough when it was just between the clinicians and the patient. When goals also had to be set with insurance company representatives and hospital utilization review authorities, the situation often became treacherous.

SHARED PRACTICE

> I've always felt like I was two people, one good, one bad. You know, like that story, what is it, Jekyll and Hyde? I remember doing those things to people, but it wasn't me. I remember the things they did to me when I was little too, but not like it was really me, like it was somebody else.
>
> —sixty-five-year-old ex-con, imprisoned twenty years for murder

Addressing Unconscious Conflicts and Conflict Resolution

One of our most important lessons was one we had to wrestle with every day—the enormous power of the unconscious in determining human events. In 1954, Stanton and Schwartz had published what became a famous sociological study of a mental institution. One of their most profound insights was about "covert disagreement" among the staff and its effect on the patients and the entire community. In their study they repeatedly noted that conflict was not so much a problem as was concealed or indirect conflict (Stanton and Schwartz 1954). Until the conflict surfaced, the life of the community would rapidly deteriorate with the most vulnerable patients erupting into agitation, excitement, and even violence. The problem could be rapidly solved by simply surfacing the conflict.

To surface conflicts we had to talk to each other a great deal and we had to have a physical space within which such talking could take place. A high frequency of interpersonal communication in a psychiatric milieu is essential if the organization is to be well-managed. Conflicts must be surfaced and resolved, and this is a time-consuming process. Unfortunately, there is never any reimbursement for these types of management activities. Consequently, as budgetary cuts become universal, this vital aspect of community functioning is the first sacrifice that is made. Without such ongoing communication, nonverbal acting-out communication fills the gap.

Decision Making

We also learned a great deal about decision making. We had all been raised to believe that the more authority and responsibility you carry, the more essential it is for you to make independent and individual decisions. Problems with this tenet rapidly presented themselves. The decisions that had to be made in the inpatient setting—like so many decisions that arise in any social setting—were extremely complicated and interconnected. No one person could imagine all of the possible alternatives or consequences of each decision. When one person alone would make a wide-ranging decision, disaster of some sort would often follow, even when the decision maker's thought processes appeared perfectly adequate. It became clear that individual processes simply are not adequate to address the needs of complex systems.

Our decision making was greatly enhanced, however, if we made decisions as a result of a group process in which everyone involved voiced their perceptions, feelings, intuitions, and judgments and then worked on integrating it all into a cohesive perspective. Belenky and her colleagues (1986) have called this "creative consensus" and have noted the tendency of women in groups to utilize this method, which demands more time, thought, and emotional commitment than just following precedent or law. When we were able to do this, decisions often became easy, even obvious.

In order to accomplish this we had to change the essential goal of every decision making encounter. Instead of basing our criteria for success on the best individual decision, which by definition sets up a competitive paradigm, success could be measured only by how creative and complete were our integrative efforts. We discovered that the only really good decisions were integrated group decisions. This required us to flatten our hierarchy of authority because the traditional authority figures, the doctors, often had only one perspective on the problem, and if too much weight was given to their take on the issue, the problem tended to get worse instead of better. This method appears to be more time-consuming in the short run, but because it tends to avoid creating so many other problems it ends up actually being time-conserving. In situations requiring rapid action, individuals would make quicker decisions, but as we came to appreciate the superiority of group decisions, we learned to make individual decisions that had more temporary and less far-reaching consequences, thus enabling us to return to the group for more demanding decisions.

We also learned that the outcome of problem solving was much better if the problem solving method involved everyone who was already or would be affected by the problem. This meant that we often included the patients as an integral part of any decision making process that was relevant to their lives. Conflict had to be expressed openly and respectfully and was to be resolved at the level at which it occurred. The community would govern itself as much as possible, given external constraints. Dissent was to be permitted, even against authority, as long as it did not lead to violence.

Often, we were forced to make attempts to balance the needs of the group against the desires of the individual. We saw that it was vital to satisfy individual needs as much as possible, but this had to be limited by any danger that individual desires posed to the well-being of the community. We learned that having a rigorous and demanding process is much better than trying to establish an arbitrary rule for every different situation. Compulsive rule-making is simply too limiting and tends to overly restrict the freedom of all because of the boundary violations of a few.

But practicing "creative consensus" is not easy for a group of individualists. We had to learn to tolerate ambiguity, confusion, suspended judgment, and ambivalence. We had to stop thinking in terms of "right and wrong," "good and bad," and "either/or," and instead feel our way toward decisions that were always compromises, never absolutes. We found that in dealing with human beings the best process is always one of juggling, of balancing, a never-ending but shifting dance. Only in the avoidance of extremes was there any chance for real change, for real growth.

Group Consciousness

When we were effective something mysterious happened. *Groupmind* is the word that has been used to describe the concept of a supra-individual nature and independence of the collective mind of a social group. The concept goes back at least to Hegel, the German philosopher who thought that individual minds are active participants of a larger social mind, a concept that influenced Marx and Engels (Hewstone et al. 1989; McDougall 1920). It was Durkheim, however, who probably first used the word group-mind, or the term collective consciousness. He suggested that large groups of people sometimes acted with a single mind and that rather than being merely collections of individuals they were linked by some unifying force that went beyond any single individual. This force was so strong in some groups that the will of the individual could be completely dominated by the will of the group (Forsyth 1990).

The development of the concept was arrested in the 1920s under the fierce attack of Floyd Allport who fiercely believed that "the actions of all are nothing more than the sum of the actions of each taken separately" and that the behavior of groups could be fully understood by the behavior of the individuals within a group (Forsyth 1990). And yet "the groupmind concept still seems to lead a ghostly life in the thinking of many social psychologists" (Collier et al. 1991). This is because the study of the individual alone has never fully explained the behavior of groups. In fact, as we are learning from studies of the physical universe, increasingly complex systems develop emergent qualities that cannot be understood by an analysis of the individual parts, and each level of complexity develops its own processes and rules for functioning that are quite different from its individual parts (Capra 1996).

After years spent analyzing the ever-changing process of groupmind that occurs whenever a group of people come together for any length of time, we recognized that this collective identity was inevitable. Our only real choice was whether to allow the effects of this social influence to remain unconscious or to make it conscious. The unconscious functioning of the group-mind can lead to "groupthink."

One of the more problematic aspects of group behavior occurs when a group is under pressure to make an important decision and resorts to what has been called groupthink. When a group has caught the "disease" of groupthink, members try so hard to agree with one another that they commit serious errors that could easily have been avoided. An assumed consensus emerges while every group member focuses on the ways they are all converging and ignores divergence. All group members share a sense of invulnerability that is conveyed by nothing except the fact that they are in it together. They come to believe that such a group of intelligent people could not be mistaken. This kind of thinking leads to decisions that spell disaster (Forsyth 1990; Janis 1972).

The alternative was to attempt the more rigorous practice of group consciousness. Faced with the seemingly impossible dilemmas that our patients often confronted us with, our individual decisions were ineffective. But when we were able to engage in the process of consensus, we could occasionally sense a groupmind force, a kind of group consciousness that was somehow bigger than all of us and yet emerged out of our joint action. The best formulations and strategy came out of these moments. This sense of collective consciousness waxed and waned, but we would all felt safer when it was present and we all worked to restore it if we became fragmented, by talking together and confronting conflicts together. These experiences helped us to recognize the magnitude of our connectedness to each other and admit that we could not function adequately without the other, that we tended to make mistakes if we had only our individual selves to look to for solutions to complex problems. In this work, we discovered that none of our institutions had really prepared us to truly help other people, to cooperate with each other, to function as a whole group rather than an aggregate of individuals (Miller 1976).

Managing Emotions

Psychiatric patients can be highly disturbing while they are very disturbed. By definition they have lost control over some important aspect of their lives, and they are very upset. Powerful feelings of despair, hopelessness, rage, terror, shame, and guilt are the everyday aspects of a psychiatric unit and such powerful feelings are contagious. We had to learn how to tolerate strong emotions and how to transmute those powerful emotions into energy that could be used in service of healing rather than destruction. No individual can handle the magnitude of these emotions. One of the major tenets of the therapeutic milieu is the use of the entire community as a container for overwhelming emotions. We learned how profoundly important it was to "bring it to the community," to repeatedly look at the larger picture rather than attributing individual motivation for all discord. Maintaining a focus on one-on-one interactions could, in fact, escalate a crisis. When emotional storms were brewing and tension in the community could be palpably felt to be growing, then it was time for a community meeting to surface the conflicts and plan steps for the restoration of peace.

The Problem of Violence

We had always shared an extremely important distaste for violent acting out. We did not find violence interesting, intriguing, entertaining, or challenging. We found violence frightening, disturbing, damaging and disruptive of the achievement of our goals. We did not allow people into the unit—

patients or staff—who were violent and if someone became uncontrollably violent he or she was transferred to a more confined setting. But, a large gap usually exists between violent thoughts and violent acting out and we had to learn how to help people deescalate from violence rather than encourage more violence. In doing so, we had to develop skills as arbiters, diplomats, and peacemakers.

Violence of any sort from anyone was not to be tolerated. Neither authority nor insanity was to be a sufficient excuse for violence, whether physical, sexual, or emotional, verbal or nonverbal. Self-harm, although now comprehensible in theory, could not be tolerated in practice. Since we saw ourselves as interconnected, harm to one was viewed as harm to all, and an injury to the community as well. Self-harm would no longer be considered a personal right, but simply another form of interpersonal violence that had to be prevented

Simultaneously we had to learn how to avoid being bullied by patients or each other. Once bullying starts it never stops without force, and the sooner it is stopped, the better. Violent acting out could easily result in ejection from the community, but we tried to provide a clear and coherent way back in if the person was willing and able to control the behavior. Sometimes the violence was due to the uncontrollable nature of some forms of mental illness in the acute stage. If this was the case, then we put the person in a more confined and structured setting and allowed him or her to return once better control had been established. If the violence was an effort to manipulate and control other people, then the message was clear: "Shape up or ship out." Sometimes, such a person would test us to see if we really meant what we said, and we would have to go through the entire ritual of discharge, transfer, or involuntary commitment before they became convinced. Later, if they sought readmission it would be with the understanding—and willing acceptance—that this would not reoccur. It was impressive to see how many violent people could control their violent behavior to self and others if that was the only way they could be accepted as a part of the community.

Boundaries, Both Large and Small

We had to learn a great deal about limits—physical, psychological, social, and moral limits. We learned that even the most controlled of people can erupt if they do not have enough physical space, and we learned that human beings perform better and are better behaved when their physical surroundings are comfortable and attractive. We learned that human beings need settings that maintain a connection with the natural—with trees and flowers, sun and sky, and other animals. We learned that every human being remains, at heart, a territorial animal—we each require our own, inviolable space, surrounded by possessions that confirm and support our unique identity. We learned that all of us—patients and staff—needed frequent opportunities to connect with each other, we needed the freedom to make our own choices about who we would connect with most strongly, and we needed other people to comfort us when we became very emotionally upset. But we also recognized that we needed other people, to help us understand when we have crossed the line into too much connection, into overinvolvement with others. We saw how confusing and how easily violated is the boundary between closeness and sexual intimacy and how destructive sexual energy can be when it is not bounded.

We also learned about boundaries between our small, multiple, and ever-changing social worlds created on the unit and between our small society and the bigger societies of the hospital, our professions, and the larger world within which we were all immersed. Human beings are startlingly proficient at creating cliques, at forming in-groups and out-groups. Being a part of an in-group is defined by its relationship to the out-group and being a part of a group can be tremendously reassuring and comforting. But we had to learn how to disrupt in-groups when they became destructive to others, how to remind people constantly of our shared humanity without losing the energy, shared commitment, and focus of viable in-group functioning.

And we had to learn how to disrupt our own sense of being an in-group enough to participate in the larger hospital culture. We learned how extraordinarily difficult this is to do if the larger culture does not share the values of the subculture. We discovered how easily our flattened hierarchical and democratic structure came into conflict with a more rigid, patriarchal, authoritarian structure and how easily the authoritarian structure attributed these conflicts to "personality" differences rather than to differences in fundamental values and meaning systems.

Living-Learning Environments and a Role for Creativity

Over the years of building, we increasingly developed respect for the role of nonverbal creative expression in managing our emotional lives. We watched with wonder as problems that seemed unresolvable in the context of individual, verbal therapy seemed to dissolve under the influence of psychodrama, art, movement, and play. We laughed with a mixture of embarrassment and delight when the art therapist would magically and correctly analyze our doodles at a staff meeting and marveled at the overwhelming transformative power of drama when the psychodramatist pulled one or the other of us into her group to serve as an auxiliary. We were awed when stiff bodies and masked faces were changed into fluid movement and laughter under the influence of the movement therapist. And, it was common for important insights, revelations, and important exchanges to occur in the context of a recreational outing, a Ping-Pong game, a shared movie, or a sports encounter. Patients routinely and spontaneously composed poetry, kept journals, wrote letters. Other patients convinced us that music was often the only thing that brought them relief from their internal anxiety and agitation. We had no way of explaining why creative expression was so important, but its vital role in intrapsychic and interpersonal change was perfectly obvious.

An essential part of training for staff and for patients was psychoeducation and the dissemination of information. We all needed a way to think about our problems, we needed a shared vocabulary and a unified framework within which strategy could be carefully formulated. Therefore, the entire community needed to provide an ongoing, ceaseless educational experience. Every interpersonal occurrence had to be seen as an opportunity for growth, in Maxwell Jones' terms a "living-learning situation" (1968a). The unconscious had to be made conscious, but people must learn how to do this and this skill does not come easily in our present social environment. We used any means we could find—writing, art, drama, poetry, dance, sports, movies—to help people put their experience into words. Only with words would they be able to put their lives into the narrative form so that the past could take its proper place and leave the present and the future alone. In formal psychoeducation groups, written assignments, readings, and videos, we taught the patients the language of trauma theory.

A vital part of the educational or reeducational experience had to focus on recapturing the enjoyment of life. Most of our patients entered treatment with thoughts of suicide as symptomatic of their overwhelming despair and hopelessness about life. Frequently they had lost the capacity to laugh, to play, or to relax in the comfort of other people. Some of them addressed the therapeutic situation with such extreme compulsivity that therapy itself became another symptom of compulsive behavior. They needed to learn how not to work so compulsively if life was to have any meaning again.

An Environment for Us All

And in practice, everyone needed to have a shared commitment to all the spoken and unspoken community values. We discovered that we needed to rigorously define and repeatedly renegotiate what we believe in, how our beliefs are or are not reinforced by what we say and what we do. We saw that apparent challenges to authority often occurred when our values had become inconsistent with our practice. We learned that when we gave our patients and each other permission to point out our own hypocritical behavior as a system instead of an individual problem, the incidence of acting out, backbiting, splitting, and all forms of underhanded manipulation, plunged.

We realized, however, that these values had to be learned and that learning is frequently quite slow and based on experience. Therefore, what was important was the commitment and the working towards the incorporation of these values, not their absolute attainment. Human beings are flawed, learn by trial and error, and require a long time to unlearn bad habits and substitute good habits. Therefore, in practice what was most important was seeing change unfold, seeing progress. As staff members, functioning as part of the community for many hours a day, we knew how difficult consistently living up to these standards would be. We knew we would fail at times.

The problems were even more difficult to surmount for the patients because they had several disadvantages: They were already habituated to abusive environments and would inevitably attempt to re-create them in our setting; and they would have very little time to incorporate the norms of our miniature society because the length of time they could stay on the unit was diminishing rapidly due to changes in insurance reimbursement. Patients who had received months of hospitalization in the past were now allowed only days. Nonetheless, we thought it was far more important to establish the values and admit to our failures to live up to them, than to pretend that values were not important, or worse yet, to pretend that we were living up to values when we were not. If nothing else, this would help to undermine the all-too-human tendency to idealize and become dependent upon authority, regardless of the abilities or character of those assuming such authority.

We learned a great deal about who could fit into our system as a patient or as a staff member and who could not. The outstanding requirement was a willingness to learn and to change. As long as someone was committed to growth and to becoming a part of the community, then we engaged in a process of mutual accommodation. Those who had the most difficulty fitting in were those who were so rigid that they could not accommodate to our system at all, those who were dishonest and placed their own personal interest above those of the patients or the community despite frequent confrontation, those who had unresolved childhood issues of their own that consistently and unremittingly interfered with treatment, and those who lacked a sense of humor. Even in those cases, we rarely had to reject people from the system—they rejected themselves, because ultimately they would find the pressure to change and to honestly confront their pain too uncomfortable. As long as they remained a part of the community we tried to work through the problems with them.

Over time, we realized that we had had a unique opportunity. In creating our own small community we had been able to establish our own norms, our own explicit and implicit standards for community behavior, some of which conflicted with and some of which were congruent with the larger, overarching community. The differences were fairly obvious. Emotional expression was valued more in our subculture than in the larger community. Emotions were seen as possessing vital information that needed to be accepted and understood. Communication between people was to be open and frequent, but even confrontation was to be done with kindness and compassion. Success was to be defined on the basis of integration not competition. Arbitrary decision making was frowned upon and was to be replaced by careful and balanced problem solving. Rule making was not to be substituted for communication and negotiation in each particular and unique situation. Boundaries between people were to be respected. Boundary violations required discussion, renegotiating, and a contractual agreement for the consequences of future violations, not punishment. Violence was not tolerable and would result in extrusion from the community until it ceased. Relationships were to be defined, protected, and respected.

The result of this attitude and practice was that many of us made enormous professional and personal changes. Essentially, that is what a "therapeutic community" is—a place in which every member of the community has an opportunity to straighten out the kinks in their lives within an atmosphere of mutual support and tolerance. Punitive measures were not necessary. Once people became a part of the community they generally wanted to remain a part of it—staff and patients. They sought out the esteem of their neighbors and would try to address areas of conflict. As long as they sensed that there was an honest willingness to accept them, even with all their foibles, then they had an incentive to work harder, to do better, to be kinder and more tolerant. The staff had to convey this attitude to the patients, and the leaders had to convey this attitude to the rest of the staff. Congruence and consistency was absolutely necessary, and lapses in consistency had to be explored, understood, and finally put to rest.

We learned all this in a setting that placed a very low value on competition. Since our philosophical position was fundamentally grounded in a belief that our system had to function as a whole, with every part of the whole as integral, there could be no "winner" and "loser" without damaging the functioning of the whole. Our working metaphor was based not on a battlefield image but instead on the more essential workings of a living system like the human body. The brain is important, but what good is a brain without a digestive tract, or a liver, or a circulatory system? Such a metaphor implies a shift in other aspects of practice among people. It means that there must be a measure of agreement among all essential components of a system before successful change can occur. It means that each component of the system must recognize and fulfill his or her own unique contribution without feeling the need to prove he or she is superior to another.

The role of the brain in the body is a complicated one. But perhaps the most important and unique function of the brain is as an *integrator*. The brain takes all the information that comes in from the outside and internal sensors and integrates it into a meaningful whole, balancing various priorities. The brain can override lower brain and body function when it is in the interest of survival, but the brain cannot function without the lower brain and the body. The parts are totally interdependent. This is a good metaphor for leadership in any system. The job of the leader is not to compulsively exercise authority or wield power over others. We learned that the role of the leader is to integrate the various sources of information within a system into a coherent whole that informs practice. The leader is a "central switchboard," balancing many priorities in service of the overall system and, when necessary, overriding other decisions in the service of system survival. In this manner of functioning, power is an outgrowth of the working of the entire system, not any individual member, and all parts of the system share in the power.

WHO WE TREATED

> I was only six, I think, when he started coming in my room at night. One day I tried to fight back and he took my puppy and bashed in his head with a rock and told me that if I didn't shut up he'd do the same thing to me. I never talked about it again and I'm still scared to tell.
> —thirty-seven-year-old corporate executive with bulimia,
> self-mutilation, and an alcohol problem

In the early stages of developing *The Sanctuary*, we remained in a general hospital setting as a general psychiatry unit. We catered to a middle-class population in a semirural area. Admission was strictly voluntary. Rather than locked doors and restraints, we used the strength and power of relationships, peer pressure, and social expectations to achieve our goals.

Locked doors convey messages to frightened people. It is the social confirmation of their worst fears—that they are "crazy." Locked doors tell patients
that they are helpless prisoners who cannot be expected to control themselves. Through locks and bars the message is conveyed that people will be
violent and they often will comply with this social expectation by acting
violently.

We accepted only those patients who could be safely maintained without
the restrictions of locked doors or restraints. Although this excluded a fair
number of psychotic patients, we did treat people who suffered from schizophrenic and bipolar disorders, as long as they could be managed in our setting. We treated men and women, adolescents and adults. Most of the adults
we treated had jobs and families. Many of them had achieved a high degree
of success in their professions and then had become incapacitated by some
kind of symptom. In 1991, we moved our unit to a private psychiatric hospital and became a discrete program specializing in treating adults who had
been abused as children and we named it *The Sanctuary*. In practice, our
population did not change very much. We saw the same variety of symptom
presentations. The only change was that patients had often self-identified
themselves as suffering from trauma before they entered the hospital, and
because we were a specialty program we began treating an increasing
number of these patients who had failed in other settings.

The range of symptoms was quite wide.[1] Virtually everyone was
depressed and/or suffering from overwhelming anxiety. Unable to sleep,
plagued by overwhelming fears and a dark foreboding, they often entered the
hospital suffering from sheer physical and emotional exhaustion. The severity of the symptoms on admission increased over the years as it became
harder and harder to even get admitted to a hospital because of insurance
limitations. In the early days we often saw people before they had reached
bottom. Later, patients often had to have attempted suicide before hospitalization would be approved by the insurance company. Many of them had
complicating medical problems as well. Other common causes for admission
were self-mutilation or a life-threatening eating disorder. Some people came
in because they were engaged in all kinds of self-destructive behavior—
shoplifting, promiscuity, reckless driving, failing to get medical care. Others
sought admission because they feared losing control over their impulses to
hurt others, most frequently, their own children. Many of them used drugs
or alcohol as a secondary problem—if it was viewed as a primary problem,
often a fairly arbitrary decision, their insurance companies would not
permit them to remain on our unit. Our average length of stay never got
longer than about sixteen days. But that meant that some people stayed for

three to four weeks and others only stayed overnight. As a staff, we felt the ideal length of stay for our treatment regimen was about three weeks, the first week for people to learn the ropes and immerse themselves in the psychoeducational material related to trauma, the second week to focus on modifying the problematic behaviors and learning new skills in modulating their emotional responses to others, the third week to prepare to resume their normal life and to consolidate the gains they had made.

We were comfortable with relatively short lengths of stay because we did not want people to become overly reliant on an institution or be separated too long from their social support system, their jobs, or their schools. At the same time, we were under no illusions that recovery from what was often a lifetime of symptoms could miraculously occur in a matter of days. We anticipated that many people would need rehospitalization as life crises occurred or as crises occurred in outpatient treatment. We did not consider this recidivism. We classified someone as a recidivist only when they repeatedly sought hospitalization without showing any improvement. We told patients that we would far rather that they called us *before* they made the suicide attempt, or before they cut themselves again, or prostituted themselves again, or drank again, rather than after the fact, and that we would consider that progress.

Over and over, in any number of ways, we reiterated our primary assumption—that people *can* and *do* recover from these disorders and that we were only interested in treating people who wanted to do so. If they wanted to stay sick, symptomatic, and self-destructive, then they could go somewhere else to do it. This may sound harsh, but only in clearly stating this position and living up to it could we convince people that we were truly committed to health, not to enabling and supporting pathology. As we became increasingly aware of the high incidence of childhood trauma and its role in the etiology of psychiatric dysfunction we became simultaneously more despairing and more hopeful—despairing that we could ever truly fix the problem using a model of individual treatment, and yet hopeful that if we could mobilize the internal healing resources of people who were injured and the external healing resources of their community, then we could see much greater change than just attempting to ameliorate the nebulous "illnesses" of the psychiatrically impaired.

Since it had already been established that about 80 percent of our original, and then 100 percent of our population as of 1991, was traumatized, we did not need to make a big deal about it. Early in the development of the sanctuary model, the patients, for the most part did not know that we had made this major shift in our paradigmatic way of thinking about psychiatric disorder. We just began enlarging our history taking to include a more thorough evaluation for a past history of trauma. We did not focus exclusively on sexual abuse. In fact, sexual abuse was the hardest thing for us to mention. It took time for us to become desensitized to the issue so that we could openly discuss it as a possibility.

We asked about combat experiences, physical assault, domestic violence, crime, car accidents, traumatic surgical experiences, childhood illness and parental absences, witnessing violence, death of a close relative, and any number of other painful, damaging, or humiliating experiences that people manage to survive. Our questions were fairly open-ended, such as "What was the worst thing that ever happened to you?" or "Describe the scariest time of your life." "How were you disciplined when you were little?" "What would happen at home if you were really bad?" Gradually we learned what various kinds of previous trauma look like, how they are transmuted to reappear in their present disguise.

Partial amnesia for the traumatic experience was typical. People remembered that they had been through a traumatic experience but remembered only a part of it, or had no feeling about it, or did not even know that they did not remember it but had obvious gaps in their recall when asked about the event. Many of them revealed that they had a suspicion that there was more but that they could not remember. Sometimes, they denied an experience, but even when asked the question became visibly agitated, scared, or defensive, an uncommon response for a truly negative answer. Total amnesia for some events was also common, but we could not know about that at the time of admission. The presence of the many forms of dissociative experience usually became known only over time, when twenty-four-hour-a-day therapeutic contact made hiding, covering up, and denial much more difficult to sustain.

As we became more familiar with the entire clinical picture of posttraumatic stress, we more easily diagnosed hyperarousal, hypervigilance, flashbacks, numbing of emotions, dissociative states, and differentiated these symptoms from psychosis. All of these symptoms are characteristic of someone who has experienced an overwhelming fright and all are very difficult to fabricate. We can lie, but it is much harder to make our bodies lie. Gifted actors spend a lifetime learning to simulate powerful emotional responses. Rapid heart rates, rapid respiratory rates, dilated pupils, profuse sweating, hair standing on end—these are all difficult to fake. Highly functioning people who were otherwise comfortable in their social skills would suddenly be cowering in a corner, terrified, crying, clinging, appearing to be about age four. To the extent that they could remember the episode afterward, they would feel overwhelmed with embarrassment and shame, and not at all pleased or satisfied that they had gotten some attention.

Sexual abuse was a particular problem. We didn't necessarily directly ask about it, but we kept hearing about it nonetheless. Sometimes it was a father or a mother—but abuse at the hands of a close family member tended not to be offered spontaneously in the history. More often at the initial interview it was adult rape, incest with stepfather or brother or uncle, molestation by a teacher, a Boy Scout leader, a minister, a priest, a music instructor, a baby-sitter. It became apparent that virtually any role that an adult could fill for a child could be used to betray the confidence and trust of the child.

This was a very hard reality to swallow. Assault, robbery, humiliation, ridicule—all of these were at least within a contextual frame that, if not manageable, were at least conceivable. Certainly, television and motion pictures had been visually immersing us in those kinds of trauma for a very long time. But grown men and women raping children? Nothing had prepared us for this. In fact, we had been taught that memories of childhood sexual experiences were largely wish-fulfilling fantasies. And it was tempting, very tempting, to shift back to fantasy as an explanation. Such a backward shift, however, posed notable intellectual problems not the least of which was the fact that those explanations used in the past had proven to be ineffective in helping our most problematic patients.

Borderline Personality Disorder

Many of these sexual abuse victims had serious psychiatric problems, and yet they were not psychotic. They often self-mutilated themselves, frequently on their breasts or in their pelvic region, as well as on their arms and legs. Many had been raped as adults as well. They tended to have extremely disturbed, abusive relationships. Their sexual adjustment was often very distorted. Commonly they were either totally abstinent and terrified of sexual contact or promiscuous without ever truly enjoying it. They had multiple physical complaints and surgical procedures directed at their genital and pelvic region, and often their gynecologist reported negative findings in the face of severe and chronic pain. Eating disorders were very common including overeating, alternating with bulimia, interspersed with episodes of starvation, and a preoccupation with body image. They often had weird, psychotic-like symptoms and heard voices, or saw things that were not there, or acted in bizarre and spaced-out ways. They had established problematic relationships with people in their social lives and then with us. At first they were very good and compliant, the ideal patient (child), and then, at the slightest sign of rejection, they became unreasonably hostile, angry, rejecting, and inconsolable. They were either all-good or all-bad, as were their relationships, as was the entire world. We called them "borderline personality disorder," but we were not entirely sure what this meant, except that treatment was very difficult if not impossible and that the origins of the problem probably lay in the mysterious past, although biochemical and genetic defects could not be ruled out.

On the other hand, they shared symptoms very similar to other trauma victims. They showed physiological hyperarousal and hypervigilance. They were unable to self-soothe or to modulate emotional arousal. They had difficulty managing anger and as a consequence often failed to self-protect adequately while acting aggressively toward others. We began to understand that much of what we had been calling psychotic symptoms were actually the dissociated memories of previous experiences. The hallucinatory voices they heard were related to the voices and sounds surrounding the sexual abuse situation. The hallucinatory visions were fragmentary memories of the trauma. The paranoia was fear combined with a temporary inability to separate the past and the present. Their apparent lack of awareness of their own behavior and the subsequent failure to take responsibility for it was related to the fact that they were relatively unaware of much of what they did in another state of consciousness. The self-mutilation was a form of self-control, a problematic form of self-soothing, an addictive behavior that had worked in the past under severe stress but had taken on secondary meanings and uses over time.

As we began to change our way of addressing their problems, they changed as well. Before this, we had termed these patients, "borderlines," "manipulators," "attention-seekers," "hysterics"—all a way of saying that our helping efforts were thanklessly frustrated. When we began to understand that these patients had suffered extremely abusive and depriving situations as children, had developed certain coping skills to survive, and had remained arrested in an earlier stage of development because of an extremely damaging, and often very secretive home life, our attitudes toward them changed dramatically. We became less offended, less threatened, by their symptoms. Now we could understand what they were doing, what they were trying to tell us about their past lives. And we could explain back to them what it was all about, why it all did make sense, given the context. Once they were able to understand, they were able to begin the long process of gaining some compassion for themselves and their own suffering. Using this bridge of compassion they could start the process of rebuilding, of starting to mature again from the point where their growth and integrity was stopped.

Multiple Personality Disorder

Another group of patients initially were extremely confusing. Dawn was the first of these that I knowingly treated. These are the people who suffer from multiple personality disorder, now known as "dissociative identity disorder." It sounds so exotic when you first see it or hear about it, as in *The Three Faces of Eve* or *Sybil*. It's actually not very exotic or incomprehensible at all. It does, however, throw a very big wrench into the way we understand the mind and human identity. Our existing philosophical, medical, and legal paradigm is based on the presumption that we have one fixed identity—a "unity of consciousness" (Tinnin 1990) that transcends the localized organization of the brain's function. When we say "I" we refer to this unity, this self-sense, this consciousness. We can, at least at times, admit to the existence of an "unconscious" self—a part of us that motivates our behavior outside of our awareness. But the idea that we could have separate identities or aspects of our self—or ego states—that can operate autonomously, and even in opposition to each other—is extremely disconcerting to our usual model of the mind. The existence of several "personalities" within the same person raises extremely difficult questions for many of our integral social systems.

Despite our several centuries old and now voluminous documentation of the existence of people who suffer from the active presence of two or more very separate personalities, some professionals still deny the existence of such a phenomenon, as if it were a matter not of scientific observation, but of religious belief. This is unfortunate because people who suffer from these disorders lie along a continuum that includes all of us. A true unity of consciousness is likely an extremely rare phenomenon and may actually be present only in those people on whom we confer a superhuman or divine attribution.

As we have come to recognize from dealing with the most extreme end of the continuum—multiple personality disorder—everyone has experiences in growing up that are fragmenting. In any home, in every school, certain impulses, desires, abilities, and tendencies are discouraged and others are encouraged. What happens to the "self" of the little boy who likes to play with dolls but who is forbidden from doing so? Where does the little girl who likes to rough-house, and play with her own genitals, and explore unknown places go when she is punished for touching herself, forbidden to go out alone, and prevented from playing sports? Children learn to simply turn off what they want to do and are forbidden or prevented from doing.

With enough love, guidance, forbearance, and redirecting, child rearing can be accomplished so that the effects of the cut-offs are minimal and the desires can be channeled in ways that are self-enhancing. Aspects of ourselves then can lie dormant until we are old enough or have the freedom enough to safely act on them. The adventurous child who had to perform intellectually for his parents gives reign to his adventurous self at age forty when he goes on an around-the-world ocean journey. The A student who gave up her scholarly aspirations to devote herself to her husband and five children finally satisfies a long suppressed inner self when she returns to college at age fifty. These and millions like them are examples of people whose "selves" did not have an opportunity to become more integrated until midlife, and yet their lives before the change may have been richly rewarding and satisfying.

People who suffer from multiple personalities are people who have been born with the same multi-potential as everyone else. But they did not have the childhood that other people had. Their childhoods are steeped in astonishing, repetitive, and erratic sadism at the hands of the adults they must depend upon. These children use whatever abilities they have in service of survival under the most desperate conditions a child can face. Their abilities raise serious questions about the mind/body dichotomy, about our latent psychic abilities, about what we are truly capable of accomplishing when we really put our mind (minds?) to it. Researchers report cases of different allergies, different responses to drugs, different physical disorders, different eyeglass prescriptions and opthalmological measures, different handedness, and different autonomic system responses to various stimuli (Kluft 1996; Zahn et al. 1996). Our present model of the connection between mind and body cannot explain these phenomena. While in alter personality states, people suffering from multiple personality disorder have been known to accomplish amazing intellectual and physical feats that cannot be explained with our present models of the mind.[2]

But for most of the time, life for people suffering from these disorders is miserable, chaotic, and perplexing. We learned that helping them learn how to help themselves was a tricky business. For people who have dissociative disorders like multiple personality disorder, dissociation has become the one way they can cope with stress. So anything that increases stress creates more dissociation. Engaging actively in psychotherapy is stressful. It's a problem—how to treat people with these disorders without making the situation worse. Though under certain stressful conditions they can accomplish feats of skill, strength, and ingenuity that defy the abilities of most of us, they may be unable to do the most basic tasks such as socialize in a group of people, enjoy simple pleasures or efficiently perform everyday tasks. This high-lights the severe developmental impairments that characterize the back-ground of someone who develops this disorder. A major focus of therapy is re-membering—putting the fragments of separate personality states together with a narrative of memory associated with feeling. But the feel-ings of terror, pain, grief, despair, hopelessness, helplessness, and rage are overwhelming and exceedingly difficult to face. Consequently, there is a temptation to remain preoccupied for too long with the manifold nature of all the different personalities while neglecting to focus on the necessary integration. At the same time, progress cannot be made unless the "host" self becomes familiar with and is ready to accept the various aspects of the other personalities that exist within the body. With experience we learned an important lesson. If, under our care, the person's symptoms kept getting worse, then there was probably something wrong with our approach.

The Men and the Perpetrators

Our unit has always been a mixed gender program. We wanted the setting to be as natural as possible, and in the real world, men must interact with women, and women with men. Early in the process of our own expansion, we had divided up the world into the good guys and the bad guys. Our patients were the good guys; the bad guys were the perpetrators who had hurt our patients. It was a fairly straightforward and easy distinction. Except that it turned out to be wrong. The men who came on our unit sometimes found it easier to talk about their own perpetration then their victimization. You can be "bad" and still be a man. But men are not sup-posed to be victims—being victimized is a girl thing. We had to deal with the fear and rage that the women felt toward any man they had to share space with who admitted to some past history of hurting other people. At first, the men who came on our unit told their stories of past abuse, partic-ularly sexual abuse, only with great reluctance. Gradually, as the staff became more comfortable listening to those stories, the men more easily spoke of their experience. We learned from men very graphically, that women can be perpetrators too.

And to our surprise, opening up the subject of perpetration and its ori-gins in abuse among the men opened up the subject for the women as well. Some of them began, with great shame and guilt, to reveal their own guilty secrets about hurting someone in the past. For us, this muddied our world view considerably. We had to contend with our own tendency to be judg-mental, to lay blame, to want to punish or seek revenge, while at the same time, forgiveness was not ours to give. Each individual had to be held accountable for what he or she had done. The individual history of abuse was the explanation, the reason for the perpetration, but it was not an excuse. Mothers and fathers who were a danger to their children had to be reported, and we expected them to report themselves, and they usually did so. People who were in danger had to be warned. No more were the good guys good, and the bad guys bad. What it finally boiled down to is that "hurt people hurt people" and if we wanted to stop people from getting hurt, then, as a society, we were going to have to stop hurting children.

The Strong and the Brave and the Astute

We also began having some very humbling experiences. In describing who we have treated I feel compelled to state that we have treated some of the strongest and bravest and cleverest people we can ever hope to meet. As we began listening to their childhood stories of survival with respect instead of disbelief, we were stunned by what these people had survived, and to some extent, overcome. Without even recognizing what they were saying, our patients would often recount tales of heroism and self-sacrifice that would make it into the evening news if the tales did not involve the secret perfidy of the family. And even in the midst of their own hurt, their own private craziness, they would often reach out to another person in the community, putting their own needs aside for the moment, exercising an understanding, wisdom and compassion that is sadly lacking in much normal social dialogue.

We learned graphically and repeatedly that our patients were not weak or fragile. In order to survive, they had developed strengths we could not even imagine and we could rely on these strengths through the therapeutic journey. Regardless of how terrified they became, how much they said they wanted it to stop, how often they accused us of abusing them for this or for that, nothing we could do would come close to replicating what had already been done to them, what they had already survived. This meant that we could challenge them, we could dare them to try something different, we did not need to be scared of their apparent weakness, fragility, or even their threats. We could encourage the strength and intelligence that was very evidently there, rather than play to the weakness. This is a lesson no one had ever taught us in our training programs. These people were injured, yes. But they were also tough, resilient, and often ingenious. The problem was that all these positive traits were aimed in the wrong direction, aimed toward maintaining "sickness" instead of seeking health, and our systems of treatment had been covertly supporting and even encouraging this "sickness."

STARTING THE PROCESS OF RECOVERY

I can't do this. I can't take any more pain. I just want to kill myself and get it over with. I wish he had just finished the job.

—forty-year-old woman, stalked by a stranger,
then raped, beaten, stabbed, and left for dead

Safety: Community Management of Destructive Behaviors

Any complicated procedure is a bit easier when broken into definable pieces. When it comes to recovering from traumatic experience, various writers have attempted to assign stages to recovery. For our purposes, the most useful description has been that of Dr. Judith Herman who broke treatment down into three stages: safety, reconstruction (remembrance and mourning), and reconnection (1992). No matter how these stages are defined however, it is clear that interpenetration of all the stages occurs, and recovery proceeds along a continuum of experience.

We knew that the most important thing we could do, the absolutely essential ingredient for recovery, was our insistence on safety. Violence to others was forbidden; violence to self was given an explanatory meaning. Self-destructive impulses were explained as the desperate attempt to signal distress, a nonverbal way of sharing an unspeakable story. Because telling the story in words is necessary for recovery, patients had to make the transition from action to verbalization.

We also framed self-destructive behavior as a form of addiction that people would need to actively withdraw from if they were to move on in treatment. This addiction was seen as powerful, physiologically insistent, and difficult to manage in any other way at first. We warned people that as they started to change, to give up their self-destructive behavior, they might begin experiencing overwhelming feelings and distressing flashbacks.

Most of them were already experiencing terrible despair and anxiety as well as flashbacks. The idea that abstinence from self-mutilation, compulsive promiscuity, risk-taking, or any other problem behavior, would lead to even worse symptoms was not exactly welcome news. This is why it was crucial to have an explanatory system that could help people understand why this was so important, why it is absolutely necessary for the brain to absorb and integrate dissociated material, this time in a context of safety. We had to convince people who had quite reasonably learned to be distrustful of accepting comfort from other people that we could be trusted to be different.

We were essentially asking them to trade an addictive behavior that worked to relieve their pain, at least temporarily, for the comfort and safety of other human beings. We were asking them to trust that relationships with other people could provide the same degree of emotional comfort and physiological relief as did their tried-and-true addiction. To expect them to take this apparently illogical course of action, we had to recruit their cognitive capacities into the process by educating them about trauma. And to do that we had to know something about what had happened to them in the past, something about the traumatic experiences they had endured as children. The behaviors that were most problematic for us, and probably for most communities, were self-mutilation, suicide threats and gestures, traumatic reenactments that involved other members of the community, behaviors that reflect the failure to use anger to protect self and others, and problems related to physical symptoms.

Self-Mutilation

People who self-mutilate engage in bizarre acts. Seizing razors, knives, jagged shards of glass or metal, they deliberately cut themselves. They may burn themselves with cigarettes or put their hands on stoves. They may pull out their hair, pick at their skin, insert painful objects into their body orifices. Any part of the body that can be reached is a possible target, including breasts and genitals. Sometimes, the person can articulate the reasons behind the choice of body part—a sexual abuse victim may slice up her pelvic region—but at other times it is the wounding that is critical, not the particular part. Like so many aspects of complex human behavior, self-mutilation is "overdetermined"—that means there are many levels of meaning that simultaneously explain the behavior. Nonetheless, until we understood the relationship between previous trauma and self-mutilation, we were not very successful at altering the behavior.

Self-mutilation is not about suicide. It is the traumatized person's way of trying to manage overwhelming negative emotions while simultaneously expressing, nonverbally, the extreme rage, despair, and agony of the tormented child. People who self-mutilate have learned that if they hurt the body, they will experience a temporary relief from a state that is described by some as one of hyperarousal and acute distress and by others as a state of numbed emptiness. Usually, people feel little or no pain while they are cutting. It has been suggested that this response is due to an endorphin response and that the repeated use of self-mutilation as a coping skill may alter the endorphin response and thus become an addictive behavior that is reinforced every time it works (Richardson and Zaleski 1983, Van der Kolk 1987a; Van der Kolk et al. 1989). The cutting does not make the person feel good—it simply makes life bearable for another hour or day. But the self-mutilation is also a form of traumatic reenactment. The victims frequently wound themselves at the same real or symbolic place that their perpetrator hurt them. The visible gashes, burns, and scars are bodily expressions of a much deeper inward pain that is visible only to the victims. In their desperate and largely unconscious attempt to communicate their distress to the world that lies beyond the boundary of their skin, they reenact the trauma by inflicting more trauma upon themselves.

Adults who self-mutilate are strongly ashamed of their behavior, but they are helpless in the face of it. They feel compelled to inflict pain upon themselves by a force they do not understand and cannot control. Just as an alcoholic must stop drinking in order to move farther down the road to recovery, so too must a self-mutilator learn to resist the impulse to cut. This is difficult for several reasons. First, many patients self-mutilate when they are in a dissociative state. Under stress they enter a trance state, another part of themselves or an alter personality inflicts the wounds, and they come to their senses without recall for what transpired.

Second, it is difficult to give up one coping skill until you have found an alternative that is just as effective. Unless you have been abused, it is difficult to understand how cutting yourself can be a coping skill, but the combined effects of the endorphin response and the sense of control one can exert over one's own feelings of inner turmoil and helplessness is seductive. For most distressed people under normal circumstances, comfort comes from the caring concern of other people. But people who have been victimized as children have learned that they cannot trust other people, that more pain and betrayal is the only result of giving up self-dependence.

Third, most people who self-mutilate, have been doing so for a very long time. As a result, behavior has acquired secondary and tertiary associations that may be difficult to give up. They may have learned that if they cut themselves and call their therapist, or go to an emergency room, that they can predictably get touched, bandaged, and cared for even if they must put up with their caretakers' anger, frustration, and discouragement. When human beings are starved for human attention and human touch, this can be a powerful motivating force.

We discovered that our attitude and behavior in the face of self-mutilation was critical if our patients were to make progress in treatment. We evolved a position that simultaneously condemned the behavior while supporting the person involved in the behavior. We honored the behavior for the role it had played as a coping skill that may have helped the patients avoid worse fates, but we made it clear that there were now other options open to them that were constructive, not destructive. We viewed self-mutilation as an act of perpetration against the self and against the community that must be stopped before healing could commence.

This mandated a withdrawal from self-abusive behavior and our job was to help our patients through this period of voluntary detoxification. No reconstructive work could begin until they had demonstrated to themselves that they could handle intense emotion constructively. Using a detoxification paradigm was helpful. People generally recognize that getting off drugs or alcohol is a difficult and painful but time-limited experience. We routinely informed patients before they even entered our program, about our policy on self-mutilation and got their consent before agreeing to admission. We used and enforced verbal and written contracts about self-mutilation that provided negative consequences for continuing the behavior. If a self-mutilation episode occurred, the patient was given an "intensive refocus assignment" which required them to write down what had happened, what they thought had triggered the behavior, suggestions for other things they could do to cope, and an exploration of how the behavior was impacting on them and those around them. These assignments helped reduce the automaticity of the behavior and made it a habit that was subject to change. The assignments also provided a way for the patients and their therapists to look at the circumstances that had provoked the episode and begin to think more clearly about how to exert control and self-protection that was not self-destructive.

Sometimes, patients were extremely ambivalent about stopping the self-mutilative behavior. Not only are habits difficult to break, but sometimes the behavior becomes incorporated into other aspects of identity to such an extent that the person has difficulty deciding how to relate to others without the behavior. On such occasions, the self-mutilative episodes tended to be dramatic, excessive and very public. With such resistances in place, it was often useful to surface the behavior as a problem for the community, rather than an individual issue. To do this, a community meeting would be held to discuss how the patient's self-destructive behavior was impacting on everyone else. As the other patients vocalized their feelings ranging from sympathy to anger, the patient could see how connected to and what a powerful influence he or she actually had on the rest of the community. Patients who have been victimized do not like to see themselves as perpetrators and viewing their self-destructive behavior in this light often produced a cognitive dissonance that provided an opportunity for change. Using these approaches, the patient would either successfully stop the behavior or discover that he or she was not yet ready to make such a commitment to treatment. Either way, the issue was clearly surfaced and put into an entirely different perspective. No longer could the self-mutilation be kept a secret. It had become a social affair.

Suicidality

Part of the art of psychotherapy is learning how to manage different kinds of suicide crises. Our understanding of trauma shed new light on the many reasons why our patients were often chronically suicidal. And some of what we learned about management of these situations put us in potential direct conflict with the existing legal paradigm that holds us responsible for the lives of our patients.

There are many reasons for suicidal thoughts and behaviors. Some people become acutely suicidal as a result of severe, biologically based depressive disorders, and must be protected, even forcibly protected, from hurting themselves. While suicidal they are in a kind of delirium—their brain is malfunctioning. Other people have a similar state of brain dysfunction as the direct effect of drugs or withdrawal from drugs. They also need to be protected by any means necessary.

For many other people suicidal preoccupations become a way of life and a way of relating to other people. Many victims of childhood trauma live with a pervasive despair that waxes and wanes but is never really alleviated. Their suicidal thoughts do not necessarily come from an acute biological cause—although they are certainly prone to suffer from severe depressions as well. These suicidal thoughts can be an expression of many other ideas and feelings, singly or in combination. For someone who has been exposed to repeated experiences of traumatic helplessness, suicide may be for them the one way they believe they can still control their destiny. For someone who has never had a moment's peace, suicide can represent a longed-for calm, an end to strife. For someone whose experiences with other people are based only on the expression of extreme emotions or behaviors, suicide threats may be the only way they can get any sense that they are cared for by someone else. For people who have never been permitted to express anger without being abused, suicidal behavior may be the only way they have available of saying to their social group: "I am furious"; "You let me down"; "I hate you." For someone who feels overwhelming guilt about their own abusive behavior towards others, suicide may be what they feel they deserve. For someone steeped in fantasies of revenge, suicide may be the fantasized way that they will finally get even.

Children exposed to overwhelming trauma often fail to develop normal coping skills. As they grow up they tend to use the only skills they had as children, such as dissociating, or running away, or fighting back. If these coping skills cease to work or are prohibited by external circumstances, desperation and despair may drive them towards suicidal behavior. For most of these people, at least in the beginning, suicidal threats or attempts are a serious cry for help to someone in their social group. They are quite literally saying "I can no longer live this way." Unfortunately, their threats and gestures will often be interpreted as manipulative. If we use manipulative in its original meaning—the skillful use of tools—then it is accurate. Patients who display this behavior are trying to convey a powerfully "worded" message to anyone who cares to listen. As representatives of the social group, we decide how we are going to respond to the message.

Traditionally, the response to suicidal behavior is to judge that the person is insane and to assume responsibility for them—medically and legally—until they have come to their senses. The problem is that most of the suicidal behavior that we saw did not come about because people were insane. They made a decision that killing themselves was or might be the best possible course of action. In taking responsibility—medically and legally for them—we were saying to them that we were able to provide a better course of action then their own, that we could protect them from themselves. The problem was that—we couldn't. While they were hospitalized, our efforts to protect them from themselves could easily be perceived as coercive and potentially abusive. And they could only remain in the more secure confines of a hospital for a brief period. Our ability to protect them, therefore, was largely illusory and served only to fuel the unrealistic expectations of our patients and provide grist for the legal malpractice mills. Many therapists and physicians are driven into coercive behavior, not because they believe it will help the patient but because it is the only way to protect themselves. This has been a chronic dilemma for psychiatry. Until someone who is sane and suicidal decides not to kill themselves, we can do very little to help them. In taking away their right to make decisions for themselves, to even manage their own possessions, we were in danger of further reinforcing the helplessness that already existed and of conveying a message that we had power that we really did not have.

We discovered that, if we were to be truly responsible, we had to be honest with our patients about the limitations of our power. If we had judged that they were suicidal, but not insane, then we had to tell them that we could not rescue them, that only they could rescue themselves. As in the case of self-mutilation, we framed suicide attempts as a form of perpetration directed at the self. As we came to understand the victim-perpetrator-rescuer triangulation, we realized that we were not doing our patients a service if we played any one of these three roles. They had been victimized, they had incorporated an identification with their perpetrator, and they were alternately waiting for a magical rescue and furious when it failed to emerge. When we became too enmeshed in their traumatic reenactment we would first be viewed as "rescuer." When we inevitably failed to rescue them from their inner torment, we would be seen as perpetrators. When we reacted negatively to being treated as perpetrators, suicidal behavior would emerge, and we would become victims as the patient held the real or symbolic knife to his or her own throat, perversely enjoying our terror, as their perpetrator once had enjoyed their fear and humiliation.

There is no winning role in this lethal game. We struggled to learn to resist becoming trapped in any of these roles, while continuing to safeguard the well-being of the patient. It was a tricky business. If someone is suicidal and refuses help, only three options exist: They control themselves, they commit suicide, or they are forcibly restrained. If we responded to every suicidal gesture or threat with the traditional restrictions of mobility and privileges, then not only did the patient miss substantial parts of the program but they quickly learned that such behavior can provide a substantial feeling of power over others. For people who are accustomed to powerlessness this feeling was very seductive but as a result, they failed to learn to manage overwhelming feelings in more positive ways. Additionally, the law is quite restrictive about the circumstances under which you can take the right of self-determination away from people. Even if we did seek involuntary commitment, and managed to get it, the commitment would only last for three days without substantial evidence that suicide was an imminent possibility. At the end of the commitment, responsibility once more was returned to the patient, and from their point of view, the parental figures had let them down once again—no one was strong enough to successfully win against their self-defeat. As such scenarios unrolled, we found ourselves hostage to a traumatic reenactment scenario in which the patient, like their perpetrator before them held us hostage to threats of death.

On the other hand, if we ignored suicidal gestures or threats, then the patient learned that even threats to life could not provide them with the help they needed and therefore the only option left was a more serious suicide attempt. In the inner fragmented world of the patient, the helpless adult was crying out for help in managing the angry and destructive child within. If we made light of these signals or reacted punitively, the adult was left helplessly abandoned and unprotected.

Faced with these dilemmas and the many meanings that can be attributed to a suicidal act, we realized that there could be no single response to suicidality. Every suicidal gesture or threat needed to be heard as an important communication from the nonverbal self of the patient. We had to find ways to give that self a real voice. And in order to do that, we had to figure out what the behavior *meant*. If the suicidal behavior was of recent origin, it often meant that a serious depression had taken hold of the patient and we needed to begin antidepressant medication and keep them protected from self-harm. But acute suicidal behavior could also arise in the context of the recovery of traumatic memories that the patient found so unacceptable or repulsive that the accompanying affect was just too much to bear. Still other patients became acutely suicidal when paralyzing feelings of guilt over a remembered act of commission or omission, emerged into consciousness. In such cases we responded with a brief but concentrated form of psychiatric intensive care that had different objectives depending on the patient. Some patients in such a state needed a rest. They needed us to restrict their activities and keep them away from interventions that would escalate their despair until the suicidal feelings came under their control once again. Other patients needed to immerse themselves further in the therapeutic work, often through an increased involvement in art therapy, psychodrama, movement therapy, or videotherapy so that they could more quickly put the overwhelming feelings into narrative form and complete the story.

But understanding was not sufficient. We also had to provide a strong and positive moral position about the value of life. We came to the conclusion that "no therapy is or can be effective unless the individual renounces self-imposed death as an alternative to life" (Foderaro 1996). To take such an unbending position, we had to be convinced that recovery from trauma was possible, but that it also was a choice, and that each individual has a right to make that choice. The corollary of that was that we had choices too. We were concerned with every individual patient, but we also had a responsibility to ourselves and to the community.

On occasion, a patient steadfastly refused to make a commitment to life and to relinquish suicidal behavior. Instead, they demanded increased time and attention from the staff and from other patients for their suicidal threats and acts. It became clear that such behavior was a powerful defense against making any progress in treatment and that as long as we played along with this, we were being victimized by the patient's acts as was the entire community, since resources had to be taken away from everyone else. At this point, we changed our role and saw ourselves as having a responsibility for protecting ourselves and the entire community from acts of further perpetration. Just as the patient had choices to make, so did we and we could choose not to continue working with them. Such chronic behavior became grounds for discharge or transfer to a more restrictive level of care. Frequently patients tested us to see if we really meant it and when they found themselves promptly transferred to another hospital, to another more secure unit, or simply sent home, they rapidly caught on to the fact that we meant what we said. Not only was this a forceful and direct message to the rest of the unit, but when the patient was ready to return, they returned on a very different basis and became much more amenable to treatment. This was a powerful intervention for the recalcitrant patient and for the entire community. In saying "no" to acts of continued perpetration and exploitation—even the exploitation that comes from assumed weakness and sickness—we were modeling behavior that our victims had never seen—someone standing up to a perpetrator and protecting those who are more vulnerable.

Managing Traumatic Reenactment

The concept of traumatic reenactment provided a powerful tool in understanding individual and group interactions on the unit and provided a relatively nonjudgmental way of understanding negative and obstructionistic behavior. Since we repeat our past behavior automatically and unconsciously, we knew that everyone who entered the unit would be subject to this principle. If their past had been characterized by caring and rational interactions, then that is what they would replicate. But if their past had been traumatic, then the trauma would be repeated. We cannot help it. We are bound to tell the story of our unresolved past through our behavior in current relationships.

As we became more skilled at recognizing these unfolding dramas, we were able to anticipate and predict what our patients would do, based on their previous relational experiences. We were able to assure them that this was a normal and expected part of treatment. If they had learned as children to cope with abuse by being obedient and compliant, then they would behave this way toward us and the more hurt and disregarded they felt, the more compliant they would be. If they had learned as children that they could decrease the amount of pain they experienced by resisting authority, then we could count on them to start fights and to strongly resist and misinterpret our efforts to help. If they had learned as children that there was nothing they could do except "disappear," then they would dissociate under circumstances of even minimal stress. We could count on almost every patient to misinterpret our behavior and to be fearful of confronting us with any inconsistencies or perceived unfairness in a direct way. Instead, we knew that interpersonal problems would be largely expressed through problem behavior, not through adult problem solving skills.

Essentially, we knew that every patient represented a split self—a functioning, reasonable adult, and a hurt and angry child. Increasing psychiatric dysfunction occurred as that child gradually came to dominate the thoughts, feeling, and actions of the adult. Our job was to promote integration between the two. We had to help the adult become a better parent for his or her own child-self, instead of trying to parent the child-self ourselves. This is the point at which many therapists get into serious trouble with these patients. The damaged child within the adult becomes easily visible as the relationship between therapist and patient grows. The therapist responds as any responsible adult would in the face of a needy child, and tries to parent.

This is doomed to failure. Throughout our entire lives, we each must contend with our own inner wishes for someone to take care of us, to make life easier, to protect us from harm. Some people experience this wish overtly, and consciously know that they have dependency needs. Other people find this unacceptable and defend against these needs by denying them and insisting that they do not need anyone, while encouraging other people's dependence on them. But the reality is, we all begin as children, and we never leave that feeling of childhood helplessness totally behind. The better the parenting has been for us as children, the more capable we feel of taking care of ourselves, even under conditions of stress, as adults. Likewise, the worse the parenting has been, the more inept we are at taking care of ourselves, at taking care of our own children, and the more we long for someone who can rescue us, make it all better, undo the past, and allow us to start over again.

For people who have had truly terrible parenting, this struggle is constant. They alternate between desperately wanting someone to make it all better, and fiercely disallowing help or comfort from anyone. Their struggles look bizarre and nonsensical only as long as we fail to understand the circumstances of their early childhood development. By the time these adults reached us as psychiatric patients, their habits of interrelating to others and to themselves had become extraordinarily fixed and resistant to change. Their whole lives and definitions of reality had become structured around traumatic reenactment, and they did not even know it. Once we learned about their past, we could reliably predict how they would behave, how they would relate to us and to each other, what they would do in the typical situations of life experience.

Once we were able to understand and even predict their behavior, then our job became much more difficult. It demanded something different from us. This social predictability is not limited to psychiatric patients. In our given roles, we are all that predictable. It does not take long before we can predict with some degree of certainly just how the other person is going to react, what they are going to say and do, in any significant relationship. This is part of why relationships are simultaneously so comforting and so easily boring. People are largely predictable if you know enough about their past.

Our reactions to our patients prior to understanding traumatic reenactment were predictable too, given our role as caretakers, experts, and authority figures. If they were hostile to us, we would do something hostile back while pretending that we were not being hostile, because after all, they were "sick." If a patient threatened self-harm, we would respond by taking charge, use our authority to restrict his or her movement and freedom, without holding the patient responsible because he or she was "mentally ill." Boundary violations would be inconsistently addressed because, after all, what could you expect from "disturbed" people? Violence could be explained, and therefore tolerated, by their "inability to control impulses." Anything that we could not understand was attributable to their "craziness" not our ignorance.

Traumatic reenactment meant that our patients' disturbed behavior needed to be interpreted as a replay of past damaging events that could communicate information that we needed to know, if we could just interpret it correctly. Even more important than our interpretation was our response. We had to attempt the difficult if not impossible task of changing our own habits of interacting with patients. As far back as 1927, Trigant Burrow had observed, "In its individualistic application, the attitude of the psychoanalyst and the attitude of the authoritarian are inseparable" (Burrow 1927). We discovered the same phenomenon in our psychotherapeutic environment. The temptation to use and abuse our authority in the face of aggravating behavior was enormous. It is small wonder that psychiatric treatment has been riddled with accusations of abuse and with the overuse of seclusion, restraints, and overmedication. It is exceedingly difficult to be faced with an abusive, yelling, screaming, demanding, hostile, accusatory, threatening, stubborn, or resistant patient without acting in kind, particularly when you have the power to stop the behavior immediately even if it means using punitive measures. It requires restraint, patience, calm in the face of stress to think before you act and to carefully plan constructive rather than authoritarian and potentially destructive responses.

And yet, changing the response is essential. Patients who have been traumatized in childhood have experienced abusive authority. They expect it,
they demand it, they create situations in which it will emerge. Such
responses establish set responses on their part that demand no change in
their behavior and therefore no increased anxiety, and no confrontation
with the past. The abuse of authority simply serves to prove their position
that trusting other people is hopeless, the situation is hopeless, and they are
hopeless. So everything stays exactly the same. But to bring about change,
we were required to change our responses, to lay aside the brute power of
our authority, and try other methods instead.

We found a dramatic metaphor most helpful in this regard. We saw that
as soon as patients entered our system, they would start to construct certain
life scenes, using us and the other patients as players in their personal
drama. They would cue us for specific responses in their set piece. If we
responded on cue, the tale would unfold as it had always unfolded for them,
and the action would culminate in another tale of abuse and failure, as
interpreted by the main protagonist, the patient. We would feel as if we had
been players too, manipulated against our conscious wishes, to become
abusers, neglecters, or powerless bystanders. The patients would cue other
patients as well, so that the victim-perpetrator scene would be reenacted for
the entire community. We had to learn how to be stupid about our cues. We
had to learn how to identify that we were being cued and then not respond,
in order to redirect the entire action of the scene. And we had to make the
entire scene conscious to the protagonists. This cueing was largely nonverbal. It came through gesture, tone of voice, a look, a behavior, all of which
conveyed volumes of information to the onlooker and yet which were
totally outside of the conscious, verbal awareness of the protagonist.

When such a dramatic crisis occurred, we first had to do whatever was
necessary to restore safety and order to the community. Only very rarely did
this require us to use brute force. Acts of violence are usually the culmination of an escalating level of conflict, and as we learned to recognize growing conflict before it reached the point of violence we were able to defuse
most crises before they reached that point. We each learned how to mediate
these situations individually by demonstrating verbally and nonverbally
that we understood that this escalation indicated that the patient did not
feel that he or she was heard, and that we were willing to listen. Usually this
was effective in bringing about a change in the dramatic scene.

For more difficult problems, we would "stop the action" by using a mechanism we called "staffings." After discussing the situation among ourselves,
all of the team members involved in treating the patient would gather

together with the patient and review the critical incident. We would tell the patient how we felt we were being cued to respond. Then we would ask if this kind of thing had ever happened to him or her before. Inevitably, the patient's verbal self would have begun to catch on and would see that indeed, this had happened to them frequently, even in every interpersonal interaction they had been involved in throughout their lifetime. Then we would ask the critical question, "Do you want to change the outcome?" Sometimes they were too overwhelmed to do anything and we would tell them to think about it and return to us later. More typically, they would agree that they very much wanted the outcome to change and then together we would work on creating a plan of approach that would help them to change these automatic reactions. Once this pattern of behavior had been examined and articulated, it no longer could be automatic. Instead of being some autonomous, stubborn character trait, it became a dramatic behavior that could be changed. No big deal, just another bad habit to be broken.

Not everyone was ready for this. We learned that "readiness" is important. These syndromes are not really "sickness" if we define sickness as being beyond the person's control. As in suicidal and self-mutilative behavior, we *can* alter destructive behavior, but not until we choose to do so. It is the choosing that is so difficult. This requires an existential leap of faith, a trust that if they give up the familiar habits of a lifetime and try something new, that someone will be there for them, someone will hold a social safety net, a ring of security strong enough to safely contain their fear, pain, anguish, grief, and rage. Patients must be convinced that in choosing to do something differently, their survival will not be threatened. Since all the bad habits are based on coping skills that they initially developed in the service of survival, their minds associated giving up the bad habit with a terrible sense of danger. This sense of danger can only be overcome by helping people use their reasoning skills, and reasoning skills work only when we are not overly stressed. Therefore, before they can be expected to give up coping skills that they perceive have kept them safe, they must learn other ways to manage stress. Each of us can manage a certain degree of stress by developing better individual coping skills such as exercise, meditation, writing, and other creative outlets, but when stress is severe, we need other people to help us modulate our overwhelming feelings. As a result, a great deal of work goes into helping people get ready to change.

Many patients would enter our unit, test out our system, and decide that they were not ready to change yet. We would tell them exactly what we thought was going on, give them some instructions as to what they had to do in order to "get ready," and invite them to return if they were ready to make a commitment to change. We would tell them very clearly that they could get better, but that to do that, they would have to be willing to stop hurting themselves or other people, they would have to be willing to learn to tolerate pain and fear without hurting themselves, they would have to be honest with themselves about their past, and they would have to trust that we did not want to hurt them but that we were not perfect, would probably repeatedly let them down, and that they would have to learn how to tolerate that as well. In exchange, we would do our best to be honest with them, to be reliable and predictable, to deal with conflicts openly and fairly, and to not repeat their past with them. Many patients who were initially totally resistant to our interventions, returned later, lowered the barriers, and worked intensively until they had changed.

We also learned that an entire community can become involved in reenactment behavior that then had to be confronted as a group problem, not as an individual problem. Sometimes the entire patient community would unconsciously collude together to avoid dealing with the pain of individual therapeutic work by focusing on irritating externals such as the behavior of a staff member, or the food, or inadequate hot water supplies. At other times they would similarly collude to avoid progress by scapegoating another patient who also was avoiding change by his or her willingness to be a scapegoat. Similarly, we discovered that as a staff community, we often behaved in the same way (Bloom 1997).

But change is difficult for even the brightest and most willing of us. Doing things differently is disturbing at a very fundamental level. We base our sense of what is real in the world on habit, and changing these habits—even when they are bad for us—disturbs this sense of what is real, concrete, and predictable. At the same time, we are the most curious of all creatures, and we thrive on change. As a consequence, we are always caught in this conflict between needing predictability and needing stimulation. But the more traumatized you have been, the more likely you are to avoid change, because you learned as a child that as long as danger was predictable you could survive, but anything unpredictable could mean death. This is one of the saddest aspects of childhood trauma—how much it robs the child of spontaneity, playfulness, and the ability to change. We were happy if our patients could have even one experience of safely changing, of altering their reality without suffering dire consequences. We were hopeful that doing it once could lead to doing it twice, and then three times, and then more. More times than not, this hope was borne out. But such progress was usually a three-steps-ahead-two-steps-backward pattern. You can teach an old dog new tricks—but it takes more time.

Anger Work

People who have been the victims of violence frequently lose the capacity to self-protect or to protect others from harm. One of the focal reasons for this deficit is their difficulty in managing anger. Our normal capacity for anger is aroused when someone has crossed a boundary that we find unacceptable. When this occurs, we give off clear messages that such an incursion is not permitted, much like an animal growls when another of its kind gets too close to its territory or its body space. But interpersonal violence is a breach of boundaries and frequently associated with rage on the part of the perpetrator. This rage is particularly intimidating to children who are physically helpless and much smaller than the angry adult. Often when children try to protect themselves with their own anger, the perpetrator responds with an escalation of rage and abuse. Children in these situations learn two lessons, often simultaneously: 1) If someone has power over you, do not ever show anger since it may make the situation worse; 2) If you have power over someone else and are angry, do not worry about controlling it.

The consequence of this early training is that people who have been exposed to unmodulated rage as children have difficulty throughout their lives managing anger in a normal way. They are either too passive and unable to mobilize their anger to protect themselves and others who depend upon them, or they are too aggressive, fly into rages, and are unable to exert self-control. Others alternate between these two styles. This helps to explain how the woman who is so mildly compliant and passive at work can become a terrifying and abusive mother with her children, and how Mr. Milquetoast meekly follows his boss's orders and then comes home and beats his wife. The inability to manage anger is a serious detriment to interpersonal relationships. Many victims of childhood abuse are terrified of their own anger and will do anything not to express anger. Having seen the distorted mask of rage on the face of their perpetrator, they fear becoming like that, as if an angry demon resides inside of them that they must always control.

We discovered that it was extremely important for us to teach our patients how to modulate their own anger more appropriately. They had to learn to tolerate other people's normal expression of anger while protecting themselves from abuse. Anger is one of the most obviously physical of all the emotional states. When we are angry, it is as if our bodies demand some kind of release of the tension. People who have been exposed to abuse are often extremely constricted emotionally because of their fear of this physical feeling. Such emotional constriction can result in a variety of stress-related physical symptoms. We learned that our patients benefited when they were encouraged to go into a special room we had outfitted, accompanied by a staff member. In the room, the walls were covered with carpet, and there were bataka bats and a punching bag, a mattress and pillows. There they could safely discover that they could experience anger, and could physically demonstrate it and manage it in a way that did no harm to anyone including themselves. Then they would be urged to put it into words, to give voice to those angry feelings so that the important information that anger supplies us with would not be lost.

The goal was not one of simple release. Emotions are not toxic substances that can be purged. Our goal was always to teach people how to better manage their normal human emotions. It was never the emotions themselves, but emotional suppression or over-expression that caused problems. People who are overly constricted need to express their overwhelming emotions because they are so afraid of them. They need to discover in a concrete and tangible way that these are simply normal feelings that come—and that go—as long as you don't hold on to them.

Learning to manage rage attacks is more difficult. We found that the best way to understand these kind of experiences was as adult temper tantrums. Roaring in rage can be a heady experience for an adult, carrying with it a satisfying sense of power and control when other people become intimidated. When we reframed this behavior as childish tantrums it was harder for people to maintain the covert sense of pride and power they often feel in being able to scare other people. Videotaping someone in the midst of an angry explosion can provide important feedback as well. Few people like the way they look when they are "throwing a fit." Ultimately, overly angry people needed to learn how to talk before losing control. Tantrums are often characterized by the active and determined suppression of normal anger until one final straw pushes the person over into a loss of control. By tracing back this kind of a progression we could often help the person learn how to express the anger so that it didn't turn into a tantrum.

The Body

It became apparent to us that trauma does indeed do terrible things to the body's physiology. Many of our patients had developed various kinds of medical disorders that complicated the treatment of their psychiatric problems. Chronic pain was a problem, and we had to struggle with differentiating between pain associated with structural or functional physical problems and the pain associated with "body memories." These somatic memory experiences were easily mistaken for signs of physical disorder and misdiagnosis in this population is very common. When a body memory occurs, the victim actually experiences pain, so his or her distress is quite real. It was difficult even for us to resist the urge to consult a gynecologist for every bout of stabbing pelvic pain, or a neurologist for the severe and persistent headaches that often accompany memory recall.

On the other hand, we had to be careful not to falsely attribute physical complaints to body memories and thereby miss an acute problem. We had to frequently remind our medical consultants that our patients were no less susceptible to "real" physical illness than any other patients. Many patients who extensively utilize dissociation, automatically do so whenever they experience pain. This can be dangerous since pain is an innate self-protective mechanism that warns us when something is wrong in the body. As a result, patients with dissociative disorder can have physical problems that need medical attention but get neglected because they are able to ignore the pain and discomfort. Patients who have been sexually abused will often refuse to seek gynecological help until they have an acute, and sometimes, life-threatening physical problem. Patients who have been traumatized by early childhood medical or surgical procedures may avoid seeking medical help that they vitally need.

Many patients had become physically and/or psychologically addicted to various pain or antianxiety medications, and we had to confront the addiction and the way they used medication to prevent themselves from feeling, not just physical pain, but any disturbing emotion. Giving a drug to someone who has psychological pain that can only be relieved by psychological and behavioral change is bad treatment. But likewise, withholding a needed medication from someone in serious physical pain can be abusive. That judgment call is tricky and each person's problem needed to be carefully evaluated individually and longitudinally.

Many of the patients needed antidepressant medication and antianxiety medication in order to do the necessary work that we were encouraging. Antidepressants were often extremely helpful and the newer medications had relatively few side effects. The antianxiety drugs could provide relief for the severe distress of anxiety but many people developed tolerance to these drugs and needed more and more drug to achieve the same effect. There can be a fine line between necessary use and abuse of the antianxiety drugs, so each case needed careful and regular evaluation.

Over time we came to learn that dysregulation in childhood appears to create physiological dysfunctions in the body that can persist in adulthood and be very resistant to change. Many patients recovered from their traumatic experiences, returned to a high level of function or achieved such a level for the first time, placed the traumatic experience into a narrative form, were able to put the memories in the past where they belonged, established healthier and lasting interpersonal relationships, but remained vulnerable to the physiologically disorganizing effects of stress. One of the most important lessons we learned from this work is how important it is for us to stop child abuse in childhood rather than try to fix what is already broken in adults. Adults certainly can recover and live full and satisfying lives, but they often must unfairly contend with the continuing physiological disturbance that early trauma leaves in its wake and that so far, modern medicine has been only partially able to relieve.

Changing Fixed Beliefs

Achieving physical, psychological, social, and moral safety in any community is a difficult and demanding task. Our belief system was not wholeheartedly embraced by our patients. To do so meant that they needed to change many of their fundamental assumptions about themselves, other people, and the world around them. These assumptions had guaranteed predictability in a hostile environment and provided a way, albeit a recurrently damaging way, of structuring relationships and reality. In pointing out to our patients that they were not so much sick as injured, we wrestled with the issue of blame. The idea of sickness places the origin of the problem within the defective patient, whereas an injury model connects the suffering of the patient to external events often deliberately perpetrated against them by another responsible human being.

A current notion says that psychiatric patients are always looking for someone to blame for their problems and that when they find someone, they experience immediate relief of their symptoms whether or not the alleged scapegoat has really done something to them. This notion is completely inconsistent with my experience of thirty years. Depressed and anxious psychiatric patients blame themselves, not other people, for their problems. Patients labeled as "borderlines" will often blame other people for their distress but just behind this blaming is a profound sense of worthlessness, a boundless hatred of the self, which they believe is the real reason for others' rejection. As a result, the more they blame others, the worse they feel about themselves and the greater the symptoms

According to various studies that have been done, blaming others often makes people feel worse, not better (Tedeschi and Calhoun 1995). Blaming others can increase the sense of helplessness that already accompanies the traumatic experience and result in an increase in psychological distress. Psychiatric patients *strongly* resist any interpretation for their distress other than their own failure. In the immediate present, they may blame staff for not satisfying their needs quickly enough, or their spouse for not responding to their wishes, or their children for getting into trouble, but push beyond this and the reason for all this rejection is that they are basically unlovable. And who initially found them unlovable? Their primary caretakers, their mother or father, grandmother or grandfather, uncle, stepmother, stepfather, or sibling who abused them, allowed them to be abused, or failed to protect them from the abuse of others. Without a great deal of therapeutic work, patients never cite the failure and responsibility of the caretaking adult; they were abused because they were bad and because they deserved abuse.

And why do they cling so strongly to this belief system? Why do we need to spend so much time understanding and interpreting the resistance to understanding childhood abuse? Why are so many memories of abuse dissociated, rejected, and denied? Because maintaining attachment relationships is more important to human survival then anything else. Human beings will sacrifice their own lives to protect the people to whom they have a primary attachment. Children, even abused children, have a primary attachment to their caretakers and we know that abuse—because it is a dangerous situation—enhances attachment. These primary attachment relationships and the powerful emotional connections that maintain them do not just evaporate because a person reaches legal age.

A primary caretaker can be long dead and in the grave, but this does not terminate the relationship or the strong emotional charge attached to it. People resist blaming their primary caretakers mightily. In fact, they will do anything, including commit suicide, to protect and defend the sanctity of those relationships. As long as they can convince themselves that the fault was theirs, that if they had done or been something else, better and more obedient children, or less pretty, or fatter, or whatever, then the abuse would not have occurred, then they do not have to deal with their own helplessness as children, and they do not have to deal with the inexplicable hatred and evil that was manifested toward them at the hands of people they loved. Human beings will do *anything* to keep from knowing all this. Anything.

RECONSTRUCTION: THE STORY EMERGES

Remembrance

Dr. Herman called the second stage of treatment "Reconstruction" (1992). In this stage, the victim of trauma reconstructs the trauma as a narrative story that can become part of the individual's biographical history instead of haunting the present. Accompanying this narrative is the inevitable sense of grief that accompanies coming to terms with an overwhelming traumatic loss. Survivors work very hard to avoid touching this deeply sensed grief, and the resistance to healing can be understood only by recognizing and respecting the magnitude of this psychic pain. For the therapist and the patient, this is often the most emotionally demanding stage of treatment and is key in understanding the process of recovery and the importance of creating a sanctuary environment.

Once patients had some degree of control over their addictive and self-destructive behavior and felt safe with themselves and with us, the traumatic memories began to emerge. Flashbacks and nightmares often appeared, increased in frequency and intensity, as patients began to review the most painful parts of the past without the "anesthesia" that the self-destructive behaviors had provided. At this point, they often appeared worse than when they first came into the hospital. Their anxiety changed from free-floating states of discomfort interrupted by episodes of acute panic unattached to any meaning, to consolidated states of terror that became attached to an actual memory from the past. As the patients struggled to tolerate the intense and disorganizing emotions, dissociative episodes frequently increased. We were able to see people's defenses in action as the extraordinary mechanism of dissociation protected them from knowing too much, too fast. They went in and out of trance states as the level of fear and despair waxed and then waned. Throughout these episodes, we worked at keeping them "grounded," helping them to come out of trance and stay in reality with us, as much as possible. Gradually they gained some control over their own dissociative processes as they learned what triggered the altered states, what internal stimuli signaled that they were beginning to dissociate, and finally how to prevent themselves from spontaneously dissociating. In order for people to stop dissociating they must learn to tolerate formerly unbearable feelings and this learning requires a high level of social support. One patient compared it to jumping off a burning building—possible only if there is a circle of people below firmly holding a very large net.

As we allowed this process to unfold, we realized many things about our own mistakes in the past. Because we previously had no way of understanding this process of reconstruction, we had usually interrupted the process prematurely. In retrospect we could see that patients often had entered these states but we had misinterpreted what was happening. We had become frightened by what we perceived as a deterioration in their status, assumed that they were experiencing psychotic symptoms, and had usually responded by administering tranquilizing drugs in our misguided attempts to stop the symptoms that were so distressing. Certainly, the symptoms were distressing to our patients and many times they welcomed the promised relief of medication. But the symptoms were just as distressing to us. The contagion that accompanies the expression of such raw pain, is difficult to bear, even as a witness. As the disconnected emotions and memories pressed for recognition, the medication was increased until the patient became a walking zombie. Complicating the clinical picture had been the fact that the patients frequently reported hearing voices which historically have been considered a sign of psychosis. Only now do we recognize that many patients with dissociative symptoms report hearing voices as well. All too often, these patients were labeled as chronically mentally ill, given high doses of medication, and hospitalized frequently for episodes of what were perceived to be acute psychotic episodes. They often posed the most difficult management problems for us because aside from their apparent psychoses, they also self-mutilated, acted out violently and were resistant to most forms of intervention. The picture was often so confusing that we would end up calling them "hysterical psychotics" or "pseudoschizophrenics" and then later "borderlines" to indicate the overlap in symptom patterns.

Treatment progress altered dramatically when we changed from responding to the symptoms as a sign of increased illness, to containing the symptoms as our part in helping a patient through a difficult stage of recovery. Now the psychoeducational material that we had been providing for our patients since admission took on new meaning. They were experiencing exactly what we had been preparing them for in the lectures and groups. Many of them already had years of experience with flashbacks, nightmares, and hyperarousal, but previously these symptoms had been associated with the overwhelming terror of feeling as if they were losing their minds. The theory they had learned provided them with a bulwark against that dimension of the fear, and a reason to hope that learning to tolerate the distress could lead to relief. We reframed the increase in symptoms as progress, the natural outcome of coming to terms with a past reality. We explained that although the trauma had occurred years before, it had been experienced only by a part of them, by a nonverbal self that was arrested in time, trapped in the past. This nonverbal self had allowed them to grow up without as much interference as would have occurred without this protection, but the price they paid was self-fragmentation. If they were to heal, the verbal self had to experience—for the first time—the traumatic event with the accompanying overwhelming emotions. Only then could the patient put the event into a narrative form so that the traumatic experience could become a true memory, safely stored in the past, no longer able to nonverbally direct and control behavior.

We stayed calm in the face of inevitable emotional storms. Lacking the descriptive powers of a novelist or dramatist, it is difficult to convey the enormity of this process. Many of the people we treated were high functioning and successful adults who were accustomed to being in charge of their minds and their emotional states. Under the pressures of reconstructive work, they found themselves immersed in the raw emotional states of childhood, unable to think clearly, perceiving physical sensations that were exceedingly vivid and yet unrelated to any event transpiring in the present. The events that they were feeling, seeing, smelling, hearing, and sensing evoked a wide range of noxious emotions including overwhelming shame. They needed people in their environment to simultaneously validate their adult sense of self while making allowances for the dependency, vulnerability, and neediness that their childlike self temporarily required. We had to help them keep themselves safe, to tell them when to rest, to encourage them to go further, to reassure them that the terror would pass, to respect their need for privacy so they could manage the shame and to help them rejoin the community for the same reason. To accomplish all this, we needed structures that would allow the nonverbal self to get the attention it needed and deserved without so dominating the entire community that other people's treatment would be jeopardized or that the individual would be exhausted, humiliated, or further traumatized.

We encouraged patients to take a number of different routes, all designed to give the nonverbal self an opportunity to "tell the complete story." In art therapy and specific trauma art groups, patients had the opportunity to "draw the story." Often, they consciously denied that they had anything to draw, that they knew anything about what had happened to them, while their hands were busily drawing out detailed pictures about critical and obviously traumatic events. In movement therapy they were urged to move body parts that were frozen, to make gestures and total body movements that were rigidified and in doing so, they experienced the movement as messages from their nonverbal, body self. In psychodrama, they asked to be the protagonist of a part of their personal drama and to recruit other members of the community to play critical roles as well. In dramatically recreating their story they were able to actually see and experience the gaps in their story, their unexpressed feelings, the internal contradictions and conflicts, all in a concrete and tangible way. They could see directly how other people reacted to specific and now conscious cues that they were giving. We encouraged them to write and write and write.[3] They could keep their writing private or they could share it with their therapists, but they had to read it themselves. Interestingly, the most resistance often arose about reading their own material and if they did not read it, the writing was not as effective (Vogel 1994). Writing may serve as a basic brain integrating mechanism, but this may only be effective through the process of reading what one has written. Otherwise, writing can just become another redundant, repetitive, and relatively useless activity.

The use of video dialogue as developed by Dr. Lyndra Bills and Dr. Louis Tinnin, was quite helpful as well. Patients told their story on camera and then engaged in a dialogue with themselves by switching tapes and taping themselves responding to the first tape. Different personalities, parts, or aspects of the self could be made more concrete through this technique. It was also something people could do as a self-help tool to promote integration of dissociated aspects of the self (Tinnin and Bills 1994). We provided daily individual sessions so that people could have a designated time, place, and person with whom they could work on specific memories, feelings, or issues. We provided them with contact people from the nursing staff so they would have other people to consult in-between the formal groups and individual sessions. We encouraged self-help through reading, writing, drawing, and videotaping outside of the group sessions. We encouraged people in the community to help each other by listening, talking, sharing, and by setting limits on each other's demands.

We discouraged uncontrolled or exhibitionistic reexperiencing, viewing this as just another way of hurting oneself. If a person was still engaging in self-destructive behavior we discouraged any form of memory work, insisting that they had to prove to themselves that they were physically safe in the present before they could safely confront the past. If self-harmful behavior restarted after reconstructive work began, we urged the patients to slow down, to use their own difficulties in managing self-destructive impulses as a signal that they were moving too fast, pushing themselves too hard. If people with dissociative identity disorder wanted to get to know their alter personalities, they were encouraged to do so within the confines of a safe and scheduled session with staff, rather than allowing themselves to be vulnerable and exposed outside of a safe setting. By modulating where and when they could be overtly symptomatic, people learned that they could gain control over behaviors that they thought were uncontrollable.

We did not have to interpret these memories for the patients, nor did we have to use hypnosis or drugs. We simply told them that they would remember what they needed to remember in order to heal when they were ready to let themselves know. But we made it clear that this reconstructive work could not take place effectively until they had made themselves safe, until they had taken enough control over life-threatening impulses so that their lives were no longer at risk.

As with any medical illness, diagnosis is made based on signs and symptoms. Based on our patient's signs and symptoms, we suspected that certain events had transpired. For instance, sexual problems often indicated a past history of sexual abuse. But we believed that it was important for our patients to find their own past, uncomplicated by our vision of their history. Most of the times, the patients' memories confirmed what we had suspected all along. But sometimes we were surprised by a different perpetrator or by a different trauma. And sometimes the trauma had nothing to do with interpersonal violence. One patient with multiple personality disorder, who had also been a victim of child pornography and sexual abuse by professionals, appeared to have had her first personality split at age three as a result of serious childhood surgery when her mother was not permitted to stay with her. The mother of another patient had been hospitalized for a prolonged period when the child was less than two years of age. Another patient had witnessed the slow death by cancer of his father. Childhood trauma cannot be defined by adult standards. Any disruption in or threat to attachment relationships can be a traumatic experience for a child.

As their minds struggled to make sense of what had happened to them, often at the hands of people they had depended upon, our patients would alternate between acceptance and denial of their memories. We noticed that the closer the relationship had been with their perpetrator, the harder the material was for them to accept. In the process of recall, a stranger's face would be substituted for a father's, or an aunt's face for a mother's. But they could not rest until they had gotten each memory sorted out in their own minds. Frequently, they would go in and out of dissociative states as the material became too threatening, too much to bear. From the outside the process appeared to be like someone struggling with various pieces of a jigsaw puzzle, moving the pieces around until they made some sense in time and space. Throughout this period we provided steady encouragement and support. An escalation of self-mutilation or other self-destructive behavior often signaled the emergence of new memories that the patient was refusing to admit into consciousness. Such an escalation usually signaled that the patient was struggling not to identify a perpetrator as someone to whom he or she was attached. Improvement in symptoms only occurred when the worst had been told. At some point, all the emotional abreaction stopped, the patients calmed down, began to sob, and could coherently narrate the story of what had happened to them.

Criticism has been leveled at therapists about their credulity in believing these stories—at least the stories about sexual abuse. Research indicates that memories of trauma appear to be "engraved" in the mind. Drs. Bruce Perry and Jennifer Pate who study children with post-traumatic stress disorder have made the point that "[c]hildren and adults who have been traumatized have affective or emotional memories indelibly implanted into their brain stem and midbrain" (Perry and Pate 1994). But as soon as the traumatic memories are taken out of the nonverbal realm and given words, they may be as subject to distortion as any other memories. We were in no position to affirm or deny the specific details of recall. It was not our job to seek external validation for these stories, although many of them had already been validated by some other witness, family member, or previous legal proceedings. When confronted with a tormented and fractured human being, we looked at the whole pattern of their lives—their symptoms, their previous history, their level of function, their relationships, their social network, their weaknesses, and their strengths—and then correlated those patterns with our own personal, professional, and community experiences. With sufficient experience in looking at the whole system that comprises a person, an experienced clinician develops a sense for stories that make sense and stories that do not fit together or are incomplete. For us it was enough that the symptoms were abating and their life was no longer in immediate danger. This improvement did not take place until the patient appeared to have their memories in order, until the stories made sense in the larger context of their lives. Only then were they able to rest. There was some relief at having uncovered a mystery, a darkly held secret, and finally discovering a personal truth. But this relief gave way to the profound grief that accompanied the recognition that someone else had stolen off with a childhood that could never be restored.

Grieving

There is much to grieve for when you have suffered abuse as a child. Humankind has always sought comfort in the myth of a golden age, when all was right with the world. So too do individual humans need a sense that there was a time when all was well, when they were loved, cherished, and protected, a time of safety and predictability that could come again; a time of innocence when all was right with the world. This feeling is the steady building block upon which we stand for the rest of our lives and to which we return for the means of self-comfort. It is upon this corner stone that we build our sense of self-esteem, confidence, and sense of mastery in the world. Children who are abused or neglected are deprived of this very basic foundation. Part of the reason why we resist remembering the reality of many of our childhood experiences is that we do not want to remember what it was really like, how helpless and lonely we often were. The worse the abuse or deprivation, the more powerful the defense against remembering and feeling the weight of this sadness.

The loss of anything resembling a happy childhood would be sufficient to explain the grief of reconstruction, but frequently survivors must face many other private griefs. Loss of a sense of peace and tranquillity, loss of specific kinds of physical functioning, loss of opportunities to be or do what you really wanted, loss of a belief that the world makes sense or that your life makes sense, loss of important life events because of amnesia or addictions, loss of the time, money, relationships, experience that the symptoms demanded—the list could go on and on. What is inevitable is that every victim of trauma must face this grief before he or she can move on, and most of us will do anything we can to avoid the pain of mourning.

Part of what makes the mourning experience so difficult is that the survivor is so utterly alone. When someone dies, socially approved and supported rituals give definition and structure to the expected period of grief. We know quite concretely the dimensions of the loss that we experience. We often share that loss with other family members or friends. For survivors, their grief cannot be easily shared. The losses have often occurred decades before, are denied by important family members, are misunderstood by friends. There are no socially approved and supported rituals. There also is usually no sense of justice restored. In most cases, the perpetrator "got away with it." The lack of repentance, remorse, atonement, or restitution on the part of the perpetrator can arrest the process of mourning in an endless quest for vengeance or for justice. This is why it can be of so much benefit to have the support of other survivors through this difficult period. They often do understand in a way no one else can.

The Role of the Family

An important and often neglected part of reconstructing the past is remembering the good times along with the bad. We often would see that patients were unable to remember anything good about their childhoods, anything truly worthy about their parents until they were able to give voice to the bad. Frequently they would first come into treatment idealizing a family of origin that certainly was far from ideal. Their mothers, fathers, siblings were all perfect—they were the sick ones, they were the problem. As they remembered the reality of their experience, their family would become the "family from hell." This seemed to be a painful but necessary corrective to the total self-blame with which they entered treatment. They needed to see that they had been victimized by a sick system, that they had once been helpless and innocent children whose trust had been betrayed. Armed with this insight, they were much better equipped to take responsibility for the destructive actions they had taken as adults, and only then were they able to make changes in the present. And then, as they became able to put their narrative into perspective, the family came into better focus as well.

In many cases they were gradually able to describe their perpetrator not as an evil Satan, but as a wounded, hurt, and angry person who sometimes lost control and sometimes could be loving and funny. This change often indicated a real maturing of perspective as the childhood terror gave way to a more realistic appraisal. Sometimes families are truly sadistic, even psychopathic, but far more often the situation is distinctly more complex. We found that as survivors became more compassionate about their own suffering they were able to begin the process of struggling to understand how their own families had passed on a legacy of pain and trauma. When multigenerational family histories were available, we were usually able to trace the traumatic affect back to some understandable, "socially acceptable" life tragedy such as war, immigration, early death of a parent, concentration camp experience, disease, or disaster, some overwhelming experience that had produced a significant distortion in the intergenerational transmission of healthy attachment relationships.

This is part of the reason why any confrontation with the family of origin should be delayed until late in the therapeutic process, when the survivor is well along in outpatient treatment and the process of recovery. If family members are confronted prematurely, pointless and unnecessary rifts in the family can end up harming the already tenuous attachment relationships that survivors often cling to in the early stages of recovery. We learned to carefully weigh the benefit of confrontation against the risk. During the stage when the patients had managed to mobilize rage against the perpetrators, they often became flushed with a sense of personal power, and pushed for a premature confrontation. We discovered that it was important to try and prevent this from happening. Too often when actually in the situation and confronting the perpetrator, his or her continued denial would puncture their recently achieved sense of empowerment, plunging them into even deeper despair.

Sometimes, confrontation is unavoidable. This is likely to be the case when the confrontation occurs before hospitalization or when some present danger exists in not confronting the situation, for example, where the patient or other children are still being abused. In such a case, patients often needed more support, including sound legal advice, in order to proceed. Current involvement in violent relationships interferes with therapeutic work that is focused on the past. In these circumstances, reconstructive work may have to be delayed until the immediate crisis is past and dealt with adequately.

Family-of-origin work can be extremely helpful if the family is able to provide support and validation of the patient's experience. In many of our cases, family members had long known or suspected the origins of the psychiatric dysfunction. When they were able to talk about it, share experiences, express anger, remorse, guilt, and grief, the benefits for the patients were often enormous. The patients' symptoms would often be relieved, and recovery accelerated much more rapidly than when the families were not positively involved.

We saw that families could move on, even with the perpetrator still connected, if there was honesty and true remorse. Forgiveness could not be unilateral. The patient who had been hurt by a family member could not be expected to forgive the perpetrator until the person admitted to guilt, experienced remorse, and asked for forgiveness. Such a process can take many years, but we frequently underestimated the power of family loyalty and attachment. When a family accomplishes this process they change, mature, become more humble and more human. We saw many sad occasions, however, when this proud sense of loyalty and the profound need for human attachment was perverted in the service of maintaining secrecy and destroying the perceived "squealer." When this happened, the survivor was isolated, targeted for abuse, lied to, and betrayed repeatedly. These cases were often the most potentially lethal and difficult to manage. There are few social stimuli as powerful as the age-old method of shunning. Over time we became impressed by the awesome power of a family united against the betrayal of secrets and the magnitude of the tragedies that ensued.

We never recommended suing family members as a constructive solution to any problems. Too often, the goals and methods of the legal system are contradictory to the goals and methods of recovery. Although some survivors say that they felt they could not rest until they had received some kind of justice, our concern was always that the civil system does not necessarily lead to justice for the survivor. It can and often does, however, perpetuate the abuse. Legal cases drag on for many years, and throughout that time the survivor cannot move on and put the past in the past. In too many instances a legal case is simply another way of staying attached to the abuser and of reenacting the abuse. Again, legal action may be unavoidable if a danger to others remains. If this is the case, the survivor will need a great deal of support and will have to be far enough along in recovery to withstand the rigors of an adversarial system. Too often in such legal confrontations the perpetrator's continued denial can arouse murderous impulses, grave self-doubts and an undermining of important therapeutic work.

During critical stages of recovery involving the family-of-choice is vital. Sometimes patients came to us with an admission complaint of child abuse and only later did we discover that the patient was currently involved in an abusive relationship. It is not possible to recover from past abuse as long as a person is being abused in the present. Our rule of safety required, then, a focus on stopping the abuse in the present. Sometimes children were being abused or were in danger of being abused or neglected which meant we had to call the appropriate agencies and report the abuse. Whenever possible, we urged the patients to report themselves or other perpetrators in the family. We saw this as an essential part of recovery as they simultaneously learned how to self-protect and protect their own children. Other times, it became clear that the patient would have to leave the abusive situations and we needed to help them make a liaison with shelters for battered women and domestic violence agencies. We learned how frightening a step this is. Trauma-bonding means that our patients were dependent upon those abusive relationships, just as they had been dependent on their abusive family members, and getting out of those relationships, left them feeling terribly abandoned. Often they needed a great deal of time and encouragement to establish an adequate support system before they left and after, to help prevent failure.

Other survivors had managed to make relatively healthy relationships. But often, by the time they had deteriorated to the point that hospitalization was required, their family members had become exhausted, frightened, threatened, bewildered, and angry. Living with someone who is psychiatrically disturbed is usually extremely stressful. These families needed as much help understanding what was happening to their loved one as the patients did. As they became educated about trauma we could help direct them toward more helpful forms of interactions with each other. Frequently, opening up the door to talking about childhood trauma provided a way for the other family members to begin talking about their own traumatic experiences and how those experiences had affected their families. If a spouse, child, friend, or any significant other was willing to be involved, learn, and provide support, improvement was quicker and more efficient. Holding family sessions, even for relatively young children, can be enormously reassuring for the kids. We learned that the children had been living with a more-or-less dysfunctional parent for varying lengths of time and had suffered the consequence of this to the dismay of the parents. Teaching children something about what was happening, conveying an understanding of what they and the family had been going through was something we could do in service of prevention. Children inevitably blame themselves, just as our patients had done when they were children, and removing the burden of blame from them can be healing for the children as well as the parents.

Learning to Play

Childhood abuse robs people of their childhood. It also steals off with their capacity to enjoy life. The formal term for this is "anhedonia," the inability to experience pleasure. Many of our patients entered our unit as the most serious people on earth. They even worked at playing. They could not laugh, relax, find even the most simple of enjoyments. Many of them recounted tales of childhood in which play and laughter were greeted with punishment. With such exposure, one learns rapidly that having a good time is not such a good idea. This is most unfortunate because we discovered that one of the best prognostic features was having—and using—a sense of humor.

We had to actively encourage people to give themselves pleasure. Survivors often live Spartan lives, with even their indulgences and addictions affording them little real pleasure. Frequently when we asked people what they enjoyed doing, they would look back and reply "nothing." This is a common finding in depression, but this was even more pervasive a phenomenon than depression and reached back much farther than acute depressive symptoms. So one of our functions clearly was to create an environment within which fun could occur. By definition, you cannot make fun happen, you can't schedule it, or put it in the diet. It is a spontaneous, creative event. All we could do was provide the space, the time, and the permission for fun to happen. We showed movies, we put in a Ping-Pong table, we clowned around ourselves, we played jokes on each other and them, we hung up funny pictures, we supported and encouraged their creativity and playfulness when we saw it. When an environment is not overly constricted, people are often very, very funny, and comical things occur in any community. We showed that we enjoyed ourselves when these things happened and that we took pleasure in their pleasure. Often, there is a very fine line between laughter and tears, but people must have an experience of pleasure if life is to have meaning, if all their grieving and anger and torment in recovery is to have a purpose.

RECONNECTION

As Dr. Herman says, "Having come to terms with the traumatic past, the survivor faces the task of creating a future" (Herman 1992). This is the stage she has called "reconnection." After people have filled in the holes in memory and have grieved for all they have lost, they must create a new life for themselves, a life that is no longer tightly organized around trauma and traumatic reenactment. This movement from a trauma-based existence to health does not occur suddenly and the future groundwork for this work of emancipation is being laid from the moment treatment begins. Here I will focus on ways in which the intensive experience of an inpatient unit lays this groundwork for the reconnection stage of treatment, a process which will continue long after discharge from the unit.

Earlier, I talked about the normative aspects of repeated traumatic experience—how through interpersonal trauma and traumatic reenactment a person's entire life can become organized around trauma so that the individual experiences highly abnormal feelings and views of reality as normal. We discovered that one of our most important and long-lasting functions was re-education. Because we had access to patients for twenty-four hours a day, often for several weeks, we were able to immerse them in an environment in which the basic understanding of human nature, about what had happened to them, and about assumptions and values were radically different from their "normative" paradigm.

The depth of the human need to make sense of the world around us cannot be overestimated. We are a labeling, categorizing, reasoning animal and we must define and redefine our reality and compare our definitions with those of our peers. Our mind drives us to do so and will not let us rest until we have fit what we know into a system of meaning. For victims of childhood trauma, the system of meaning they have been forced to create is highly dysfunctional and undermining to adult, mature decision making and problem solving. But, that is all they have available if their abuse and neglect have been severe and methodical.

We provided patients with a way of comprehending what had happened to them, an integrated framework that incorporated their own personal traumatic experience into a larger medical, psychological, social, and political context. Within this context they began the long and arduous process of making sense out of their personal and collective tragedy. This helped them to mobilize their cognitive and reasoning capacities in service of altering behavior. People who have been traumatized often experience a paralysis of will. The enforced helplessness has left them with a perceived inability to change anything in their lives. When we could reason with them, and demonstrate that this paralysis of will was actually related to past childhood experiences with helplessness, they were often able to mobilize the adult capabilities that resided within most of them in service of helping the helpless child within them to mature.

We provided the educational information, but the social situation created the opportunity for rehearsing change. As patients became conscious of the role they had been playing in their own traumatic reenactment scenarios, they needed other people to interact differently with them. In allowing this to happen, patients experienced the help, support, and encouragement that can safely be derived from connection with others. They found that other people were able to help them manage and contain their emotions and that this could be a far more satisfactory exchange then cutting or burning oneself, for instance. In the interpersonal interactions that were constantly occurring, patients had an opportunity to learn new patterns of attachment, patterns far less abusive than the normative patterns they had learned as children and carried into their adult life. Each time they altered a fixed behavioral sequence, they were able to see where that sequence led, often to a much more gratifying outcome than their usual habits of relating. This rehearsal of new ways of thinking, feeling, acting, and interacting could occur only within a rich social context in which connecting to other people was given a high priority.

This rich social context was the community itself, in its entirety. From the moment they set foot on the unit, the patients entered a socialization process that was directed by both patients and staff. Twice a day the entire patient community would meet together along with as many staff members as could be present. This meeting was designed to provide a focus for the entire group and was an opportunity for people to raise issues to do with community problems rather than specifically individual problems, although there was always a dialectical movement between the personal and the social. Patients who had been on the unit before or who had been there the longest, along with the staff, were the carriers of the culture. They informed new patients about the overt and the covert rules and expectations of the community.

An essential component of the culture was the emphasis on emotional expression and talking. From the time they entered, patients knew that their job was to "tell their story." As each told his or her story, other patients offered feedback, but they also heard themselves. For many patients, these were stories that had never been told, secrets that had been locked up for decades, weighing them down. In the sharing of their stories patients would receive emotional support, acceptance, and validation. But they would also receive reinterpretations and corrections of some of their own fixed assumptions. And they would hear other people's assessment of their behavior at the time of the traumatic experience. Most of our patients were harshly critical of the role they had played in the abuse situation. They tended to make unrealistic appraisals about the degree of control they actually had at the time. The staff and other patients were able to challenge these distortions and tended to be much more compassionate and understanding of them then they ever were of themselves. In this way they began the slow process of reconstructing a different view of the self.

Staff and other patients served as coaches for changes in behavior. When a person manifested an inability to self-protect in some way—which was inevitable—that behavior could be immediately questioned or challenged and suggestions could be offered for alternative behavior. Opportunities constantly arose for Maxwell Jones's "living and learning situations." Confrontation had to be balanced, however, with kindness. Such an approach has been called "carefrontation" and begins with the premise that "people need help, not punishment from other people" (Wheeler and Baron 1994).

Part of the intrinsic difficulty of practicing in this way is the sharp contrast between our way of approaching people and their problems and the approach of many of the institutions to which our patients were bound to return in a short time. Our shared assumptions, goals, and values were notably different from the families, offices, schools, and other systems within which our patients would have to survive once they left the hospital. As Maxwell Jones had warned "The therapeutic culture in a psychiatric hospital may, and probably must, differ to some extent from the culture of the community outside, but to deviate too far is to court disaster" (Jones 1968b). This discrepancy was openly discussed. We made no bones about it—our unit was a sanctuary, a temporary refuge from all they would still have to deal with at home. Our rules were different and were meant to be different. We wanted to give patients a taste of what it could be like, but the burden was still going to be on them to keep the change going. They could only do this by building up support systems at home that were more similar to the quality of the relationships they were learning about in the hospital. Outpatient treatment would be necessary once they left the hospital, but it was not enough. They would need many other ways to reconnect with others and with new kinds of people, not people who were there simply to play roles in their traumatic reenactment.

Our goal, over and over, was to *normalize, normalize, normalize*. A psychiatric label is a heavy burden to carry.[4] And psychiatric labels often become self-fulfilling prophecies. If a patient's social group expects them to "be bad," they will definitely "be bad." If a patient's social group expects them to dissociate, throw hysterical fits, create a hundred personalities, they will do so. All of us are strongly influenced by social expectations and social pressure. We do not create pathological behavior, but any social system can encourage it or discourage it. We wanted people who had become desperately isolated to reconnect, and to do that, they would have to recognize that everything that they had or would experience was a part of human reality, part of the tragic nature of human existence. Their behavioral disorders were understandable and expectable under the conditions of abnormal stress to which they had been exposed. But now they were free to make choices, to rejoin the human race, to be more like other people, to fit in, to benefit from their own abilities, to have fun. It also meant that they had to stop running away, stop acting like hurt children, and start assuming more responsibility for directing their own lives. We endeavored to show in a thousand different ways that there is no dividing line between us and them, between psychiatric disorder and health, between good and bad. All is along a continuum, and we are each capable of making decisions in the present about where we want to be on that continuum, even if we were unable to do so in the past.

But, if they were going to do that, if they were going to normalize and cease living in the past, then they were going to have to give up being a psychiatric patient. They could remain a person with specific vulnerabilities, but they were not a disease. In some way, somehow, they were going to have to transform their post-traumatic pain into a strength instead of a weakness. Dr. Herman has described the need of some survivors to develop a "survivor mission" and says, "These survivors recognize a political or religious dimension in their misfortune and discover that they can transform the meaning of their personal tragedy by making it the basis for social action. While there is no way to compensate for an atrocity, there is a way to transcend it, by making it a gift to others. The trauma is redeemed only when it becomes the source of a survivor mission" (1992).

We believe that this is a vital aspect of recovering from trauma and reconnecting with the living. It is akin to the Alcoholics Anonymous Twelve Step program in which the recovering alcoholic is required to help other addicts. Following the rejection of social psychiatry by the psychiatric professions, bringing social or political issues into the private and individual world of the psychotherapeutic session became unacceptable. With the exception of religious counselors, religion and values were to be kept out as well. We have found this fragmentation impossible to maintain. It is impossible to focus on child abuse, domestic violence, and all forms of interpersonal violence without understanding the social and political context within which such violence is maintained, supported, and encouraged. We try to help our patients see that their traumatic experiences are part of a much larger picture of the traumatic exploitation of human beings around the globe and that what they learn to heal themselves needs to be applied to their families, their friends, and the larger social systems within which we must all live. The purpose of this theoretical and philosophical position, is once again, reconnection. We saw that our patients' inner fragmentation was a mirror reflection of the fragmentation within all of us, and of the fragmentation that is visible in every social system we have created.[5]

We came to understand that an essential part of recovery for our patients, ourselves, and our communities is a reconnection with the political, a willingness to shoulder the responsibilities of citizenship that accompany healthy life in a democracy. Without political action and political change, without dramatic limitations on the capacity of so few to abuse so many, our work is meaningless. Unless we are simultaneously involved in healing *and* prevention, we become parasites, feeding off the remains of what the abusers have left behind. Years ago, the slogan "If you're not part of the solution, you're part of the problem" became popular, and as is the case with so many folk aphorisms, a much deeper wisdom resides within that simple phrase. Psychotherapy is pointless unless it leads to change, and in an interconnected, networked world, individual change must be linked to reverberating change in the web of social and political connections within which we are all embedded.

HOW WE TOOK CARE OF OURSELVES

Oh, yeah, sure, you'll be there for me, just like my mom was when my brother started putting those things inside me and when my uncle raped me, and when my father beat me, and when she let all the rest of them get me. What a bunch of crap you all are.

—twenty-six-year-old victim of child pornography with multiple abusers

When, as a staff, we moved toward a trauma-based approach, we found it to be a vast improvement over our previous style of professional involvement. We felt that we understood far more about how people become disturbed, why they do the things they do, and how to address those problems in a vastly more constructive way. The results were obvious. Patients whom we had considered untreatable, became treatable. Patients whom we had never understood became understandable and when we understood them, they improved. On the whole, our patients were far more empowered, less demonstrably "sick," more responsible for themselves, and more solicitous of each other. They achieved a level of improvement that far surpassed our own previous results in treating similar kinds of problems. But at the same time, the work placed more demands on us than we had experienced in the past.

Judith Herman has made the point that psychiatry's understanding of trauma has been discovered and lost repeatedly over the centuries (Herman 1992). So too has knowledge of the social aspects of psychiatric care been discovered, forgotten, and rediscovered. Because we are simultaneously involved in both areas—creating a social environment and doing so with a trauma-based approach—I clearly understand why these two aspects of our group understanding keep getting lost. They are extremely difficult to consistently create and maintain. Understanding people who are emotionally and behaviorally disturbed as victims of previous trauma demands an empathic connection that is painful and emotionally draining. The powerful negative emotional charge that pervades a psychiatric unit is contagious and hard to resist. Listening to the bone-chilling stories of abuse that children experience is exhausting, overwhelming, devastating, and harrowing. Compassion fatigue or vicarious traumatization are virtually inevitable.

Compassion Fatigue

Regardless of our professional training, nothing really prepared us to share the relentless and overwhelming nature of post-traumatic emotional states. The patients needed and deserved an empathic response. They needed other people to help them feel safe, to restore their sense of trust in others, to willingly help redirect their traumatic scenario. This is the social response that had failed them as children and could not fail them again. But there was an unending stream of them, and only a few of us. We found that the only real protection against this kind of toxic exposure was diffusion, spreading the overwhelming emotion over a group large enough to detoxify it. But we have all—patients and staff alike—been reared in a culture that shuns group approaches to anything.[6] We have been taught since childhood to compete when we are in groups—that winning, and beating the other guy is all that is important. Even in team sports, individual achievement is the pinnacle of success. Nothing should interfere with our individuality. This philosophical paradigm put us at a distinct disadvantage when it came to working with these patients.

We had to learn new skills. Just as we encouraged our patients to lower their defenses and trust other people, we had to do the same with each other. We were forced to recognize that we too brought our own unresolved conflicts and past traumas into every setting and that these conflicts could get in the way of good therapy. For our community to stay healthy, we had to expose ourselves to each other's criticism and judgment and hope that the other would be kind and compassionate. If we did not take care of each other, we could not take care of our patients.

The Responsibility to Care

Looking back now, we realize that we needed to develop and hone abilities that were not emphasized in our training but have been looked at by feminist scholars. In her research on the study of normal moral development, Carol Gilligan studied the moral development of women and noted that there are gender differences. Women tend to make moral judgments based on context more than on abstract rules. The judgments that women make focus more on care and responsibility for others than abstract criteria of right and wrong (Gilligan 1982). This point was driven home to us over and over. Our clear-cut sense of right and wrong was destroyed in the context of trauma. Behavior that we had formerly clearly defined as wrong turned out to be in service of adaptation. Behavior that we had defined as right turned out to be an exploitation of our position of authority. Rules had to be based on the needs of the particular individual at the particular time. More general rules often tended to be destructive to the growth and flexibility of the individual and the community. And yet rules and structure were clearly vital if we were to maintain a safe and healthy community. We discovered that establishing a living process for constantly negotiating values-based rules was more important than being bound by lists of inflexible and rigid laws.

Continuity of Care—Sharing the Burden

In dealing with patients who had been severely traumatized we learned at least one consistent lesson—the individual model of psychotherapy may be necessary but it is certainly not sufficient. When we first began inpatient work, although our approach was more social than most settings, we still placed a high priority on daily individual psychotherapy sessions with our patients. Individual psychotherapy can be extremely helpful for many people. But for the most complicated, difficult-to-manage, and pained people, no one person could encompass their needs, and trying to do so could rapidly lead to therapist burnout and therapeutic mistakes. Nor could any one therapist develop an expertise in all of the techniques that a trauma survivor may need to use in order to heal. After all, PTSD changes the body, the thinking, the memory, the feelings, and the belief systems. We found that outpatient therapists began to frequently use us as consultants who could provide tangible relief to them when their patients became acutely distressed and help them to extricate themselves from therapeutic impasses. For the most difficult patients, using more than one therapist was extremely useful, as long as the two therapists shared the same basic philosophy and did not permit splitting or fragmentation of the treatment.

Treatment was most successful when a true continuity of care could be provided by the inpatient team, the outpatient therapist, the family, and any other significant people or social institutions, such as schools and church groups. This raised the whole problem of the appropriate nature of confidentiality. When is confidentiality an obstacle, rather than a support, of treatment? We let our patients know that we felt that sharing information was vital if they were to get proper care and then let them decide if they were comfortable with this. As we knew, fragmentation is the hallmark of trauma, and if the treatment program was fragmented as well, healing could not occur.

Communing Through Laughter

Edward De Bono, who has written extensively on cognitive processing, has said, "Humor is by far the most significant activity of the human brain." Certainly, we would rate no stress management tool higher than a sense of humor—for our patients and for us. The more utterly humorless a person was, the worse their prognosis. There was simply no way to deal with the tragedies that assailed us on every front without laughter. Eco observed, "The comic is the perception of the opposite; humor is the feeling of it." Only with humor were we able to lurch ourselves and our patients out of the miasma of anger, grief, and abject misery that can easily prevail in an environment such as ours. In studies of resilience, humor is one of the qualities that comes up over and over as necessary for people to be able to rebound from adversity (Tedeschi and Calhoun 1995; Wolin and Wolin 1993). "Gallows humor" is typical of many people who work in service professions—emergency room personnel, fire fighters, and police officers. We needed to learn how to laugh at ourselves and help our patients laugh at themselves: "Anyone who takes himself too seriously always runs the risk of looking ridiculous; anyone who can consistently laugh at himself does not" (Havel 1990).

Of course, humor in the form of sarcasm, ridicule, and in-jokes can be used as a weapon. People who have been victimized as children often have problems with humor because laughter was viciously used against them within their families. We had to be sensitive to this aspect of trauma. We had to learn how to judge when our play had gone over into cruelty, as perceived by the patient, and make amends if necessary, or at least explanations. As people healed they could begin perceiving humor as a form of intimacy and playfulness rather than attack.

Sometimes the community would play jokes on us. Our unit was situated on one side of a glass-enclosed central courtyard and the entire hospital community had to walk through hallways along the other three sides to get to the dining room. One day at lunch, our patients surreptitiously scurried out into the courtyard. Several of them knelt down, while others scrambled up on their backs and shoulders, supported by several chairs confiscated for the purpose. Holding aloft urinals filled with water, they formed a human water fountain as they recirculated the water from member to member. Their play was a gift to us, a precious confirmation of their willingness to allow us to help them heal.

Power Distribution and Leadership

There is no hope of creating a better world without a deeper scientific insight into the function of leadership and culture, and of other essentials of group life.

—Kurt Lewin 1943

We live in a democracy. Democratic principles are a fundamental part of our belief system. But in practice, we have relatively little training throughout childhood in democracy. In most cases, the more abusive the home, the more rigidly authoritarian is the structure of the family. For our patients, authority is abusive but is actively sought and even demanded. We needed to construct an authority system that would provide order and structure but that would not be abusive and would enhance both individual and group function.

The question of power distribution and leadership has been an ongoing concern in the literature related to the therapeutic milieu. Gregory Bateson, in evaluating the early therapeutic milieu that Harry Wilmer had created, noted, "There is no rule to what the psychiatrist ought to feel. The only rule is that of integrity" (Wilmer 1958). Maxwell Jones said that the most basic function of the leader is to create situations that promote social learning (Jones 1968b). "There are many leaders of various professional and treatment groups within the hospital, and their contributions have to be brought into harmonious whole. The most important attribute of a leader in this context is his capacity to preserve the wholeness of an organization, while at the same time encouraging flexibility, self-examination, social learning, and change" (Jones 1968b). He said the leader had to "lead from behind," helping other people to look at themselves and their feelings when it is appropriate, and encouraging new leaders to emerge (Jones 1968b).

Thomas Main described the change that he noted in the leadership structure as he helped to create a therapeutic milieu: "The anarchical rights of the doctor in the traditional hospital society have to be exchanged for the more sincere role of member in a real community, responsible not only to himself and his superiors, but to the community as a whole, privileged and restricted only insofar as the community allows or demands" (1946). Much has been made in the literature on the therapeutic community about the presence of a "charismatic leader" and how the community tends to fall apart if the leader leaves. This may not be intrinsic to the therapeutic milieu itself, but may reflect the innovative role in the larger culture that the milieu repeatedly struggles to create, often against strong resistance. When the sociologist Max Weber classified leadership, he suggested that during times of change and innovation, power and authority tended to be exercised through charismatical leadership rather than through the traditionally sanctioned distribution of power. This charisma on the part of the innovative leader was accompanied by the positive moral commitment of the followers and both were required if traditional power was to be challenged (Manning 1989).

At present, our social systems do not encourage the development of the kind of leadership these writers have described. Medical school does not prepare physicians to be these kinds of leaders. As Maxwell Jones noted, "In our present society the highly trained professional who attains a leadership position automatically acquires authority, responsibility, power, and prestige. To share such privileges and status goes against the formal training and culture of the medical world" (Jones 1968b).

One author (Helgesen 1990) describes the typical "ecological focus," a concern for the group as a whole, that she attributes to women leaders. These women often describe their leadership style as a "web of inclusion" in which leaders do not see themselves at the top of a hierarchy but in the center of a web of connections. In such a system, leadership is characterized more by facilitation, extracting, directing information, and transmitting data outwards, than by competitiveness. The authority in the web can be just as powerful as in a hierarchy, but manifests itself in very different ways.

In another interesting description of leadership, Clastres (1987) discusses Native American chieftainship and says that the Indian leader demonstrates three essential traits: The chief is a peacemaker, the group's moderating agency; he is a giver, generous with his possessions; he is a good orator. He points out that tribes often have two leaders, one who takes over during times of military need, whose style is much more coercive, but whose power is withdrawn as soon as the immediate need is past and the external threat has been met. When peace is restored, coercive power ends.

All of these descriptions are useful in establishing a framework for the kind of leadership necessary to properly manage a program such as *The Sanctuary*, whether the leader is a physician or nonphysician, a man or a woman. I learned that the leader must constantly remember that he or she is the embodiment of the unit values, the primary carrier of the culture. This demands a level of integrity, as Bateson pointed out, that is sometimes very hard to bear. In the establishment of a new setting this often does require the presence of a "charismatic" leader who can provide the necessary excitement and energy to overcome the force of institutional inertia and to attract the kinds of people who are willing to take on the enormous commitment of time and resources necessary for start-up (Jones 1968b; Sarason 1972).

We created multiple levels of leadership, a long-standing recommendation of the therapeutic milieu. Although I was the medical director, leadership function was largely determined in a team setting with at least two other key managers who had been chosen by me. At first, the division of leadership functions occurred out of necessity, given the enormous amount of labor that goes into starting a new program. Over time we learned that this system of multiple leadership functions simply worked better, allowing for far more flexibility and interchangeability of role responsibilities. This made the system less dependent on the presence of any one person. Additionally, decisions made by three people whose abilities, training, and perceptions were different but complementary, proved to be far superior to individual decisions. As more people joined the team we were able to expand decision making to include them.

Patients and staff bring with them, into any interaction, all of their past history with authority figures. And the leader, of course, has been powerfully influenced by his or her own experience with authority. Because few of us were raised in systems that encouraged a "web of inclusion" we had to learn a new way of relating to each other. To do this, we attempted to overcome fixed, hierarchical perceptions and expectations of leadership. Hierarchical leadership encourages an unhealthy degree of dependency and discourages group problem solving, the lack of which can be lethal to the operation of any integrated system. This was a barrier that had to be repeatedly overcome. "Subordinates" had difficulties learning to assume responsibility, to speak up, to challenge authority, and to defend their own perceptions. Likewise, those in authority had a hard time learning to delegate, to subordinate their own wishes to those of the group, and to "lead from behind."

To be consistent with the relational principles that we were trying to convey to our patients, we had to be concerned about relationships ourselves, among each other. In a fixed hierarchical scheme, if someone is not doing a job properly, he or she can be viewed as a part of a machine, a part that is not functioning adequately and can be replaced. In a web, no part of the web can be damaged without damage to the entire fabric. The result is that we had to learn how to confront, manage, and resolve conflicts with each other. Over time it became perfectly obvious that the principles set forth by Stanton and Schwartz in the 1950s were just as pertinent in the present—any unsurfaced conflicts on the part of the staff would manifest in the patient community (Stanton and Schwartz 1954). Whenever there was a conflict in the community we had to learn to look at what was going on among ourselves, how we were failing to provide adequate leadership for the community. Not only did we have to nurture change within our patients; we also had to nurture and insist on change within ourselves. Any inconsistency in that position, any hypocrisy, would be immediately seized on by the patients as a reason to delay addressing their own problems.

Once a workable system was established, we discovered that the greatest source of stress for the leaders did not derive from internal problems. The biggest problem was dealing with the world outside of the community. Maxwell Jones had talked about this phenomenon as well: "I was in the almost untenable position of having to look in two ways at the same time: to defend the unit from its detractors outside, and, at the same time, to remind the unit staff and patients of the reality of the outside world" (Jones 1968b). For the leaders, the constant sense of responsibility was a steady, heavy stress. We learned that the health of our system would always be limited by the health of the systems within which we were embedded. As long as our values, goals and practice were in conflict with the the hospital, the mental health system, the health care system, insurance companies, or managed care companies, we would always be in a constant state of preparing for attack, with the occasional border skirmishes draining off energy we needed to deal with the problems presented by the community. Our manner of dealing with issues of power, authority, competition, and discipline were always in conflict with some of the most basic assumptions of our society. And yet in practice, the conflicts that arose with these other systems were never attributed to actual differences in basic values but to "personality conflicts" between our leaders and the leaders of the larger organizations.[7] It was as if the basic value conflicts were secret and could not be discussed, reminding us of the secret conflicts that characterized the families of our patients.

Given the covert, or sometimes overt adversarial nature of the larger institutions, many times our leaders had to compromise with the larger system in order to guarantee our survival. That sometimes led to anger on the part of the members of our community who felt that we had compromised too much. We were then forced into the untenable position of defending policies we did not support. Our usual course of action was the most difficult one: we simply told the truth, that we were often forced to make choices between two conflicting values, integrity and survival.

We learned that like the Native Americans, we needed two different leadership styles. In times of threat or crisis, taking the time to deliberate and reach consensus decisions can be quite dangerous. We also knew that decisions made during times of stress are often not of the same high caliber as those made during times of calm. Therefore, those in positions of responsibility were urged to make the best decision they could make in terms of ensuring safety during a crisis. These decisions could be quite coercive and therefore contradicted our basic values system. After the crisis had deescalated, we were free to change decisions that had been made at the time of crisis, while still affirming the decision at the time. Coercion was to be used only as long as a threat existed. This dual role is quite difficult for one leader to assume, because very little in our social conditioning prepares us to be flexible enough to lead from the top under some circumstances and lead from behind or from the center under other circumstances.

In the practice of psychotherapy and medicine as a whole, relatively little attention has been paid to "taking care of the caretaker." Nor has much attention been paid to the toll that leadership takes on the a leader. The hierarchical paradigm for leadership divorces leadership from the responsibility to those who are led but is also tremendously isolating and emotionally unsupportive for the leader. Leaders are subject to the constant attack and criticism of those who are led, while superhuman attributes are often unconsciously applied to the leader. Given all of our history, authority figures are understandably feared more than they are loved, needed more than they are appreciated or understood. The expectations put upon leaders are often quite unconscious and outside of the realm of negotiation or even conversation.

I had the luxury of leading a group of relatively mature people who were able to discuss and negotiate conflicts. Nonetheless, the burden of leadership was more than I had ever imagined. From talking to others and from reading about the experiences of leaders, I believe I have gone through a process that is symptomatic of the dilemma of being caught between paradigms, as we somewhat erratically and unpredictably shifted between a hierarchical and a web model of leadership and control. In the beginning of our creative process, most of my energy was consumed with beginning the program, training the staff, working collaboratively with a very creative group of colleagues, and treating the patients. Before long, however, my role shifted and as representative of our program, more of my time had to be spent dealing with the external world. In this role, I usually felt like an emissary from an alien culture, attempting to inform people about our language and customs, about which they were very suspicious and generally hostile. We represented change, and humans usually greet change with distrust.

As an alien, I could never really relax and could never feel truly safe. And, it was essential that I take responsibility for keeping my alien culture safe. Therefore, I had to do whatever it took to provide the host system with what it wanted to allow us to live. In the hospital world this meant that we had to feed the hospital with dollars. As far as the hospital was concerned, I was an effective leader if I made money so that the hospital could survive and didn't cause any law suits. Returning to my culture, our ethical system demanded that the need for dollars could never interfere with helping traumatized patients. I had to mediate between the real and the ideal—a reality I could not avoid if we were to survive, and an ideal that was the reason I was doing all this in the first place. At the same time, as leader, one of my essential roles was to manage overwhelming feelings and to protect my staff from feeling helpless and overwhelmed so that they could remain functional for the patients. I understand now how easy it is for a small, counterculture system to become paranoid and cultish. This is what Maxwell Jones warned about when he said that it is potentially dangerous to be *too* deviant from the external world. I found the ethical dilemmas to be the most consistently draining aspect of leadership and only possible to tolerate because our values were, in fact, consistent with the long-established psychiatric tradition of the therapeutic milieu.

I was progressively isolated because even my closest colleagues could not fully understand how alone I felt, and yet I could not tell them and fulfill what I perceived, rightly or wrongly, as my role. Nor could I find any true allies in the host culture as long as I maintained values and beliefs that were alien to them. As the alienation progressed I found myself gradually drawing away from my staff, as they understood less and less of my frustration, just to find some peace. They became angry and hurt with my distancing, which I perceived as self-preservative. I suspect that it is at this point that many groups and social movements may splinter. Certainly, we would have if we had not had fifteen years of experience, trust, respect, and enjoyment in each other as well as a commitment to the work and the values we believe in. But this is astonishingly hard work.

WHERE WE FAILED

A twenty-seven year old man was found dead of a gunshot wound to the head today, an apparent victim of suicide. He was awaiting sentencing for the sexual molestation of his two young daughters.

—Newspaper account of prison guard who had been molested
by a police officer as a child, gang-raped by some prisoners at work,
who later was convicted of molesting his own daughters

Burnout

We have had a very good program and have helped a great deal of people, but I would be dishonest if I were to leave an impression that there were no problems. One of the most critical issues is that of staff "burnout." We have not found a solution to this problem, and if anything it is getting worse. The reasons for this are complex. I have wondered if there may not be a limit to the amount of traumatic exposure a caregiver can tolerate without relief, a bit like radiation exposure. I have used the metaphor of toxic exposure to describe the experience of patients who have been exposed to overwhelming trauma. Bearing witness to the retelling and reliving of these experiences, every day, all day long, is also toxic.

The group setting, weekends, days off, and vacations provide some relief. All staff members needed to be urged to attend to their own needs for recreation, attention to health matters, and personal growth and development. One of the reactions to this toxic material can be to become overly self-sacrificing, which encourages faster burnout. Certainly, clinicians who practice in a setting such as ours have much more ongoing support from a wider group of people than most individual practitioners. On the other hand, the exposure is greater because of the large numbers of patients being treated. Coming close to this material also stimulated the awakening or reawakening of any unresolved traumatic issues in one's own past, and therefore staff members had to be encouraged to pursue their own personal therapy when needed. The use of humor in the setting was a powerful prophylaxis against burnout.

Again, a significant part of the difficulty in preventing or managing burnout has to do with the larger sociopolitical setting. Changes in the health care environment have made psychiatric work much more stressful than it used to be. Clinicians now have significantly less control over important treatment issues and are regularly told by anonymous callers from managed care companies what they can and cannot do with their patients, who is allowed to be admitted and who must stay out, when patients can leave and when they must be discharged. Their position, of course, is that they are not dictating treatment, they are just dictating reimbursement policy, but the outcome is the same.

The stress of constantly—and I mean every day, all day long—wrestling with ethical dilemmas cannot be overestimated. "The insurance company says it will not pay, but I am still afraid this person is a risk to himself. Do I send him out so he does not incur more bills and therefore more stress? But if I send him out he may hurt himself again. And if I make the decision to send him out, I am liable for the decision, not the insurance company." If you keep the patient in the hospital, then not only are you failing to protect yourself, but this guarantees the wrath of the hospital administrator, the patient's family who is stuck with the bill, and the patient, who cannot afford to pay on his own. The stress is compounded by the fact that the clinician is helpless to effect any change in this system which has gotten out of control. If you argue with the managed care companies you can become secretly "blacklisted" and will have more difficulty with every patient that they review.

Even more worrying is the effect that this managed costs environment is having on the health of our program. The level of stress threatens to reach intolerable limits. An interconnected system such as ours can work only if there is a high level of intercommunication, and communicating with people takes time. And there is no more time. Over a recent four month period our admissions and discharges increased by almost 65 percent and our average length of stay decreased by over 30 percent. This means that the pace has increased dramatically while, at the same time, staffing has been cut. Because it is so difficult to get approval to come into a hospital, people are being admitted when they are already in a crisis, even though for many of them earlier admission could have averted the crisis.

Like most hospitals around the country, our hospital has had to rapidly downsize in the past year resulting in the hasty deconstruction of long-standing professional and social systems. As a result the entire organization is experiencing signs of stress. One of the results is that most open units have reverted to locked units. It takes more staff to keep a psychiatric unit unlocked because communicating with patients must supplant the use of physical means of control. It takes more staff to allow patients the freedom to eat their meals in the cafeteria, so now most patients are confined to the locked units. So far, we have kept our doors unlocked, but it remains an ongoing issue of contention.

Our social workers, who used to provide individual, group, and family sessions in the past, now have no time for clinical work because they must prepare insurance reports and converse on the phones with insurance reviewers who often demand a review every day. Because we could not increase our staff, other staff members have had to add to their own work. As a result, staff members are staying overtime, without pay, to complete their work and that is cutting into the private time they need for recuperation. Free-floating anxiety, chronic feelings of anger, fear, depression, guilt, and loss are admitted to by everyone as well as increased marital, relational, and parenting stress. There has been an increase in physical symptoms and actual episodes of illness. Since the staff members universally pride themselves on their commitment to the patients and see this commitment not just in professional, but in moral and even spiritual terms, the ethical dilemmas are producing even more stress. This is an environment that is very conducive to burnout.

Additionally, these changes have brought a virtual end to much of the innovation in the mental health care field that mushroomed in the 70s and 80s. Like our traumatized patients, the entire psychiatric health care field is now more concerned with survival, than with creating, evaluating, and maintaining healthy environments. The constant stress of being forced to resolve impossible ethical dilemmas, of never knowing whether our program will survive past tomorrow or next week or next month, all in a context of helplessness, is a more powerful contributor to chronic burnout than any amount of close involvement with our traumatized patients. So far, we have failed to figure out a way of reducing the magnitude of these problems.

Damage of Developmental Trauma

Although our rate of success with very difficult patients is much greater now than it was before we made a shift to a trauma-based approach, we do not succeed with everyone. And we do not succeed rapidly. The reasons for this are many. Sometimes we fail because developmental trauma has done overwhelming damage to critical physical and psychological systems that we lack the power or knowledge to reverse. We have all grown desperately aware of the need to prevent this damage, rather than simply trying to treat people after the damage has been done. Patients often remain vulnerable to stress even when they have made great improvements.

We can help most of our patients begin the process of healing, but their wounds are inflamed again when they return to the situations that brought them into the hospital and frequently, the gains they made are torn down. Our patients rarely get sufficient time to adequately build up their strength. Sending them home too soon is similar to sending a cardiac patient, who has been kept in ICU for a month, back out to work digging ditches. Outpatient therapy helps, but it is not enough. We need a network of good partial programs, intensive outpatient programs, modified work schedules, halfway houses, transitional group homes that include families, in-home visitation programs, support groups—a web of connection and healing. Although some of these programs still exist, changes in the economic climate have eliminated many of the safety nets that were available. Failures in the larger system leave patients, clinicians, and the public with the impression that the patients are hopelessly ill when it is the larger system that is a failure.

Our Limitations

We have all been raised in a patriarchal, hierarchical, individualistic, fragmented social system. We strive to achieve the practice of a different paradigm, but it is hard to maintain this practice. Under stress we revert to our earlier training and have to slowly pull ourselves up and out again. Sometimes we are better at it than others. Sometimes we remember to resolve conflicts with each other; sometimes we don't. Sometimes we use group support; sometimes we don't. All I can say with certainty is that when we do remember, when we are able to achieve the practice of a different paradigm, we feel better, patients do better, the community is healthier and less violent. But sometimes we don't have the energy to keep it going steadily.

This, perhaps, is our largest area of failure so far: that our challenge to the existing paradigm is like a cry in the wilderness. Clearly we are going against the flow of events in health care. We want to succeed and cannot do so without a great deal more help and support from the social systems within which we are embedded. Just as our patients need safe environments, compassion, encouragement, and social support, so do we. Think of it as an energy flow that has to keep circulating for the entire system to stay "lit up." But within our present paradigm, there is always one or more blocks to the flow of energy, and without that sustenance people—and systems—burn out.

WHERE WE SUCCEEDED

To express my feelings in words about my experience at The Sanctuary seems almost impossible. This is the safest place I've ever been. You all have been the family I've always needed. Although the therapies have taught me a great deal, it is the sharing with the community that has been most beneficial to me.
—Read to the community before discharge

Patients Have Changed

On the other hand, we would not continue to do this work under such adverse conditions if it were not personally and professionally rewarding. The reward has come largely from our patients. They have told us what our treatment has meant to them. They have told us that we have helped them save their lives. We can see many of them, over time, becoming good parents, going back to school, taking on more responsibility at work, becoming socially active, helping other people, making creative contributions in the arts. They have inspired us with their courage, commitment, and perseverance.

We Have All Changed

Our exposure to people who have been severely traumatized has had an enormous personal and professional impact on all of us. Our horizons have broadened. We now understand much more than we ever did about human nature, human tragedy, and human perfidy, but also about courage, perseverance, and moral fortitude. We value connection much more than we ever did and have become convinced that we are moving toward an ecological paradigm that, if fulfilled, can mean a much better life for men and women on earth in the future. This hope and vision has given our life and work a far deeper meaning and purpose, a confidence and surety that was formerly lacking.

Survival, Growth, Propagation

We have survived and grown together for more than fifteen years. We have seen people join us, grow, change, and move on, following their own destiny. People who have trained with us have taken up positions of responsibility, and we can share proudly in some of their accomplishments. And we have helped a few other programs—in the United States, Canada, and Great Britain—get started on the right foot, as they develop in their own way, using a model that we have helped articulate.

WORK TO BE DONE

> But what's going to happen to my kids? How can they ever get over what I did to them?
> —thirty-six-year-old survivor of at least three generations of sexual abuse, who deliberately scalded her son and sexually molested her daughter

Survival Under Conditions of Abuse

A great deal of work remains to be done. The most essential priority at present is simple survival. Our challenge right now is to survive and even grow under conditions that are not conducive to either. The status quo at present is to cut back spending, programs, and personnel in the mental health professions and to focus strictly on biological treatments such as electric shock treatment and medications. Psychotherapy is under attack, and the kind of therapy we are proposing—social therapy—is not even possible except in a very limited way. As long as we remain committed to this work we are bucking the status quo and will continue to do so. We have to figure out how to continue to do that without self-destructing.

Building a New Generation

Our work does not really mean much if it is the product of a unique group of personalities working in a specific place during a specific time. To be truly meaningful, our work has to be transmitted to a new generation of people on our unit and be tried out and modified to fit needs outside of our immediate center.

Finding More Effective Self-help Treatment Modalities

But, regardless of how effective we could be at disseminating this information and getting people to seek treatment, there could never be enough individual therapists or psychiatric programs to treat all of the traumatized people who have been already hurt or are in the process of being damaged now. We have to find more effective, communal solutions to these problems. Healing must become a self-help process that everyone freely engages in without stigma, that simply becomes a part of health maintenance. The knowledge that we have about managing difficult problems and difficult people has to be more widely disseminated and available for anyone's use, because all it takes is one problem person in a group to splinter the group process.

Prevention

Individual survivors transform their personal tragedy into a "survivor mission." Groups of traumatized people frequently manage the same transformation. It is vital that the knowledge we have gained in our work lead to *prevention*. We now can see that a substantial proportion of psychiatric and social disability and dysfunction is a result of *totally preventable* experiences. Never before in history has such a large body of scientific data supported this finding. The struggle, suffering, and sacrifice of our patients and all victims of violence, can have a greater meaning and purpose if it leads to the prevention of those same disorders in children yet to be born. Prevention cannot occur without significant changes in *all* of our social systems and in the very way we think about those systems and the problems they struggle to define.

CONCLUSIONS

Our growing understanding of trauma profoundly changed our attitudes. The change, however, was subtle, a change at the level of basic assumptions, not technology, and therefore difficult to articulate. Our program director said it best when he observed that we had stopped asking the fundamental question "What's wrong with you?" and changed it to "What has happened to you?" (Foderaro 1989). The first question implies an individual perversity of judgment and behavior. It is the implicit question we ask of anyone demonstrating behavior that diverges from the accepted norm. It is the first in a long series of questions, attitudes, and behaviors that sets us upon the course of detaching ourselves, distancing ourselves from other people, setting them outside of the realm of human discourse, allowing us to avoid sharing in their experience of separation and suffering. "What's wrong with you?" allows us to continue to believe that "bad things happen only to bad people," providing us with a comforting sense of control, thereby avoiding the uncontrollable nature of human existence. Disturbances of the mind have always terrified witnesses, and as a consequence, the mentally disturbed are always "the other."

But if these are—or were—normal people who were badly hurt and reacted normally to abnormal situations, then this *could* happen to us as well. If the bad guys are discovered to be abused children, raised in a context of violence and betrayal, who learn to distance themselves from others and focus on their own survival, then it becomes more difficult to keep them neatly in a box labeled "evil" and forces us to critically assess a society that allows its children to be so treated. If the "crazy" ones are found to be not really crazy at all, but reacting with previously healthy learned coping skills to unbearable stress, then the dividing line between us and them becomes uncomfortably difficult to perceive. If, as the concentration camp survivor and psychiatrist Victor Frankl has said, "An abnormal reaction to an abnormal situation is normal behavior," then an important shared cognitive schema becomes profoundly disturbed, and the clearly defined and neatly split world starts to congeal, to flow together, to merge into a whole. This is a highly disruptive experience and it should come as no surprise that it is so heartily resisted by many people in the present cultural milieu. Change is always difficult, and seeing all human beings as suffering beings walking along some long and desperate continuum of behavior challenges deeply held religious and philosophical principles. We break the entire world down into dichotomies because thinking has always been easier that way. We forget that those dichotomies are a convenient, arbitrary, and largely false portrayal of the world.

As we became more familiar with this territory called trauma, we began to realize that knowledge of childhood experience and development was absolutely necessary if we were to understand adult experience and development. We came to understand that our traumatized patients were not so much sick or crazy as developmentally arrested—stopped in time, with fragments of their personality or aspects of their development trapped in the coping skills, feelings, and behaviors of an earlier developmental period. From that perspective, violent behavior in a man looks a great deal like the violent temper tantrums of a two-year-old and the desperate clinging behavior of a woman resembles the terror of a five-year-old being abandoned in a shopping mall. Childish behavior in adults is certainly unappealing and problematic, but perhaps it should not be reified by complicated and pejorative diagnostic classifications that simply describe behavior without encompassing causation. There is something to be said for convincing someone that it is time to grow up and leave childish behaviors behind, rather than attempting to convince someone that they are special by virtue of their exotic psychiatric classification or because they epitomize evil. The continuing refusal to understand and empathize with the child in the adult, to fully grasp the importance of a developmental model of human functioning, is the adult demonstration of a prejudice against children that is deeply rooted in Western culture and that permeates and contaminates every aspect of our social lives, with far-reaching and quite threatening consequences (Breiner 1990; Miller 1983; Shengold 1989). We learned clearly that the child *is* the father to the man, and mother to the woman, and that if you hurt the child, the man or woman *will* have revenge.

Over the course of our experience we underwent another profound shift in our attitude toward the victim/perpetrator dichotomy as well. When we first began to understand the pervasive nature of victimization in our culture, we fell into the trap of neatly dividing the world into victims and perpetrators, good guys and bad guys. It was comforting, since clearly we were on the side of good. Then we were confronted with another major insult to our carefully constructed cognitive framework. Many victims were also perpetrators, frequently reenacting their own victim experience on someone else, or victimizing themselves through self-harm, or more subtly victimizing us by inducing us to collude in some way with their self-harmful reenactments. And many perpetrators were also victims, revealing horrifying but convincing tales of their own past brutalization and their fierce determination to never allow themselves to be in the helpless position again, even if it meant hurting others. Even more difficult was the dawning recognition that all of us participate routinely in this cycle of victim-perpetrator behavior until it merges into expectable *human* behavior, as the wealthy among us vote to decrease social programs for the poor, the powerful abuse the privilege of their positions and repeatedly hurt the people who depend on them, and the poor and disenfranchised self-destruct rather than organize for constructive social change.

We also learned that trauma predetermines repetition. History repeats itself, whether in the life of the individual or the life of an entire culture. But when we began to understand trauma we began to wonder whether repetition *is* inevitable *if* traumatic experience is worked through rather than dissociated, suppressed, and denied. This led us to a reevaluation of methods of healing. We came to see that human existence is, by its nature, tragic in the Greek sense, in that human beings are controlled by forces we cannot control, that reason and justice are limited, and that catastrophes occur all the time (Steiner 1961). Tragedy can only be transcended and transformed. Without such transcendence, tragedy becomes a boringly repetitious way of life, rather than an instructive and dramatic three-act play.

We came to see that our patients, through their symptoms, were constantly performing the actions that displayed their own personal tragedies. They were trying to "get attention" because their transcendence was dependent on a response from their social group, a shared experience of pain that would allow them to find a place back within the human community. They were desperately trying to engage the rest of us in a transformative ritual. It was the social group that needed to respond to their performance in a healing way, and it is this response that we had repeatedly failed to give, creating instead a society that revolved around unconscious and repeated trauma instead of change, transcendence, and transformation.

five

Toward the Evolution
of Sane Societies

One way of helping people is by reminding them that the time is getting late, that the situation is grave, that it can't be ignored. Seeing the outlines of horror induces the will to face up to it.

—Vaclav Havel, *Disturbing the Peace*

GOING BY THE NUMBERS: A TRAUMA-ORGANIZED SOCIETY

It is not my purpose to depress you, the reader, or overwhelm you with numbers. But like Havel, playwright, former political prisoner and now President of the Czech Republic, I too feel an urgency about time passing and time running out. Although we talk a great deal about violence and preoccupy ourselves with tales of terror and horror, the causes of the violence go on, seemingly unaffected by our concern. If I could have you spend just a few days on my unit, I know that like me, you would brush so closely up against the open wounds of our society, that the suffering of our children and their parents would be undeniable, that you would see the interconnected nature of our social problems and feel compelled to do something to make a change for the better. But I cannot take you into my experience with anything except words and ideas, and only with these numbers can I attempt to convince you that we are all part of a society that is organized around unresolved traumatic experience.

Violence to Children

- Hitting children is virtually universal; 25 percent of infants one to six months are hit, and this rises to 50 percent of all infants by six months to a year (Straus 1994).
- Over ninety percent of Americans parents have assaulted their children (Straus 1994). It may be called spanking, or discipline, or just a slap, but the same behavior between adults would be grounds for criminal proceedings.

- By parents' own report, 5 percent of parents punish their children by punching, kicking or throwing the children down, or hitting the child with a hard object on some part of the body other than the bottom (Lewin 1995).
- According to a recent Gallup poll of parents, 1.3 million children a year are sexually abused (Lewin 1995).
- In 1992 alone, 2.94 million cases of child abuse and neglect were reported in the United States, and in the same year, an estimated 1,261 children died from abuse and neglect. One estimate is that the rate of child neglect alone is 14.6 per 10,000 children (National Victim Center 1993).
- According to the U.S. Government-sponsored National Incidence Study of Child Abuse and Neglect, between 1986 and 1993 and under a restrictive standard of harm, the estimated number of sexually abused children rose by 83 percent, the estimated number of physically neglected children rose by 102 percent, the estimated number of emotionally neglected children rose by 333 percent, and the estimated number of physically abused children increased by 42 percent (Sedlak and Broadhurst 1996).
- In five studies of sexual abuse of women between 1940 and 1978, one-fifth to one-third of all women reported that they had had some sort of childhood sexual encounter with an adult male (Herman 1981).
- The number of children traumatized in the United States in a single year equals the number of combat veterans who served in Vietnam for a decade (Perry and Pate 1994).
- According to a Department of Justice study, for every violent and sexual offense committed by a youth under 18, there are three such crimes committed by adults *against* children and teens (Lindquist and Molnar 1995).

Violence to Women

- Gelles and Straus (1988) have estimated based on probability sampling that from 2 million to 3 million women are assaulted by male partners each year in the United States and that 21 percent to 34 percent of all women will be assaulted during adulthood by a male with whom they are intimate.
- More than 50 percent of all women will experience some form of violence from their spouses during marriage; more than one-third of these are battered repeatedly every year; 15 percent to 25 percent of pregnant women are battered (National Victim Center 1993).

- Violence kills as many women every five years as the total number of Americans who died in the Vietnam War (National Victim Center 1993).
- An American woman is four times more likely to be attacked at home by a person she knows than attacked at home by a stranger.
- Every year, domestic violence results in almost 100,000 days of hospitalizations, almost 30,000 emergency department visits, and almost 40,000 visits to physicians (National Victim Center 1993).
- Domestic violence already costs companies nationwide $3 billion to 5 billion annually in absenteeism, reduced productivity, and increased health care costs (Anfuso 1994).
- One out of every eight adult women or at least 12.1 million American women, has been the victim of rape sometime in her lifetime (Kilpatrick et al. 1992).
- In 1990, 683,000 American women were raped and of these, only 16 percent were reported to the police (Kilpatrick et al. 1992).

Violence to Men

- Self-inflicted injury among males ages 10 to 44 grew by 76 percent over the four years of a study of a Philadelphia African American neighborhood (Schwarz et al. 1994).
- In 1991, approximately 20,000 males ages 12 and over were sexually assaulted (Bastian 1992).
- Overall, in terms of the effects of all forms of violence on boys, a Massachusetts study estimated that 1 in 42 teenage boys receive hospital treatment for some form of assault (Guyer et al. 1989).
- Compared to other countries such as England, France, Japan, Canada, and West Germany, a 16 to 29 fold differential separates prime risk American males, ages 25 to 34 from their foreign counterparts (Fingerhut and Kleinman 1990).

Violence At School

- From *Time* magazine, January 25 1993, some statistics for every school day: At least 100,000 students tote guns in school, 160,000 skip classes because they fear physical harm, 40 are hurt or killed, 6,250 teachers are threatened with bodily injury, and 260 are physically assaulted. These statistics came from the National Education Association.
- A recent Centers for Disease Control report shows that the murder rate for 15- to 19-year-olds jumped 154 percent between 1985 and 1991, and the increase was largely a result of gun violence (Arbetter 1995).
- The attitudes of children may be just as frightening as the numbers of

actual incidents. Twenty percent of suburban high schoolers endorsed shooting someone "who has stolen something from you," and 8 percent said it is all right to shoot a person "who had done something to offend or insult you" (Toch and Silver 1993).

- In a 1993 national study of 1,700 sixth- to ninth-graders, a majority of the boys considered rape "acceptable" under certain conditions, and many of the girls agreed (Wallis 1995).
- One study indicated that nearly 25 percent of 2,016 college women surveyed had been raped, according to strict legal standards. Another survey revealed that 1,000 rapes were reported on college campuses during the 1991–92 academic year (Nichols 1995).
- Approximately 7,500 violent crimes occurred on 2,400 campuses in 1991–92 (Nichols 1995).
- Ninety-five percent of violent crimes on campuses involved drugs or alcohol. Eighty-six percent of college students under legal age consumed alcohol and nearly 18 percent of this group reported experiencing alcohol-related trouble with police (Nichols 1995).

Violence At Work

- Workplace violence has tripled in the last decade and is one of the fastest growing types of homicide.
- According to the National Institute for Occupational Safety and Health violence was the third leading cause of workplace death from 1980 to 1985 for men and the leading cause of workplace death for women (Duncan 1995).
- The Bureau of Labor Statistics counted 1,063 workplace homicides in 1993.
- In addition, more than 2 million personal thefts and 200,00 car thefts occur at the workplace (Dilworth 1994).
- More than 30 percent of workplace victims faced armed attackers (Dilworth 1994).
- Between July 1992 and July 1993, 2.2 million full-time workers were physically attacked on the job, 6.3 million were threatened with violence, and 16.1 million were harassed (Anfuso 1994).
- One out of every four employees was harassed, threatened, or attacked between July 1992 and July 1993 (Yarborough 1994).
- The U.S. Justice Department reports that boyfriends and husbands—current and former—commit more than 13,000 acts of violence against women in the workplace very year (Anfuso 1994).
- A National Institute for Occupational Safety and Health study shows

that between 1980 and 1990, a total of 522 deaths occurred among health care workers on the job, and 106 of these workers were murdered (Mainellis 1996).

- According to a 1992 survey of 103 California hospitals, 60 percent of the staff had suffered injuries from visitors or patients, usually from guns and knives (Wheeler and Baron 1994).
- In a University of Louisville study done in 1988, of 127 emergency rooms, 41 reported at least one verbal threat against workers a day, 23 reported at least one armed threat per month, and 55 emergency room workers sustained at least one physical assault per month (Wheeler and Baron 1994).
- The numbers are even higher for mental health professionals. Back in 1978 a study showed that 24 percent of psychiatrists, psychologists, and social workers in a metropolitan area reported being assaulted by one or more patients during a one-year period (Edelman 1978). A study published in 1992 surveying both a private psychiatric facility with an outpatient community mental health center in a middle-class urban area and a state hospital in a lower-middle class inner-city area showed that 62 percent of the 224 clinical staff surveyed reported that their physical safety had been threatened or that they had witnessed a serious injury or death (Caldwell 1992).
- Of those attacked, threatened, or harassed, about half experience difficulties at work related to the violence and about one-fourth became physically injured or sick (Yarborough 1994).
- In the mental health professional study (Caldwell 1992), of the 224 clinical staff, 61 percent reported symptoms of PTSD such as intrusive thoughts or increased emotional reactivity. Of those reporting, 10 percent would have been given a DSM-III diagnosis of PTSD. Of the 138 clinicians who reported experiencing traumatic incidents on the job, only 15 percent reported any later external review of the experience by people in positions of authority.
- Of 37 police officers involved in serious shooting incidents between 1977 and 1984, 17 fulfilled DSM-III criteria for PTSD, 17 others showed impressive pattern of PTSD symptoms, only 3 showed no PTSD (Gersons 1989).
- A study of the San Ysidro Massacre showed that 50 percent of law enforcement personnel developed PTSD (Sewell 1993).
- In one study of young adults in the Midwest, life threat, seeing others killed or badly injured, and physical assault all produced lifetime PTSD rates of around 25 percent (Breslau et al. 1991).

- Rape victims report a PTSD lifetime prevalence of 80 percent. In a national sample of women who had experienced aggravated assault, 39 percent developed PTSD (Kilpatrick and Resnick 1993).
- Of those who experienced traumatic bereavement, 25 percent developed PTSD (Green 1994).
- In the same study, crime victims showed a current PTSD rates of 12 percent from sexual assault, 13 percent from rape, 5 percent from traumatic bereavement (Green 1994).
- PTSD, of course, is rarely found alone, even in community samples. The most common coexisting diagnoses are major depression and substance abuse, as well as a panoply of other psychiatric and medical disorders (Green 1994).
- A study of 400 women enrolled in a large HMO who were crime victims showed that they had significantly worse health problems than other women in the HMO and reported symptoms across a wide variety of types of medical symptoms with a dramatically increased utilization of medical services (Koss et al. 1991).
- In a study of 200 postal workers in Northern Ireland who had been involved in robberies on the job, absence for sickness increased by fourfold following the attacks (Jenkinson 1993).
- A U.S. Department of Justice study found that as a result of workplace violence, more than 500,000 employees miss 1.8 million days of work annually, resulting in more than $55 million in lost wages, not including days covered by sick and annual leave (USA Today 1995).
- Violence, threats, and harassment in the workplace cost companies more than $4 billion in lost work and legal expenses in 1992 (Anfuso 1994).
- According to the National Safe Workplace Institute, the average cost to employers of a single episode of workplace violence can amount to $250,000 in lost work time and legal expenses (Anfuso 1994), while 111,000 incidents of workplace violence cost employers an estimated $4.2 billion in 1993 (Yarborough 1994).

Guns

- In 1968, U.S. civilians owned about 90 million guns (Zimring and Hawkins 1989). Now we own more than 200 million, and the number is growing daily.
- Of these, approximately one third are handguns and of the handguns, approximately 30 million are semiautomatic weapons (Schwab 1993).
- In various reports 6 percent to 20 percent of high school students have carried a gun to school, and in the inner city, 20 percent have been shot

at, and the numbers continue to rise (Callahan and Rivara 1992; Russell 1993).

- In 1991, of the 24,703 murders that were committed in the United States almost 17,330 were committed with a firearm, and in approximately 14,700 cases the weapon was a handgun (Callahan and Rivara 1992).
- A gun kept in the house is 21 times more likely to kill a family member during an argument (Kellerman and Reay 1986).
- A gun kept in the home for self defense is 167 times more likely to result in a suicide than in a defensible homicide (Kellerman and Reay 1986), and guns are twice as likely to be found in the homes of suicide victims as in those of suicide attempters (Brent et al. 1991).
- Of Americans today, one in 360 will die from a bullet, most likely from a 9mm automatic handgun. A person shot with a semiautomatic has on average 2.7 wounds and is three times more likely to die at the scene than if shot with a nonautomatic. In the United States, 35,000 die from bullets each year; 10,000 to 12,000 die from AIDS (Dolinskas 1995).
- A four-year study of Philadelphia neighborhoods completed in 1990 found that gun-related violence increased 179 percent. The same study reported that during the four years of the study 94 percent of men in the age group 20 to 29 had to go to an emergency room at least once with an injury, caused 41 percent of the time by violent encounters (Schwarz DF 1994).
- Firearms are far more likely to kill than nonfirearm weapons: 60 percent of firearm assaults are fatal, 4 percent of knife assaults are fatal, 1 percent of blunt weapon assaults are fatal. (Dolinskas 1995).
- For every death, there are at least 5 non-fatal injuries (Mercy and Houk 1988). Handguns are estimated to cause approximately 100,000 injuries per year, and handguns terrorize far more people than they kill (Larson 1993).
- In 1990, firearm injuries cost the nation $20.4 billion: about $1.4 billion for direct expenses, $1.6 billion in lost productivity, and $17.4 billion due to premature death. Public sources pay 86 percent of the cost of a firearm injury, private sources pay only 14 percent (Dolinskas 1995).
- In a comparison of the similar, nearby cities of Seattle and Vancouver, a citizen in Seattle had a 4.8 times higher risk of being murdered by a handgun than in Vancouver, while the rate of homicide by other means was similar in the two cities (Sloan 1988).
- In 1990, there were 10,567 homicides committed with handguns in the United States while in Canada, there were 68 (Russell 1993).

Substance Abuse

- In a classic study done by Shupe in 1954, 87 percent of 882 persons arrested shortly after committing a crime had measurable alcohol levels in their urine. A recent reanalysis showed that higher alcohol levels were more highly correlated with perpetrators of violent than nonviolent crimes (Volavka 1995).
- Overall, the extensive literature on assault and homicide indicates that assailants were under the influence of alcohol in more than half of the violent crimes (Volavka 1995).
- Experts estimated that 1 out of every 7 people in the United States abuse or are dependent on alcohol and an additional 1 in 20 individuals abuse or are dependent on other drugs (Fialkov 1992).
- One-third to two-thirds of college student rapists and approximately half of their victims had consumed alcohol prior to the rape (Koss et al. 1994).
- Sixty to seventy percent of incest victims say their fathers had been drinking at the time the incest first occurred (Crewdson 1988).
- Approximately 50 to 60 percent of women and 20 percent of men in chemical dependency recovery programs report having been victims of childhood sexual abuse.
- Approximately 69 percent of women and 80 percent of men in such programs report being victims of childhood physical abuse (Matsakis 1994).
- Yandow estimates that as many as 75 percent of women in treatment for alcoholism have a history of sexual abuse (Bollerud 1990)
- Between 60 percent and 80 percent of war trauma victims have concurrent diagnoses of alcohol abuse or drug abuse or dependency. (Friedman 1990).
- Battered women are 15 times more likely than non-battered women to abuse alcohol (Salasin and Rich 1993). Briere reported that 27 percent of sexual abuse victims had a history of alcohol abuse and 21 percent a history of drug abuse, while Herman found that 35 percent of female incest victims abused drugs and alcohol (Green 1993).
- The numbers of drug abusers rose to 80 percent in a group of female incest survivors who had been inpatients (Green 1993).
- Of a sample of 2,300 police officers, 23 percent reported drinking problems and another 10 percent said they abused other drugs (Mitchell and Dyregrov 1993).

Pornography

- In Chicago, police found that in 100 percent of cases of arrest for child pornography, photos and other evidence documented the actual sexual assault of children by pedophile pornographers (Tate 1992).
- Ninety percent of pornography is geared to male heterosexuals, 10 percent to male homosexuals, and consumers were "predominantly white, middle-class, middle-aged married males" (Kimmel 1990).
- A telephone survey of 600 respondents in 1985, however, found pornography to be quite accessible to teenagers and younger males. The average age at which males saw their first pornographic magazine was 11 years old. All of the high school male respondents had read or looked at some pornographic magazine. High school males reported having seen an average of 16 issues; junior high school males reported an average of 2.5 issues. The average age for viewing sexually oriented films was 12.5 years. Eighty-four percent of high school students had seen X-rated films, with the average age of first exposure at age 16 to 17 (Russell 1992a).
- A survey of "adults only" paperbacks available to general public readers published between 1968 and 1974 revealed that one-fifth of all sex scenes involved completed rapes and the number of rapes in the books increased each year of the study (Russell 1993).
- In 1976, one-fifth of all sex episodes in published pornography involved completed rape and the number increased each year; 6 percent involved incestuous rape. Less than 3 percent of the rapists suffered any negative consequences, and many were rewarded (Russell 1992a).
- In a content analysis of "adult" videos, 19 percent involved aggression, 13 percent sexual aggression—22 percent of these last were rapes (Russell 1992a).
- About 10 percent of the male student population are sexually aroused by very extreme violence, about 20 to 30 percent show substantial sexual arousal to depictions of rape when the women appears to be aroused, about 50 to 60 percent show some degree of sexual arousal by rape when the victim becomes aroused by the end (Russell 1992a).
- In addition to increases in themes of aggression and violence in pornographic materials, there has also been an increase in child pornography. A study in 1990 in Britain found that 70 to 80 percent of children contacting a child welfare agency had been involved in some form of child pornography (Kelly 1992).

- The U.S. Postal Service found that 80 percent of those it identified as purchasers of child pornography were active abusers (Tate 1992).
- The pornography industry generated about $8 billion in 1984 in the United States alone (Itzen 1992).
- Department of Justice figures estimate the child pornography "cottage" industry to be worth between $2 billion to $3 billion a year (Itzen 1992).

Media Violence

- Sixty percent of men on TV are involved in violence, and 11 percent are killers. Prime time television has 5 to 15 violent acts hourly and two murders a night. Unlike actual rates, in the media the majority of homicide victims are women (Gerbner 1994).
- The negative consequences of violence are not often portrayed in violent programming—84 percent do not depict any long term consequences. Perpetrators go unpunished in 73 percent of all violent scenes. (National Television Violence Study 1996)
- Children's programs are 50 to 60 times more violent than prime time shows. Some cartoons have averaged more than 80 violent acts per hour. By age 18, the typical American child, who watches 28 hours of television a week, will have witnessed 40,000 simulated murders and 200,000 acts of violence. By age 18, a child's view of the world, its composition, and the role and characteristics of women, minorities, the disabled, and other groups and individuals will be most profoundly influenced by the content of television programs (Gerbner 1993, 1994).
- Children watch an average of 8,000 murders and 100,000 other violent acts on television before finishing elementary school, according to the American Psychological Association (Toch and Silver 1993).
- In a Canadian town in which TV was first introduced in 1973, a 160 percent increase in aggression, hitting, shoving, and biting was documented in first- and second-grade students after exposure, with no change in behavior in children in two control communities (Centerwall 1992).
- Other studies of long-term exposure support a correlation between viewing TV violence and contact with the criminal justice system even after controlling for the effects of socioeconomic class, education, and race. In men, a strong correlation was found between being convicted of a crime and two of the following: physical abuse by the mother, physical abuse by the father, and exposure to TV violence (Heath et al. 1989).

Prisons

- In 1992, 13 million persons were in state and federal prisons, and the number has risen steadily since. (Forer 1994).
- According to the Justice Department, from 1980 to 1992 the American state and federal prison population soared nearly 150 percent, from 139 to 344 jailed for every 100,000 of total population—the Western world's highest ratio (Starer 1995).
- More people are behind bars in America than in any other country in the world (Forer 1994).
- In 1992 more than 100,000 children were in correctional institutions (Forer 1994).
- Despite an increasingly punitive attitude toward crime, the U.S. rates of robbery, murder, and rape have tripled since 1960 (Brill 1993).
- Prison has not rehabilitated inmates. About 80.3 percent of male state prisoners and 67.8 percent of female prisoners are recidivists.
- Of the women in prison, 75 percent of them are mothers and 88 percent of their children are under the age of 18. It is estimated that at the end of 1992, 167,000 children had mothers in prison (Forer 1994).
- In the past decade state and federal annual prison expenses have risen from approximately $12 billion to $24.6 billion with no end in sight (Worth 1995).

Economics

- The United States has the widest gap between rich and poor of any industrialized nation (Barlett and Steele 1996).
- Of people living below the poverty line, 40 percent are children (Freedman 1993)
- According to the National Center for Children in Poverty, 24 percent of all American children under the age of 6 are poor (Herbert 1995).
- In the 1980s income for the lowest 40 percent of families declined while income for the top 20 percent rose by almost 30 percent, and income for the top 1 percent rose by 75 percent. In the last decade the proportion of families moving out of poverty declined by 40 percent (Barlett and Steele 1992).
- Women are the fastest-growing class of impoverished people, heading 24 percent of all poor households in 1960 and 48 percent of all poor households in 1984 (Katz 1989).
- The increase in total salaries of people earning more than $1 million per annum went up by 2,184 percent during the 1980s while the total

dollars in wages that went to the middle class increased only an average of 4 percent a year (Barlett and Steele 1992).

- The top 1 percent of American households controls 30.4 percent of the nation's net worth. The next 9 percent hold 36.8 percent of the nation's net worth. The remaining 90 percent of American households only own 32.8 percent of the wealth (Barlett and Steele 1996).
- The corporate share of taxes went zooming down, accounting for 39 percent in the 1950s and only 17 percent in the 1980s with individuals making up the difference (Barlett and Steele 1992).
- The salaries and bonuses of the highest-paid executives in America ballooned an average of 951 percent between 1975 and 1995, or five times the inflation rate, while the average earnings of more than 73 million blue-collar and white-collar workers went up just 142 percent, not even keeping up with the inflation rate of 183 percent (Barlett and Steele 1996).
- The most important sector in international trade is not oil, cars, or planes—it is armaments. Arms sales are incredibly large—at least $900 billion annually. Some experts place the real figures for arms sales at two, three, even four times higher (Saul 1992).
- The U.S. defense budget continues to escalate even though the Cold War supposedly ended. The House recently approved funding that the Pentagon had not even requested (Dellums 1995).
- We will spend $2.5 trillion from 1995 to 2005 under Clinton's deficit reduction proposal for the military (Hartung 1995).
- In 1988, 33 percent of the federal budget was spent on armaments, while education, social services, and highway construction together amounted to only 15 percent of the budget. It is generally estimated that one-quarter of the U.S. government gross domestic product is militarily oriented. Forty per cent of all U.S. scientists are employed on defense-related projects (Saul 1992).

Everybody

- The Department of Justice estimates that 83 percent of all Americans will be victims of violent crime at least once in their lives.
- In 1984 approximately 37 million Americans experienced a criminal victimization and of these 6 million were victims of a violent crime (McCann and Pearlman 1990).
- A number of studies in recent years have shown that up to three quarters of the general population in the United States have been exposed to some event in their lifetime that can be defined as traumatic (Green 1994; Kilpatrick and Resnick 1993; Norris 1992).

- In one study of young adults in the Midwest, life threat, seeing others killed or badly injured, and physical assault all produced a lifetime rate of post-traumatic stress disorder of around 25 percent of those who had these experiences (Breslau et al. 1991).
- In another recent study 39 percent of women who were victims of aggravated assault developed post-traumatic stress disorder as did 35 percent of those who were raped (Kilpatrick and Resnick 1993).
- Post-traumatic stress disorder rarely occurs alone; it most commonly coexists with major depression and substance abuse, but it can coexist with other psychiatric and social problems as well (Green 1994).
- The effects of trauma are not short-lived. In one follow-up of a disaster, one quarter of the survivors studied showed continuing and significant psychopathology (Green et al. 1990).
- Less than 20 percent of the earth remains forested; a forested area the size of England is being destroyed each year, and the rate is increasing. Tropical forests containing 40 percent of all species on earth are being cut at the rate of two acres per second (Russell 1992b; Schindler and Lapid 1989)
- Ten thousand species of plants and animals become extinct every year. Current estimates are that one-fifth of all the species on earth may disappear during the next twenty years (Schindler and Lapid 1989).
- Carbon dioxide is being produced faster than the oceans and remaining plants can absorb it; half of the 20 trillion tons we produce each year remains in the air. (Russell 1992b).
- Soil is being turned into sterile dust that is washed or blown away at the rate of five tons *per person* per year, which will leave no soil left in a hundred years (Schindler and Lapid 1989).
- As of 1989 there were more than 50,000 nuclear weapons on the planet, with a total firepower of more than 6,000 times the firepower generated by the entire Second World War. It would only take several dozen, exploded in major American cities to stop the United States from existing as a modern society (Schindler and Lapid 1989).
- At least 22 nations have the capacity to make chemical weapons (Schindler and Lapid 1989).
- Acid rain is killing lakes and pine forests in North American and Europe. At least one-third of west German forests have been damaged by acid rain (Schindler and Lapid 1989).
- Industry alone generates 80 billion pounds of toxic waste per year (Schindler and Lapid 1989).
- Population growth curves indicate that there will be more than 6 billion people on earth by the year 2000 and 8 billion by 2025. Before

1960 basic biological systems stayed ahead of population demands but since the 1970s the renewal of life-supporting resources has continued to decline while population has increased, resulting in a downward spiral leading to increasing poverty, starvation, and social instability (Schindler and Lapid 1989).

- One billion out of 5 billion of the world's people are classified as insufficiently nourished. More than 35,000 children die *each day* from hunger-related causes (Schindler and Lapid 1989).
- In the United States, the wealthiest of all nations, more than 1 million people are homeless during a year and more than 100,000 of those are children (Schindler and Lapid 1989).
- The Vietnam War continues to affect the lives of 500,000 to 800,000 Vietnam era veterans and their families. Of the 8,861 million Jews living in Europe before WWII fewer than 600,000 escaped death, 75,000 from the death camps. The genocide of the Cambodians was responsible for 2 million deaths. Since 1975 more than 700,000 Southeast Asian refugees have come to the United States after having been severely traumatized, including being tortured. (McCann and Pearlman 1990). In the 1970s in Argentina, 9,000 to 30,000 people were tortured and killed (Staub 1989).
- An estimated total of 170 million human beings have been destroyed by wars and totalitarian genocide in the twentieth century—what Brzezinski has called *"megadeath"* (1993).

Pretty overwhelming isn't it? No wonder so many of us feel confused, anxious, and helpless. How in the world do we do anything about problems that are a catalogue of the ills of humankind, many of which reach far back into our prehistory, others of which are, apparently, an inevitable outcome of our industrialized, technologically advanced society? I will not pretend to have *all* the answers to such very large questions but I do think that our work with victims of violence have given us some hints of answers, or at least, a better way of asking the questions.

SANE SOCIETIES?

Our jails and prisons are filled with criminals. Our institutions are filled with insane. Our hospitals are filled with cripples—cripples mangled by war. Wars are made by bullies. Bullies are made by fear. And this kind of fear is made by injury to the child, physical or emotional injury when the child is too young, too helpless, to be able to protect himself.

—James Clark Moloney, M.D. 1949, *The Magic Cloak*

When I listen to the news these days, I am struck by the parallels between our national dialogue and the arguments that used to occur in our small inpatient community. For me, it is reminiscent of the daily dilemma we faced when confronted with the complex problems of our patients before we knew about the long-term and developmental effects of trauma. We were bewildered because we had no way to really conceptualize the magnitude and interconnected complexity of their problems. Many of the issues are the same. After all, the problems that confront us as individuals, as small groups and as an entire society reflect the same basic human themes. How do we connect and care for each other? What do we do with the people who cannot control their emotional states? How do we stop the violence? What is the role of authority, and how do we get others to respect it? What are we missing, failing to understand, and why is there so much dishonesty? What do we do about all the addicts? What is fair when it comes to the poor and the rich? Why is it that the more things change the more they remain the same? Why do the problems get bigger and bigger? What is wrong with America, this extraordinary land of opportunity and plenty?

These days, many voices are attempting to define what ails us as an entire society. Many of these voices make good sense and are offering valuable advice. But defining a problem is supposed to lead to problem solving and this does not appear to be happening very often no matter which institution confronts the problem. In part, this is a failure of will, a deep-running ambivalence about facing up to problems and making necessary changes. But I suspect that is not the only difficulty. More fundamentally, a coherent strategy does not appear to be available for even beginning to think about how to solve the massive sociopolitical problems that confront us.

I see now that we were functioning for years with a huge obstacle in our way. But the real difficulty lay in our inability to see the obstacle. We denied not only its importance, but its very presence. It was as if we were all together in a large room, and in the middle of the room stood a huge elephant. By now, everyone has heard the story of the blind men and the elephant, about how each one could feel only a part of the animal and in doing so, assumed that the part was the whole. But before they could even reach this point, they had to confront the elephant—they had to see it and agree with each other that something was in the room. As a social group, we have been denying that the elephant is even there. We have used a long list of half-truths or outright deceptions to convince ourselves that there is no elephant: Individualism, predeterminism, biological reductionism, social Darwinism, and original sin are but a few of these.

We seem reluctant to confront the reality of our human nature, that we are an exquisitely complex, interconnected, integrated, multidetermined, social being with extraordinary sensitivity. This emotional sensitivity combined with a powerful memory system and language-based reasoning makes us unique in the animal world. We are simultaneously connected by our biology to our animal and reptilian ancestors, by our psychology to our own past, present, and future, by our sociology to each other, and by our imagination and soul to God. What emerges out of this soup is largely determined by what happens in the formative period of our development—childhood. For all our talk about children, our lamenting, our heart-rending news stories, our Baby Gaps, abortion protests, and disavowal of murderous parents, we still don't really get it. We are the only living species that regularly and predictably maims and destroys its own young. The elephant in the room is the Child. Not Man, not Woman, not Fetus—but the Child. A hurt, angry, violent, vengeful, embittered, and alienated child, perhaps, but a child nonetheless.

From the skewed, distorted, and damaged perspective of the adult, we do our best to turn our children into what we have become. What we fail to seriously consider is that what we have become is seriously flawed, maladaptive, fragmented, and sick. By the time we are adults, we have lost a significant part of our own potential integration and then we pretend that there is no loss, that this is the way things are supposed to be. Artists, poets, playwrights, storytellers, musicians, and mystics keep trying to tell us that we are off track, that we are leaving the most valuable part of us behind, but we have a hard time hearing their messages and we tend to marginalize and criticize those who say it. Like our patients, traumatized as children, we do not want to remember what our child-self has been through, how much of value, of vital importance, has been lost along the way.

I have tried to show in a number of ways, how child development is skewed by the omission and commissions of childhood experience, how trauma alters the developmental pathways. Quite often, the results of the distortion do not manifest themselves until adolescence, when a synthesis of previous childhood identities must be merged with adult desires, impulses, and strivings. But it is virtually impossible for a helpless, dependent, angry, alienated, despairing child to turn into a capable, interdependent, self-controlled, compassionate, creative, cooperative adult. Instead, as we have seen, adults who are severely traumatized as children are frequently emotionally numb, dissociated, amnestic, hypervigilant, paranoid, self-deceptive, unable to think clearly and alternately rational and irrational, disconnected from others, inconsistent, hypocritical, cynical, alienated, antisocial, self-destructive, self-mutilative, suicidal, destructive toward others, murderous.

The hang-up, the fixation, occurs in adolescence. Traumatized children cannot make the transition; they are stuck in the cocoon. Disturbed adolescents have difficulty figuring out who they are or where they fit in the world. They have problems managing their sexual desires and aggressive impulses in ways that are not destructive to self or others. As a result they are often intensely preoccupied with sex and aggression to the exclusion of other interests. Adolescence is the time for defining career aspirations and relationships, and troubled adolescents have difficulty with both. They are unable to assume personal responsibility, balance rights with obligations, or stick to their commitments. They are moody, flighty, unpredictable, and have a difficult time maintaining focus. They have poor control of their emotional expression, particularly rage. They often attempt to exercise their will through bullying others. Their belief systems are either undefined or excessively rigid and are not integrated with their emotional lives or their behavior. They have great difficulty creating and maintaining balanced relationships and instead often become involved with relatively few people but have obsessive relationships with these few. They are preoccupied with immediate gratification of the self and exploiting others to satisfy their own impulses, with little sense of social responsibility or accountability.

Since the beginning of this great American experiment, various writers have looked at our "national character" (Inkeles 1997). As a physician, I am trained to diagnose what is wrong, rather than what's right. From that point of view, if we consider the country as a whole, at least for the purposes of imaginative brainstorming, then I would say that America is a brilliant, beautiful, talented, creative, severely disturbed adolescent who suffers from many of the symptoms of what I am choosing to call "cultural post-traumatic stress disorder." In using such a metaphor, I am making the point that we are a society that has become organized around unresolved traumatic experience. Like my patients, we are culturally fragmented and dissociated, emotionally numb, self-mutilative and self-destructive, alienated, hypocritical, murderous, and abusive. But like my patients, that is not all that we are. These post-traumatic effects are interwoven with our extraordinary energy, compassion, generosity, creativity, humor, courage, perseverance, faith, and integrity. Because we are largely blind to the post-traumatic effects, however, they corrupt us—our thinking, feelings, ability to relate, behavior, and beliefs all become distorted by this insistent post-traumatic influence. We must lie and lie and lie so that we do not see what we are becoming. Our greatest strengths become our fatal weaknesses. It is a disease, a public health menace, that has been being passed down through the generations, intertwined with all the gifts from the past. The twentieth century, the century of "megadeath," has provided a superb breeding medium for this contagion. In failing to recognize and deal with our individual and collective pasts, we become trapped in a vicious cycle of destructive traumatic reenactment as an entire social group, and we stay stuck as perpetual adolescents, doing all the disturbing things that troubled adolescents do.

What do all those statistics tell us about our society, about what we have grown so accustomed to that it no longer seems weird, sick, or crazy—if it ever did? It is my premise that trauma has been a central organizing principle in the formation, development, and maintenance of human society as a whole, not just as a group of individuals. Our small psychiatric unit must struggle every day to provide a sanctuary for a group of very injured people. In a parallel fashion, America, as the world's melting pot, has itself served as a sanctuary for many millions of people for more than three hundred years. Waves of immigrants have come to these shores seeking a better life, often leaving behind years of threats, violence, torture, and despair.

A legacy of trauma has been left for us to repair. We are quite comfortable speaking of the proud and honorable legacy that our ancestors have left for us—our system of government, our beautiful land, enormous wealth and power. But like my patients, there is another legacy, another national history lying below the surface, split-off from consciousness, denied, and taken as normal. Using this broader framework, it is possible to see analogies between the symptoms that my patients suffer and the symptoms of our national distress. I have called these the "nine a's of trauma": disrupted attachment, unmodulated affect, unmanageable anger, abusive authority, diminished awareness, multiple addictions, automatically repeated self-destructive behavior, avoidance of feeling, memory, and guilt, and massive alienation from self and others. I hope that these nine characteristics can provide us with a useful way of using the lessons of the individual to inform our understanding of the group.

Disrupted Attachment

> The past shapes the present and influences the future. To know our parents and grandparents is to know their history as immigrants.
> —Edward Wakin 1977, *The Immigrant Experience*

Odd as it may sound, every American family is rooted in broken attachments. Except for the Native Americans, all of us are the descendants of immigrants or of slaves. The only thing that separates us is whether the disrupted attachments and their attendant loss occurred two years ago, ten years ago, fifty years ago, or a century or two ago. Leaving home, land, country, family, friends is an overwhelming and terrifying experience at the same time that it is filled with wonder and excitement, relief, and hope. Survival depends on focusing on the possibilities, not the grief. But does the longing for roots for a sense of home ever really go away?

A melting pot experiment on this scale has never happened before in history. As exciting and dynamic an experiment as it is, there has to be a negative side as well. Given our peripatetic background, it is small wonder that we would become a nation of extreme individualists, always on the move, heading for any available frontier, involved in a never-ending search for that elusive "freedom." For us, this freedom is often equated with a freedom from attachment to others and a marked preference for consumer goods over relationships. All too often, freedom in America has come to mean a maximum of individual rights divorced from responsibility for others. This self-preoccupation, this fervent defense of personal space, preference for material objects over connections with other people, pervasive disconnectedness, and difficulty in maintaining healthy relationships is also typical of many individual victims of trauma.

The family is the point of attachment for human beings, and this is the first time in history, as far as we know, that family disruption has been so pervasive. The breakdown of family life mirrors the breakdown of the entire social framework of attachment as manifested in increased violence, increased poverty, increased unemployment and joblessness, increased homelessness, increased economic inequality. Its roots are in the massive changes secondary to the Industrial Revolution and the triumph of capitalism (Barlett and Steele 1992, 1996; Bellah 1973; Edelman 1987; Garbarino 1992; Gelles and Loseke 1993; Lasch 1977; May 1991).

Disrupted attachments do not just spontaneously resolve themselves. Instead, disrupted attachments in childhood create specific patterns of attachment in adults that are then conveyed via parenting styles of attachment to the next generation (Alexander 1992). In this way, disturbed relational patterns are transferred from one generation to another. Other researchers have shown that similar disrupted patterns can be transmitted through an organization as well, while one "generation" unconsciously passes on to the next, norms that alter the system and every member of the system (Menzies 1975). If enough of the population is "carrying" these disrupted patterns, then they become normative behavior. No one any longer knows that there may be another way of relating, another way of experiencing intimate and family relationships, friendships, and partnerships. As a result, emotional inhibition, isolation, alienation, social irresponsibility, and antisocial behavior can become a social norm that must then be denied and rationalized and given other names like "self-control," "independence," "skepticism," "profit considerations," and "healthy competition"

Unmodulated Affect

> The history of this country was made largely by people who wanted to be left alone. Those who could not thrive when left to themselves never felt at ease in America.
>
> —Eric Hoffer 1973, *Reflections on the Human Condition*

When abnormal behavior becomes normative, it does not automatically self-correct. Instead it becomes part of the definition of normality, which is then equated with health (Becker 1963; Burrow 1950; Fromm 1956; Horney 1937; Laing 1967; Oldenquist 1986; Scheff 1975, 1984). When attachment patterns are disrupted, emotional expression and interpretation is disrupted as well. Affect loses its signal quality for the whole group and we lose our ability to experience our emotions as the "sensitive mental radar" they are meant to be. Emotional contagion is a part of our built-in evolutionary equipment and the only way we can be around each other and not experience each other's emotions is by shutting down our own capacity for empathy and diminishing our own ability to feel and respond. We carefully teach our children to suppress affect. Boys are not to cry; girls are not to show anger; no one can deal with shame. It is unseemly, even unprofessional, to be emotional. The result of all this is not an absence of emotions, but a lack of modulation of emotions and emotional inhibition. Over time, this emotional blunting becomes normative behavior as styles of relating emotionally are passed from parent to child and the inhibition and suppression of normal emotional experience is encouraged, supported, and even demanded.

In individual victims of trauma the extreme version of this phenomenon is called "emotional numbing." Often, under these conditions, it takes more and more stimulation for people to feel anything. Some even reach the point where they will inflict physical harm on themselves in order to feel something (Glover 1992). The emotional vacuum is filled with a peculiar sense of emptiness, of anomie, discomfort, anxiety, even loneliness. But what victims of violence describe is an exaggerated version of a sentiment that rings throughout the twentieth century in the works of many of our most articulate writers, playwrights, musicians, and poets—deadness, coldness, alienation, isolation, an unutterable loneliness. Our social preoccupation with increasing levels of violence on television, in movies, and in real life may be our group effort to feel something, because our emotional numbness responds only to massive and life-threatening stimulation. People who are repeatedly exposed to the numbing effects of trauma often find that the only time they feel anything is when they are once again in battle, or pursuing a felon, or are involved in some other dangerous pursuit. The result of this numbing and disconnection is empathic failure, poor impulse control, and poor health (Pennebaker 1995).

Victims of trauma often need to learn an entire new emotional language. Their language functions and emotional lives have become disconnected. To a great extent, this is acceptable practice for all of us. We are, in fact, "emotionally illiterate" (Orbach 1993; Goleman 1995), emotionally handicapped as a culture. This disability manifests bilaterally. In the first place, we avoid maintaining attachments to other people because the intimacy of relationship triggers old memories and feelings of old hurts that are unresolved, unmetabolized and therefore threatening. But secondly, we avoid attachments because when the other party in the relationship is a member of the same emotionally illiterate culture, his or her response to our pain is quite likely to be humiliation, hostility, rejection, blaming, and abandonment. Emotional abuse is so fundamental to the functioning of our entire cultural system that we are only now beginning to define it, much less cure it (Loring 1994).

Unmanageable Anger

> In the little world in which children have their existence, whosoever brings them up, there is nothing so finely perceived and so finely felt, as injustice.
>
> —Charles Dickens, *Great Expectations*

> Nations, like individuals, need to face up to and understand traumatic past events before they can put them aside and move on to normal life.
>
> —Tina Rosenberg 1995, *The Haunted Land*

At this time in our history, the most problematic affect is anger. People who are traumatized have a difficult time managing anger. They are either too passive, too rageful, or they alternate between the two extremes. Whatever the case, anger fails to serve the purpose for which it is designed—the protection of boundaries. Violence in all its manifestations is, of course, the obvious sign of anger gone completely wrong. But there is a growing level of hostility in all public discourse as the civil society continues to break down. Simultaneously there is an extreme lassitude and passivity in the face of extraordinary boundary violations. This rage spews out on highways, in grocery stores, at the office, and at school just as frequently as it disgorges itself on television shows, in campaign speeches, and in the houses of Congress. Like so many of our developmentally traumatized patients, we no longer seem able to protect ourselves or protect those we care about without assaulting someone else.

The voices of protest that should be organizing and vociferously countering forces of intolerance, hatred, and repression are largely quiet or absent. In the absence of such boundary protection, the forces of rage are left to go on a rampage, attacking the sick, the injured, the poor, women, children, homosexuals, non-Caucasians, and anyone who fails to conform to rigid and repressive expectations. The behavior of those in prison and the behavior of those in our top offices often looks very similar, but if you have no power and fly into a rage you may go to jail. If you have the same rage and have power, you may be called strong and assertive, an aggressive businessperson, a revolutionary congressman.

When we can get our angry patients to hold still, listen to their inner voice, and look at the past, other feelings surface, feelings even more difficult to manage—guilt, sadness, despair, hopelessness, helplessness. What is it that we, as a people, are so very angry about? What may lie behind all our hate speech, blaming, and finger-pointing? Do we suffer from unconscious group guilt that we need to deny in ways similar to my guilt-ridden patients who have perpetrated against others?

What will happen if we really empathize with victims of slavery, of chronic poverty, of genocide, of nuclear disaster, of domestic violence and abuse? How will we feel when we look at the natural resources, the forests, the animals we have plundered, savaged, and lost forever? Nations have always been able to get angry—that's what wars are about. But can a nation grieve for its own lost innocence? Make confession and atone for its own acts of criminal perpetration? How can we manage the overwhelming shame that our behavior engenders? That is what our patients must do if they are to heal. We ask them to face their powerful and terrible feelings without being destructive. It takes an astonishing degree of honesty and courage. But, if my brutalized and symptomatic psychiatric patients can do it, then there is really no reason why our Congressmen, corporate executives, judges, and administrators cannot do it as well. In various places around the globe, countries who have tolerated, within their borders, terrible acts of violence and perpetration are realizing that a process is required for a country to heal. The Minister of Justice of South Africa, Dullah Omar has said, "We recognized that we could not forgive perpetrators unless we attempt also to restore the honor and dignity of the victims and give effect to reparation . . . we need to heal our country if we are to build a nation which will guarantee peace and stability" (Omar 1996). If we are to ever be safe, we must learn to deal more effectively with our anger and to do this we may have to surface our guilt and make amends to the people, and the generations, who have been hurt.

Abusive Authority

> Authority has always attracted the lowest elements in the human race. All through history mankind has been bullied by scum. . . . Every government is a parliament of whores. The trouble is, in a democracy the whores are us.
> —P. J. O'Rourke, 1991, *At Home in the Parliament of Whores*

For several decades, feminist activists, and theorists have been taking to task the white male establishment for its endemic abuse of hierarchical authority in the family, in government, in corporate offices, in schools, and in hospitals. But this abuse of authority is not the domain only of white males. The substitutive hunger for power in the face of the lack of satisfaction of other human strivings is a fundamental dynamic in human nature, and in all traumatized beings as well. Power brings with it the promise of control and mastery over those feelings deemed unacceptable feelings such as helplessness, despair, rage, and shame, a promise that may be more inherently addicting than the tangible goodies that power also can bring in its wake. Power by itself is not inherently destructive. Only when power is divorced from the responsibility, the stewardship, that accompany it does power become abusive. Once the dynamic of power divorced from responsibility enters a system, it spreads like a virulent infection, creating its own lethal offspring wherever it goes. Whether in an individual, in a family, or in a social system, the power dynamic takes on a life of its own and people lose control over the systems they have created until we lose sight of how a fair, responsible, and humane authority functions (Schmookler 1983).

Patients who have been exposed to abusive authority have difficulty managing their own lives. They are frequently obedient to people who abuse them, even when an objective observer sees an alternative to obedience. They often lack the will to exert authority over their own internal impulses and when put into positions of authority they can, themselves become abusive and demand obedience from others (Adorno et al. 1982; Miller 1983). Stanley Milgram's experiments demonstrated that it was not just the Nazis who responded unquestioningly to authority. In the experimental setting, his subjects would obey an authority and administer shocks to another person even when the victim cried in pain, even when he claimed heart trouble, even when he pleaded to be freed. In his conclusion,

Milgram warned, "A substantial proportion of people do what they are told to do, irrespective of the content of the act and without limitations of conscience, so long as they perceive that the command comes from a legitimate authority" (1969).

Legitimately constituted authority, when used by abusers, can sanction acts of violence, even acts of mass violence, can dehumanize groups of people, play upon people's fear, and thereby set in motion events that will result in the persecution of individuals and entire groups (Hirsch 1995; Staub 1989). Since authority figures have so much power to influence and even control individual and group processes, we need to simultaneously reevaluate authority in the family, our renewed wish for unquestioning obedience in children, hate mongering on radio and television, in movies and in print, and our willing obedience to abusive policies established by corporate executives, agency administrators, bankers, the military, and representatives of government.

Diminished Awareness

We live in a world where amnesia is the most wished-for state. When did history become a bad word?

—John Guare

The fear for oneself, that one can do something about. On it one can turn the light of awareness. But when one is no longer worrying about oneself, then comes the fear for other people, and after that, for the world.

—Peter Hoeg, *Borderliners*

Since the 1960s, American culture has been bombarded with evidence of the ubiquity of traumatic stress throughout the social environment. Vietnam veterans, victims of political torture and terrorism, refugees, Holocaust survivors, disaster victims, rape victims, battered spouses, and finally victims of child abuse all have testified to the universal effects of overwhelming stress, terror, and helplessness. The clear-cut evidence of man's inhumanity to man, witnessed nightly on every news program by millions of Americans, has faced many people with seemingly insoluble problems. In our apparent helplessness, many of us find ourselves becoming emotionally numb to the suffering, able to turn off the TV and turn off our emotions as well.

Add to that, family breakdown, increased unemployment, decreasing wages, longer work hours, higher prices and it is enough to make any reasonable person dissociate. As individuals, dissociation is an adaptive strategy because we feel so little personal control over these massive social problems and also perhaps because we have all "identified with the perpetrator"—few of us can figure out how to solve these problems without toppling a system that we all depend on for the essentials of our everyday existence and the maintenance of what is still the highest standard of living in the world, as long as we are able to stay above the poverty line.

The hallmark of dissociation is the ability to tolerate marked incongruity and there are some very dramatic examples of this kind of tolerance in our cultural milieu. One obvious example is our attitudes and behaviors towards violence. On the one hand, we are terribly concerned about violence and the fact that we cannot walk our city streets at night, it is not unlikely that we will be assaulted at work, our schools must be equipped with metal detectors, and no one feels safe. Yet, we continue to buy guns at alarming rates, guns which are clearly shown to kill far more family members than assaultive strangers, and we continue to psychically feed off of the nightly array of violent acts of perpetration on our television and movie screens. Even though the public continues to provide enormous support for gun control, our legislatures refuse to enact gun laws or overturn laws that exist.

There is a very peculiar dissociative break here. We are terrified of being shot, so we arm ourselves, and we get shot with alarmingly increased frequency. And yet we still accede to a gun lobby that equates the very foundation of American democracy with gun ownership. Crime rises, we put more people in prison, crime continues to rise so we build more traumatizing prisons and then let out onto the streets, men and women who are more brutal than when they entered the prison system. This is all very odd.

Another example is that of child abuse. According to the September 1996 Executive Summary of the Third National Incidence Study of Child Abuse and Neglect performed by the U.S. Department of Health and Human Services and other federal agencies, the number of seriously injured children who are victims of abuse and neglect *quadrupled* from 1986 to 1993 and this is not thought to be due to increased reporting but to a real rise in the problem (Sedlak and Broadhurst 1996). Given that we now definitively know that there are serious short-term and long-term physical, emotional, economic, social, criminal, and parenting consequences for child abuse and neglect, does it strike anyone else as odd that these figures have led to so little public concern? Why is it that most people who read newspapers or watch television can provide detailed information about the spurious "false memory syndrome," a pseudodiagnosis that has never been scientifically validated by a single controlled study, given by an organization that provides support for people accused of sexually offending against their children, while few of them will be acquainted with the fact that according to the same government study, the estimated number of sexually abused children rose from 1986 to 1993 by 83 percent?

When my individual patients are saying they want help to feel safe while they are slicing their arms with razor blades, I know that I am dealing with a severely split, dissociated person who is suffering from a trauma-based syndrome. And I know that until I increase that patient's level of awareness, he or she will stay in that dissociated trance state, because increasing their level of awareness, breaking through their wall of denial, is going to make them uncomfortable long before it brings relief. They are going to have to learn to feel again, to give up the safety of emotional numbness and rely once again on human compassion and righteous indignation.

The continuing denial of reality in my individual patients leads to increasing disability and self-destructiveness. So too, cultural denial of the fundamental organizing principle of trauma in our social makeup is particularly virulent at this time in our cultural history. It is now that we need a comprehensive, cohesive, and compassionate cognitive framework that provides us with a direction and process for strategizing about meaningful and effective social change. Pretending that the problems do not exist, or referring them back to explanations that have been shown to lead to ineffective solutions is patently self-destructive to us all.

Multiple Addictions

All sin tends to be addictive, and the terminal point of addiction is what is called damnation.

—W. H. Auden 1970, *A Certain World*

In using the word "addiction" here, I am not just referring to the biological addiction characteristic of alcohol and many drugs. I mean addiction in its broader sense, any behavior that is in some way destructive and beyond the individual's ability to control by an act of conscious will. Used in this sense, addiction is a characteristic of American culture. Humans can apparently become addicted to virtually anything—and we do. Substance abuse is a major problem accounting for billions of dollars in social expense, to say nothing of the enormous human toll in lost or disabled lives. But there are also addictions to varied forms of sexual behavior leading to disorders characterized by sexual compulsivity. Many people suffer from addictive problems related to food, leading to a variety of physical, emotional, and social difficulties. Spending is another American addiction, constructive in that our consumer spending boosts the economy, destructive in that we have an excruciating national debt, increasingly dangerous environmental problems, and a cultural milieu that generates a particularly lethal form of envy.

But perhaps our most virulent addiction, the one that affects us all, is violence. I call violence an addiction because, although we have long been fascinated by violent men and violent acts, our preoccupation with violent behavior has now reached such a pitch that it threatens the very stability of our major social institutions. Our nation was born in a violent struggle and the repetition of that struggle for survival continues today via our willingness to equate guns with safety, despite all evidence to the contrary. History repeats itself as automatically for the social group as it does for the individual.

Automatic Repetition

> Those who cannot remember the past are condemned to repeat it.
>
> —George Santayana (1863–1952)

> Every time history repeats itself the price goes up.
>
> —Anonymous

I suspect strongly that traumatic reenactment is a potent force in our national life. Automatically we repeat the past because it is a habit to do so, because we feel compelled to do so, because we cannot see any other way of doing things. There is an increasing awareness of the cycles that we become trapped in—the cycle of violence, the cycle of abuse and the cycle of poverty are good examples. But we need to get much better at understanding, analyzing, predicting, and altering these patterns.

On our psychiatric unit, the conceptual framework of traumatic reenactment has helped us to understand much of the seemingly contrary, perverse, odd, and, of course, repetitive behavior of our patients. This understanding has helped us bridge a gap between our world and theirs, a gap that was so wide before that we could not even communicate effectively about constructive change. As long as we were blaming them for a problem that they could not even see, our insistence that they change the problem was just more people saying, "It's all your fault," and they had been hearing that for years, helpless to do anything to alter the problem behavior. When we were able to say, "You keep doing the same thing over and over. It's not your fault. These habits originated in good coping skills that have now gone awry. But change is now your responsibility as well as the responsibility of the social group who failed to protect you from harm in the first place," obstacles to self-efficacy began to clear away.

This is a middle position binding together a recognition that people are injured by other people and suffer consequences of these injuries, that then compel them to go on injuring themselves. It is a way out of the false dichotomies we become trapped in when we excuse terrible behavior because a person has been victimized, or feel righteously justified in victimizing someone because they have done terrible things. In reality, "hurt people hurt people" with a regularity and predictability that is frightening. Our patients must be held accountable for their repetitive and destructive behavior or they will not alter the traumatic reenactment scenario. On our unit, if someone cuts themselves, or threatens someone else in any way, we take this behavior very seriously and there are consequences to the behavior that limit the individual's freedom to continue pursuing the destructive acts. But, they need us to know them well enough to understand the ways in which the past is connected to the present, and to see the repetitive patterns which dissociation has left them blind to. They need us to encourage, cajole, push, threaten, set limits on, and emotionally parent them while they struggle to see another reality, an alternative pattern of behavior that is a way out of the trap of reenactment. It is not possible to do this alone.

As a society, we need to view our chronic social problems from the same point of view. Problems of poverty, homelessness, unemployment, and crime eat away at our social fabric. In discussions of these problems, people of compassion stand on one side of a great divide pointing out the impossible and quite real dilemmas that the poor, minorities, homeless, unemployed, and criminal have been subjected to since childhood. On the other side of this divide are people of responsibility who insist, just as loudly, that all these disadvantages can be overcome and failure to do so is a personal failure of responsibility and should be punished. They are both right and both wrong. One side focuses on the social, the other on the individual when solutions can only come out of an integration of both points of view. Individual victims *do* need to assume responsibility for altering the patterns of behavior that lead to destructive lives. But it is impossible for them to succeed without the help and support of their social group. Punishment is not an adequate substitute for compassionate problem resolution nor is forgiveness an adequate substitute for accountability.

Avoidance of Feelings and Accountability

If we Americans are to survive it will have to be because we choose and elect and defend to be first of all Americans; to present to the world one homogeneous and unbroken front, whether of white Americans or black ones or purple or blue or green.... If we in America have reached that point in our

desperate culture when we must murder children, no matter for what reason or what color, we don't deserve to survive, and probably won't.
                    —William Faulkner 1958, Interview in *Writers at Work*

Our patients struggle mightily to confront squarely their history of victimization after many years of avoiding the reality of the past. But it is much more difficult to confront the knowledge of knowing you have done something very wrong, something inconsistent with your values and with the way you view yourself. Many times people become so overwhelmed by the shame associated with admitting the role they have played in perpetrating destructive acts against others, that their rationalization, denial, avoidance, and dissociation appear totally divorced from reality, psychotic, or just deceitful. Confrontation with one's own perpetration can be life-threatening because of the shame it evokes and for some people, the shame of even being ashamed. Gilligan points out that among the men he has worked with in prison, "This is a secret that many of them would die than reveal . . . in fact many of them do die not to reveal it" (1996). The secret Gilligan refers to is shame in the absence of either love or guilt. For our psychiatric patients there is often shame *and* guilt, also without the love, and the magnitude of these emotional states can lead to dangerous, and sometimes lethal, suicidal acts.

People engage in acts of violence as a form of real or symbolic self-defense. As Gilligan has said "all violence is an attempt to achieve justice, or what the violent person perceives as justice" (1996). In the criminal population the justification for acts of violence are often overt, rationalized, primitive and seemingly free from guilt. In the psychiatric population, the justification is often hidden behind the mask of dissociation and denial. But there is another tune being played behind all the obfuscation and avoidance of the effects of one's violence. That other tune is knowledge. Anyone who has perpetrated against another knows, at some level of consciousness, that he or she has done so and this knowledge has a corrosive effect if it remains unconscious. Some people self-destruct, others escalate their hurting of others, and still others fail to protect those whom they love, but whatever the case here is a downward spiral of hypocrisy, deceit, betrayal, and corruption that can only be healed through confession, atonement, and restitution. Such acts of contrition, however, require a social group that is willing to help the perpetrator tolerate the depth of self-annihilating shame that is the price to be paid for true remorse.

Nations also commit acts of violence in the name of national security and defense. Across the globe, there are few nations who can claim to be free of the taint of violent perpetration, either through active participation or a failure to act to prevent, acts of mass violence and genocide. The Treaty of Versailles represented the Allies' attempt to hold Germany accountable for the aggression World War I; the Nuremberg Trials represent the Allies attempt to hold Germany, through her leaders, accountable for World War II; the Truth and Reconciliation Commission in South Africa represents that nation's attempt to hold internal perpetrators accountable for acts of violence against their own group. These are all examples of large social experiments in wrestling with issues involving national acts of perpetration against individual citizens and against entire groups of people.

But we have a long way to go. How much of our national discontent, anxiety, and ongoing angst is related to an underlying knowing without knowing—an awareness of national guilt for acts of perpetration which we have actively engaged in or passively allowed? In 1995, the Smithsonian Museum became embroiled in a loud, many-sided debate about a planned exhibit commemorating the dropping of the first nuclear bombs on Hiroshima and Nagasaki, illustrating our push-pull dilemma in even coming to terms with this kind of national dilemma, an argument already over fifty years old. What national shame and guilt could be corroding our foundations if we consider, for example, acts of genocide directed at Native Americans, slavery, the fratricide of the Civil War, Vietnam, and our involvement in internal acts of violence in Argentina, Chile, Nicaragua, El Salvador, Guatemala, Turkey, and many other countries around the world? Could we be trapped in a spiral of avoidance and corruption as we enact legislation and enforce policies that make the poor even poorer, rob citizens of health care, rescind efforts directed at racial integration, undo environmental protection measures, and place unendurable stresses on American families?[1]

This is a huge and vitally important challenge that will extend well into the twenty-first century and one that we cannot afford to avoid. How do we contend with the fact that otherwise good people sometimes do very bad things? How do we evolve systems that hold perpetrators accountable for their actions without further traumatizing our social body? How do we achieve a viable system of justice that does not depend upon acts of punishment that simply perpetuate or promote further injustice?

The avoidance of such unpleasant or disturbing questions is ubiquitous and can be used by an individual, by a group, by a community, or by a nation. As we see in so many of our patients, denial can be life-saving in the presence of acute threat. But continuing to avoid reality rather than solving problems has disastrous results. Rafael Moses raises the question of what price we pay for this type of denial and asserts: "Bluntly stated, I believe that such denial brings about an impediment in the ability to face and therefore deal with the danger that is being partially denied. By not facing danger, the society, just as the person, is able to deal less efficiently than possible with the approaching threat" (Moses 1989).

Alienation From Self and Others

Alienation as our present destiny is achieved only by outrageous violence perpetrated by human beings on human beings. No man can begin to think, feel or act now except from the starting point of his or her own alienation.

—R.D. Laing

Alienation is defined as emotional isolation or dissociation, a state of estrangement between the self and the objective world or between different parts of the personality. Our patients start from a position of alienation and many of the most prominent intellectuals, writers, playwrights, and poets of the twentieth century have seen alienation as a starting point for a discussion of the plight of modern man.

For our patients, the most corrosive loss that accompanies a legacy of abuse, is the loss of meaning and purpose. It is as much a spiritual as an emotional or physical sense of loss. Proverbs 29:18 of the Hebrew Bible tells us that "Where there is no vision the people perish" and I suspect that this proverb holds true, regardless of whether it is applied to an individual or to a society.

Like our traumatized survivors of abuse, perhaps we, as a whole people, avoid the pain of confronting real horrors and thereby deny whole segments of our experience because we lack a clear vision of different world, a different way of being. Whether we call it a crisis of conscience, a crisis of meaning, or a crisis of values, we are apparently at a crisis point, a crossroads and our options are still open. Perhaps, like our patients, we have learned to be helpless, avoidant, dissociated, alienated and thus we compulsively reenact the past, because like them we have had no other way to understand or think about what our problems mean or how we got into this situation. Perhaps we all carry around a legacy of blindness about our individual and collective pasts, in refusing to see the elephant in the room our vision ahead is blocked.

If this is true, if we do in fact live in a society, one of whose central organizing principle has become the legacy of denied and suppressed traumatic experience and all that accompanies it, then much that we have learned about prevention, intervention, and treatment of the individual may have some degree of applicability to the social group as well. If our society is, in fact, organized around trauma, what are the forces in the society that permit or promote the occurrences of overwhelming stress, forces that may be controllable if we can properly identify them? Can we—together—construct a different and workable vision for the future that corrects the mistakes of the past and gradually places us on a path that leads away from the ravages of traumatic reenactment?

LESSONS FROM THE SANCTUARY MODEL AND MORAL SAFETY

Moving Toward an Ecological Viewpoint—It's All A Matter of Balance

> The Noble Path, that transcends the two extreme and leads to Enlightenment and wisdom and peace of mind, may be called the Middle Way. What is the Middle Way: It consists of the Eightfold Noble Path: right view, right thought, right speech, right behavior, right livelihood, right effort, right mindfulness, and right concentration.
>
> —from *The Teaching of Buddha*

The naturalist and biologist Lyall Watson has also been struggling with the issue of violence. He has looked at the natural environment from an ecological viewpoint and has noted that there are three principle ways in which benign things deteriorate into the malign: 1) Good things get to be bad if they are displaced, taken out of context or removed from their evolutionary environment; 2) Good things get very bad if there are too few or too many of them; 3) And good things get really rotten if they cannot relate to each other properly and their degree of association is impoverished (Watson 1995). I was struck by how useful an ecological point of view is to the way we function as individuals and as groups. It embraces the idea of balance—anything goes bad, no matter how good it is, if it is out of balance with itself, its neighbors, and its environment.

We learned that although our patients tended to look for extreme solutions to end their pain, the better road was the middle road. Our job was to help them find some sort of balance. I suspect that this is a necessary goal for the beginning of any intervention that aims at creating a safer, healthier, more loving world—balance. Without focusing on how to get to the middle we repeatedly end up enacting policy that moves the pendulum from one extreme to the opposite, but just as problematic, extreme. Right now, our health care situation is one example. In order to compensate for problems in one direction, we have succeed in producing opposite and just as destructive problems. We have not solved the problems; we have just shifted them from one group to another.

Fostering Groups, Fostering Communities

> When committees gather, each member is necessarily an actor, uncontrollably acting out the part of himself, reading the lines that identify him, asserting his identity.... We are designed, coded, it seems, to place the highest priority on being individuals, and we must do this first, at whatever cost, even if it means disability for the group.
> —Lewis Thomas, M. D. 1979, *The Medusa and the Snail*

America is the land of opportunity for individuals and I wouldn't have it any other way, except that maybe we have taken a good thing a bit too far. Our strong emphasis on the development of the individual and the role of competition in this development has brought us where we are today—for good and for ill. The problem—as in all things—is one of balance and integration. Were we to ban the creative efforts of the individual we would find ourselves in a mess at least as problematic as the one we are in today. But we could envision a future in which the best efforts of each individual are integrated into a whole. This will require compromises and limits on the part of the individual and the group but it can be done. In fact, every successful orchestra in the world does just that. I am convinced this orchestral way of functioning can occur outside of the symphony hall because I have been working in concert with a group of creative individuals for almost twenty years and the music we make together far surpasses our individual efforts.

Orchestral working and living, however, does require some important organizational steps—shared values, shared goals, and shared practices. When we first created *The Sanctuary,* it was vital for us to articulate the values that we share and it has been necessary to continuously restate those values with the formation of every new community—which is virtually every day. Every time we meet as a team we have to decide what our goals are for the meeting. As treatment providers, we must collaborate with each patient to establish the goals for the patient's stay. We also had to establish practices that would promote frequent communication, opportunities to evaluate whether we are remaining consistent with our values, methods for surfacing conflicts, occasions for laughter and debriefing after stress, and methods to deal with crises. I have had opportunities to consult with other treatment programs, schools, and churches and these processes of establishing values, goals, and practices appear to be necessary reconstitution steps for any organization. One of the most strenuous challenges for any group is overcoming our deeply ingrained tendency to compulsively compete. Any group of people must remind themselves that the goal of group formation is to integrate various points of view not to have one point of view emerge as victorious over others. This requires turning our definition of success on its head, requiring us to feel like we have failed if one singular point of view is dominant over others.

Establishing Safety: First and Foremost

The bomb that fell on Hiroshima fell on America too. It fell on no city, no munition plants, no docks. It erased no church, vaporized no public buildings, reduced no man to his atomic elements. But it fell, it fell. It burst. It shook the land. God have mercy on our children. God have mercy on America.

—Hermann Hagedorn

The first value to be established, goal to be set, and practice to be formulated is that of safety. Regardless of whether we are referring to an individual victim of violence, a small group, or an entire community, healing cannot advance unless there is an environment of safety for all community members. This is a tall order because violence seems to out of control, so beyond our ability to confront it. However, people can take back their homes, their streets, and their workplaces if they choose to do so and all over the country people are experimenting with doing just that. One of the obstacles to progress is, again, our unbalanced approach towards individual rights. To reclaim our dangerous streets we may need to enact and enforce legislation that appears to be in conflict with the rights of some individuals. It may be time for us to realize that we have a public health emergency, an epidemic of violent perpetration, that can be arrested if we have the will to do so. Remember, most of the dysfunction, adjustment problems and outright disorders, that I have mentioned in these pages, are 100 percent preventable.

Containing the Infection of Intergenerational Trauma: Investing in Families

You may house their bodies but not their souls, for their souls dwell in the house of tomorrow, which you cannot visit, not even in your dreams. You may strive to be like them, but seek not to make them like you, for life goes not backward nor tarries with yesterday. You are the bows from which your children as living arrows are sent forth.

—Kahlil Gibran

The current statistics on child abuse are terrifying in their implications and the abuse cuts across every socioeconomic and racial group. Child abuse bears more than a passing similarity to radiation poisoning, because it silently works its effects on subsequent generations, not through genetic mutation, but through the subtle but potent effect of disrupted attachment relationships.

Fortunately, it is a bit easier to alter attachment relationships for the better than it is to alter genetic structure. But it still will require an investment of time, money, and effort to do so. We can at least begin by focusing on mothers and families who are designated as being at high-risk for the kinds of problems that correlate with child abuse, problems like overwhelmed teenage mothers, single mothers who lack social support, parents involved in substance abuse, parents who have been abused or neglected themselves, families involved in domestic violence. High-risk families need to be provided with opportunities for nontraumatic attachments that they will probably not be able to find on their own. They are designated high-risk because they are already trapped in the multigenerational cycle of abuse and neglect.

We cannot wait for young, impoverished, and traumatized young mothers to repeat the past—we have to provide help for them before they get into trouble. One way to do this is through neonatal home visitation programs such as Hawaii's Healthy Start. The program is voluntary but 95 percent of high-risk mothers consent to be a part of the program. The family is assigned a home helper who stays in contact with the family for the first three years of the child's life. With this program, and many others like it, the rate of abuse and neglect has been significantly reduced at a cost that is meager compared to the long-term costs that continued abuse will lead to (Breakey and Pratt 1991). This is a program that "parents the parents" and has been repeatedly shown to be effective.

Homelessness in this nation is an absurdity. There is no excuse for a child to grow up without a home or a family. Every community needs alternative family living arrangements for parents who are faced with a wide spectrum of conditions that impair parental functioning so that treatment is provided while healthier living conditions are found for the entire family. This includes various impaired populations such as substance abusers, the mentally ill, and victims of domestic violence. A major area of community involvement needs to focus on universal access to high quality infant-toddler day care. Supplementing regular day care, each community also needs crisis child care and respite care, recognizing the reality of parents' lives and in the willingness to help, providing an alternative to abuse for the stressed family.

Despite well-intended efforts, there is so much intergenerational damage in the population that some families will be beyond help. These children will end up in a foster care system that cannot meet their needs. By definition, foster care families must deal with children who have been so neglected or abused that removal from their own families was necessary.

These children present multiple and often overwhelming problems that can only be adequately managed in the most carefully thought-out and supervised systems. Such systems are expensive and with the deconstruction of the health care environment, there are few facilities any longer available, even for the most severely damaged children. Last week I was informed that an abused six-year-old girl, who was talking about suicide, was refused admission to a major center because she "had no clearly defined plan for suicide." We have a very big mess to clean up and *somebody* must be willing to be the substitute parents that these children need.

Maybe we need to consider creating a profession of parenting so that caretakers can be trained to parent troubled children in a home setting and make enough income so that reparenting these damaged children becomes their primary occupation. Adults whose attachment relationships have been severely damaged when they were children can learn to parent adequately, but it takes a great deal of time and effort. And in the meantime, the children are still not safe. We have to plan more creatively for balanced approaches that maintain family connection but which *also* adequately protect the child. Only then can we hope to arrest the cycle of abuse.

And we must not forget the adolescents. Adolescence is the final chance for many young people, the last stop on the road prior to adult deviance. Adolescents are still flexible enough to change, grow, and overcome many developmental insults. Many families are able to raise a young child with some degree of success but then fail when the child reaches adolescence. Special therapeutic family situations must be established to deal with adolescents who are able to function adequately outside of their family of origin but who decompensate when exposed to continued family dysfunction. Here again, we must find ways to maintain connection with the families of origin while providing the adolescent with whatever he or she needs to grow into a healthy adult.

The proposed focus on high risk families is not meant to imply that inadequate parenting is a problem only of the poor and disenfranchised. The high risk approach simply reflects the long-standing medical tradition of triage, a system used to allocate a scarce commodity to those most in need. There are few families today that are not under significant stress and the very structure of modern family life lends itself to interfamilial tension, stress, disharmony, detachment, and violence. Every city, town, and village in America needs free access to community parenting centers, centers that can become a focus of community life, buildings that afford the opportunity for formal classes and informal consultation about parenting, family life, and other emotionally sensitive issues as well as recreation, cultural events, political meetings, and service opportunities (DeMause 1993; Linden and McFarland 1993). A strong community focus on parenting and education can provide a core for the reestablishment of a sense of community and the ongoing practice of democratic principles, but to be effective the entire community must be pushed, encouraged, and even coerced into participation—including the employers in the community who play such an important role in determining family health or dysfunction.

Trauma Debriefing

> Chaos, against which the only weapon God has ever given us is memory.
>
> —Steve Erickson, *Arc d'X*

Although we have complex procedures and special emergency teams to deal with physical emergencies, relatively little attention is paid to the early intervention and prevention of psychological trauma. Specially trained crisis teams need to be formed in every social setting to educate people about the primary and secondary effects of trauma exposure, to provide written information, and to encourage important health measures, such as encouraging victims to talk and other members in their social support system to listen. Trauma debriefing should occur whenever violence erupts in school, at the workplace, or anywhere else in the community. Special attention needs to be given to law enforcement officers, medical personnel, and firefighters, who risk extraordinary exposure to overwhelming traumatic experiences and death (Anderson 1995; Flannery 1990; Flannery et al. 1991).

Creating Sanctuary in the Classroom

> The adult does not understand symbolism easily. . . . The child possesses this understanding intuitively. . .this intuition of the first years of life is quickly lost and replaced by what is usually called common sense but which in reality is merely stupidity based on repression.
>
> —Georg Groddeck 1925, *The Meaning of Illness*

The school setting naturally lends itself to the creation of sanctuary-type environments (Bloom 1995a; Staub 1992a). But to turn a system around a great deal of preparatory work has to be accomplished first. It is clear that the violent and disruptive students in high school, frequently become violent and disruptive adults and that these were the same children who were misbehaving in grade school. As researchers have repeatedly demonstrated,

"The stability of aggressive behavior patterns throughout the life course is one of the most consistently documented patterns found in longitudinal research" (Laub and Lauritsen 1995).

The children who are the most disruptive in the classroom are called "conduct-disordered" children. For the most part, these problems originate in abuse, neglect, and exposure to violence at home and are often exacerbated by punitive measures in school. Schools in the past have not been successful at managing these children just as we were never successful at managing our most difficult cases before we understood more about the causes of violent behavior. These are the most traumatized children and they can be understood and managed only by having a cognitive framework that helps organize our thinking and plan coherent strategies. Our work at The Sanctuary with adult victims of trauma has demonstrated to us that victims of trauma require a balanced approach—nurture, compassion, and care balanced with a strong emphasis on self-discipline, personal accountability, and social responsibility. It is not a "hard" approach versus a "soft" approach, but an integrated approach that makes a difference. But to accomplish the development of an integrated approach, all of the members of the school community who are devising a violence prevention strategy for the school, must share a knowledge base and a set of assumptions not dissimilar to those we articulated when we established The Sanctuary.

The first goal in establishing a school as a sanctuary is reclaiming the sense of safety that is so vital if learning is to occur. The requirements are very similar to our experience in a psychiatric inpatient unit. There has to be a "zero tolerance" for violence of any kind. A variety of different measures may have to be instituted in order for the adults in the system to regain sufficient control of the physical environment for the children and faculty to feel safe once again. This may include creating special programs for the conduct-disordered children, as well as links with juvenile probation and other community resources.[2]

The safety measures are necessary but will not hold without reinforcing change in the entire context that has until now supported a culture of violence. Innovative programs and a strong commitment to addressing the needs of the most troubled youngsters can go a long way toward restoring order to the school systems. But restoring order is not sufficient. My patients cannot move further in treatment until they learn how to protect themselves and others. The cessation of overt violence does not mean that the problems have been solved. We have to learn together ways of resolving conflicts that encourage and support human growth and connection.

Children need multiple opportunities to develop attachments to other children and to adults. The emotional system of a child is still developing, and children ultimately must learn systems of internal control if they are to function adequately with others. Likewise, the overcontrol of emotions can be extremely detrimental to physical and mental health. Therefore, a vital part of childhood learning centers on learning how to manage a variety of emotional experiences both intra- and interpersonally. Can we expect the schools to solve all of our social problems? Certainly not without a great deal of help from the rest of us. But I suspect the schools could solve—or rather prevent—many of our future problems if we made some rather dramatic changes in the way we currently think of schools.

Any constructive change requires the creation of a shared vision. When we began to construct our system, we had to envision the kind of place where we wanted to work, learn, and grow. We knew that if the environment was healthy for us it would also be healthy for our patients. Likewise, if the school is an environment that promotes growth, expression, and learning for the faculty and the administrators it will also be a learning environment for the children. But just as the fundamental mission of our environment was to help traumatized adults become functioning and healthier citizens, the mission of the school is to help produce functioning and healthy citizens. This means that we always must keep in mind the ends and repeatedly check whether our means helps to further the ends. Certain similarities in the two environments emerge when ideas about creating sanctuary are applied to both.

Children need to learn the process of practicing democracy from the moment they set foot in a school. The classroom needs to be children's first experience in learning how to do group process while preserving individual integrity. This means creating classrooms that are therapeutic communities. In this model, the classroom would become a sanctuary-type environment from elementary school through high school. An essential goal of the entire classroom group would be to create a "cooperative context" for learning in which students learn how to resolve conflicts constructively (Johnson and Johnson 1995). This learning can proceed in parallel with more traditional educational goals as the social context itself becomes the medium within which the message of the educational discussion is actively learned. At any point in the school day a child or teacher could call a "council meeting" to immediately resolve interpersonal problems that are interfering with learning (Mercogliano 1995). This is part of the change in process similar to our use of special community meetings and staffings to manage particularly difficult problems. Reminiscent of our own experience with changing our system, creating schools that are truly sanctuaries will require change at the level of basic assumptions and structure and without such change, simple instrumental changes will be useless.

When self-governing, conflict-resolving, cooperative strategies for problem solving are in place, established as the social norm, and reinforced by the adults and older children in the system, children learn to resolve their own problems, think for themselves, cooperatively govern, and problem-solve without violence. In such a community atmosphere, children have the opportunity to develop multiple attachments with many different people. If these attachments are promoted early enough in a child's life, much of the damage that occurs in their families of origin can be undone or at least mitigated. In this kind of a setting, children are offered repeated opportunities to learn how to modulate their emotional experiences by turning to adults for soothing, by helping each other, and by watching the reactions of other children. Gradually, they develop self-soothing and self-control habits that are neither disturbingly expressive or overly suppressed. This self-control greatly enhances their capacity to learn.

In a more democratic and egalitarian system, children learn about authority that is based not on bigness or power but on more knowledge, more moral authority, or more leadership skills. The result of interacting with a more democratically influenced authority structure is that this becomes internalized as their own sense of authority over their own impulses. In this way they also learn how to protect themselves more effectively from abusive authority. Children who have people to turn to who can help them manage overwhelming feelings are far less likely to turn to addictive substances or behaviors. Children must learn how to manage their aggressive feelings constructively and creatively. In a community setting where open and honest communication is valued, children can see the consequences of each other's behavior and can insist that each assume responsibility for those behaviors. Children are capable of establishing equitable systems of justice and restitution that teach them important and far-reaching life skills. With effort, all of this contextual learning can occur in parallel with the required academic pursuits.

Artistic creativity and performance are necessary forms of human expression and are particularly important for children who have so much to express but a limited vocabulary with which to do so. The kinds of mental activities that are associated with creativity are essential for creative problem solving, for negotiating complex social situations, and for understanding and fully appreciating relationships. The arts give form, shape, and sound to the numinous, the traumatic, and the nonverbal, which can therefore be brought into full awareness and integrated into overall functioning. Without this we are doomed to obtain knowledge about only a very limited aspect of ourselves, others, and the world. And without this knowledge we are doomed to repeat our past mistakes.[3]

Changing the Process of Doing Business

> History teaches us that men and nations behave wisely once they have exhausted all other alternatives.
>
> —Abba Eban

The initial corporate response to violence in the workplace is usually to improve basic safety, just as creating physical safety is the first vital mission in any attempt to create sanctuary. Creating a safe workplace means setting a zero tolerance for violence whether it is physical, verbal, or nonverbal (Barrier 1995a).[4] The cultural norm must be established that violence is to be taken extremely seriously—any threat of violence whether subtle or direct. Companies that do so are establishing a different social norm and set of expectations in relation to violence, at work and at home.

But physical and behavioral safety measures, along with trying to keep violent people out of the workplace, are not enough, just as installing safety screens or locking doors is never sufficient to keep a psychiatric unit safe. More important is creating a "violence-free company culture" (Barrier 1995b). There are many different aspects to the creation of such a culture, some of which—as with *The Sanctuary*—involve setting much clearer limits and firmer expectations, and others of which place a strong emphasis on education, personal communication, openness, democratic and consensus decision making, and freedom of expression.

Our patients have taught us about the corrosive effects of power, how this corrosion spreads throughout a family, down through the generations, and consumes entire lives like some virulent cancer. I can no longer grapple with the issue of power and powerlessness in the individual lives of my patients without simultaneously struggling to grapple with the uses and abuses of power at the level of the groupmind, most obvious as demonstrated in industry, management, government, and the military. The whole issue of perpetration is at stake. It is socially acceptable to perpetrate violence against children only because we live in a culture in which the exploitation of others for one's own gain is acceptable practice. Violence is not unacceptable, it is simply regulated. Only people who have power are able to hurt other people and have their behavior condoned by the state.

Nothing has value in and of itself. It is this paradigm that allows us to base an economy on weapons, to spoil the environment, to sell dangerous substances, and it cannot easily be changed without catastrophic upheaval. This does not just occur in the context of the family—it is our existing and accepted social paradigm in government and in business.

We rationalize it. We call this abuse of power many things. We justify hurting others in the name of "freedom," "democracy," "capitalism," "healthy competition," "a free market economy," but we hurt them nonetheless. As Americans, we hurt individuals, and we hurt groups of people, and we hurt entire nations, and we even sometimes hurt the whole world—and then we lie about it to ourselves. We excuse our hurting by talking about how other people don't take responsibility for themselves, or they really want to be miserable, or their misery is their own fault, or their suffering is what they need in order to improve themselves. The excuses—or "reasons"—I hear for our shared behavior on news reports, from politicians, and in the papers sound extraordinarily like the excuses of child abusers when confronted with their behavior—"he deserved it, he was bad"; or, "She really wanted it," or, "I'm just trying to teach them what the world is all about." As long as our corporate and government leaders support, condone, and encourage a value system that promotes violent perpetration—regardless of whether that support is overt or covert—children will never be safe and the flow of patients to our doorstep will continue unrelentingly.

What is clear from what we know now is that we must change our way of dealing with ourselves and each other at every level of our society. At a fundamental level of process this means, changing our definition of what constitutes "success." In our present way of doing business, success is too often defined as winning, beating out the other guy.[5] In a world in which we recognize our interconnectedness and interdependence, success must be redefined to reflect the joy not of winning, but of integrating various points of view, solving problems, and hammering out compromises. Inevitably, this also means changing the way we deal with each other emotionally, because winning and losing implies a rise in self-esteem for the winner with a commensurate loss of self-esteem and increase in shame for the loser. Shame leads to many outcomes, most of which are detrimental to the well-being of the whole. We need to move to a cultural scenario in which we learn to protect each other from shame rather than reveling in and deliberately inducing it. This requires kindness and compassion, which are human traits that can be ignored or cultivated as a matter of choice.

When I became the leader of a group of people, not only did I reap benefits from this position, but I also assumed a mantle of responsibility for the safety and well-being of those who followed me. This is what corporate responsibility is all about. Simultaneously, I had a responsibility to those in positions of power over me, to provide them with the benefits they needed from me. Many of our business corporations presently seem much clearer about their responsibility to their shareholders than they are about their responsibility to those who depend upon then for their safety and well-being. A more balanced approach to corporate responsibility will require overturning some fastly held shibboleths about the importance of competition, obedience to the bottom-line, and the sanctity of money.6 As Michael Linton warns: "It all comes down to money in the end. The problems of the world come from our actions, and our actions, both as a society and as individuals, are largely determined by the way money works. Many trivial and even damaging things are happening—simply because some people have the money and the will to do them. In contrast, other things of real value, many essential to the survival of the planet, are not happening—simply because those who have the will, have not the money. People are working in ways detrimental to their personal health, to that of the environment, both locally and globally, and to the well-being of their community because they need the money" (1993).

Justice as Sanctuary

> Justice is conscience, not a personal conscience but the conscience of the whole of humanity. Those who clearly recognize the voice of their own conscience usually recognize also the voice of justice.
> —Alexander Solzhenitsyn

Justice is defined as the quality of fairness, the upholding of what is fair treatment and due reward in accordance with honor, standards or law. The question of what is just and how is justice served permeates much of our political and social discourse, and of course, is the main focus of concern for our criminal justice system. But justice has always been a slippery term, vulnerable to being used to condone the most infernal acts. Punishment is a penalty imposed for wrongdoing. Historically, justice has often been served through the administration of punishment. The entire notion of punishment as just, however, is a provocative one, particularly when punishment results in further traumatizing a guilty person and thus turning the administrators of justice into perpetrators themselves, along the lines of "two wrongs don't make a right." Do we serve justice when we place human beings, even though they are wrongdoers, into environments which are inherently, dangerous, abusive, unjust and hence traumatogenic?

Herman Bianchi has proposed a model for a new justice system that is consistent with what we have learned about managing traumatized and perpetrating patients. He argues for new methods that will enable people to experience the law as supportive of them and their social interactions, which will focus on conflict resolution, restitution, and atonement rather than punishment, and will involve the perpetrator and the victim in meaningful ways that stand a reasonable chance of making the situation better, not worse (Bianchi 1995).

Based on our clinical work, this approach makes more sense both for the perpetrators, the victims, and for those of us who are responsible for enforcing a system of justice. People who have demonstrated by their behavior that they cannot safely live freely with other people must be deprived of the right to do so in order to protect others. Such arrested development requires special facilities that are restrictive and sufficiently ordered to prevent the person from inflicting further harm, and that provide adequate opportunities for maturation if the person is capable of change. Reifying childish behavior to an identification with evil is an incentive to pursue the same behavior—it can create a sense of pride, not shame. Failure to manage responsibility is a sign of immaturity, of insufficient parenting, of developmental arrest, of inadequate emotional reward for engaging in the difficulties of trying more mature behavior. As such, the response should not be further trauma, which encourages such emotional responses as rage, vengefulness, projection, and blaming, but a withdrawal of privileges with clear guidelines for the type of behavior that must follow if the privileges are to be returned. Far too often, punishment has no meaningful connection to problem solving, to actual correction of the problem. Instead, punishment, while disguised as being for the person being punished, is actually a way for the punisher to vent the unacceptable emotions aroused in him or her by the transgressor or by someone else.

Much as we shun the idea, our criminals are a part of us too. If we look at our social body as being an interconnected whole, then the criminal population can be seen as a split-off, negative, shadow part of us that we deny, suppress, punish, and even try to kill. Yet in their deviance, our criminals point to the darker parts of our social world, to what happens to human beings who are reared in environments lacking in love and in moral conscience. In disturbed families, children become the "poison containers" for all the distress and disturbance that the family feels unable to manage.

Criminals become the poison containers for the distress and disturbance of entire societies, allowing the society to blame the individual criminals rather than look at the social circumstances that promoted the aberrant and destructive behavior. In a balanced approach, wrongdoers are held responsible for their behavior and so is a society which failed to sufficiently protect and nurture the child that criminal once was.

Producing an Emotionally Literate Population

> Human history becomes more and more a race between education and catastrophe.
>
> —H. G. Wells

A large body of knowledge is available about the effects of trauma, the necessary ingredients for healthy child development, the normal and traumatic processing of memory and emotions, the importance of human relationships set within a context of values, the process of cognitive development, problem solving, conflict resolution, and mediation. Unfortunately, however, few people know very much about any of this information. We spend far too much time consuming lurid news tabloids and violent entertainment. The media could and should play a vital role in making this body of knowledge available to the general public, showing the interrelatedness of this information and the complex nature of human behavior, rather than attempting to oversimplify and sensationalize. Democracy needs an educated, cognitively developed, and aware populace. Relatively few opportunities exist for children or adults to develop these skills through the national media, other than on educational television, which chronically begs for subscribers. But this means finding commentators, news anchors, and reporters who can think in broader terms than black-or-white sound bites, and media executives who are willing to see themselves as social leaders, not profiteers.

Good parenting skills do not come in the genes. If you have been lucky enough to have good parents, you will probably be a good parent yourself, as long as misfortune does not dog your tail. If you have had less than good parenting, however, then your automatic parenting will be marginally better than the generation before. There is really no reason for parents to automatically assume that they know how to parent well. If only we could change the social standard of acceptance so that adults believed that raising a child deserved as much practice and accumulation of knowledge as flying an airplane, we would all be much safer.

Getting Straight and Growing Up

We are reviving a medieval social theology in which human nature is deemed incurably corrupt in order to reconcile the poor with poverty, the sick with sickness, and the whole race with extermination.

—Howard Barker, Arguments for a Theatre

It is time for us to become serious about our problems with addiction. That means ceasing to see it as a problem of the inner city crack and heroin addicts, a problem that can be addressed by building more jail cells. Serious drug addicts and alcoholics are damaged people. Their addictions are a result of severe experiences with trauma and deprivation. Much greater efforts must be made to treat them effectively so that we stop the cycle of addiction which is profoundly intergenerational.

This means spending much larger sums of money on treatment including creating environments that are conducive to recovery, and that give addicts a chance for a better life—homes, jobs, shelters, child care, education, while guaranteeing that they stay off the drugs. Prisons need to use therapeutic community models for everyone who can be safely maintained within them. Such models have been used in the incarcerated substance abuse population with good results.[7] Some addicts may continue to need mood-altering substances for life because of basic biochemical deficits or permanent deficits resulting from child abuse. We need much more research to define just who they are and what substances do the most good and the least harm in stabilizing them. Taking our drug problems seriously also requires enforcing severe consequences for *anyone* who financially benefits from harming others through encouraging addiction.

But addictions have to be taken more seriously by the rest of us as well. Excessive alcohol, marijuana, nicotine, and even food have been proven to be bad for the health of the individual and bad for the health of the family. Alcohol in particular is highly associated with violence. And alcoholism is alcoholism when alcohol causes a problem, any problem. Again, for people to get straight they have to feel bad feelings that they are defending themselves against, and doing that requires help from other people. That is why Alcoholics Anonymous and the twelve step programs are among the only effective treatments for addictions—they provide a healing environment through the support of other people in a nonjudging atmosphere. Recovery gets a bad name from people who don't know better. The truth is, we all need a dose of recovery—the alternative is staying sick.

Our addiction to violence is perhaps, even more problematic than our other addictions. The place to start is recognizing it for what it is—an infectious disease. Violence begets violence and we minimize how important a contributor the all-pervasive social exposure to violence is in determining what kind of society we have. Our social norm, our tolerance for violence has become far too unbalanced and that change in norm *does* give permission to use violence as a way of solving problems, thus discouraging conflict resolution, impulse control, and tolerance. If we accept violence at our sporting events and the encouragement of violence on talk radio, then we should not be surprised that children turn to violence to resolve their problems.

A Bill of Responsibilities to Children

> Perhaps we cannot prevent this world from being a world in which children
> are tortured. But we can reduce the number of tortured children. And if you
> believers don't help us, who else in the world can help us do this?
> —Albert Camus

One day I was leading a psychoeducational group on the unit and the patients and I became embroiled in a discussion about the resonance between the personal and the political that they could see in their own lives. We talked about the similarities between abusive fathers and political tyrants. One patient, speaking of the injustice she had experienced at the hands of an abusive father, and the injustice she sees all around her, astutely commented that our country has gotten this far with the Bill of Rights but now needs a "Bill of Responsibilities." She was right. Our forefathers gave us a system of government that included an abundance of rights, but they did not anticipate the gradual de-linking of rights and responsibilities that has occurred in our time. When children are given privileges before they are mature enough to manage the responsibility of the privilege, disaster often ensues. In families this is bad parenting. It is time for us to be more firm in a resolve to link the acquisition of rights to the development of the ability to handle responsibilities based on behavior and performance, not on chronological age.

What should such a Bill of Responsibilities contain? It must begin with responsibilities toward children. Adults have a responsibility to provide children with a safe environment within which they can reach their full potential. This means that a child needs food, shelter, clothing, love, education, and freedom from violence. We have an abundance of research showing that children require loving and compassionate, nonviolent attachments if they are to mature properly. Likewise we have an abundance of evidence that large numbers of children do not even get enough food, much less love and guidance. And then we puzzle over the sources of crime.

The root cause for violence, the lowest common denominator, is the violence perpetrated against children. And this includes all forms of violence—allowing children to go hungry in the midst of plenty, denying them adequate educations, permitting homelessness, withholding medical care, failing to support overwhelmed families, and tolerating corporate and governmental policies that make good parenting virtually impossible. Nothing will change for the better until we take seriously our shared responsibility for the well-being of *our* children—*all* of our children.

The U.S. Advisory Board on Child Abuse and Neglect made a list of important recommendations in its 1993 report, drawing some of the language from the United Nations Convention on the Rights of the Child. This is their proposed declaration:

- Respect for the inherent dignity and inalienable rights of children as members of the human community requires protection of their integrity as persons.
- Children have a right to protection from all forms of physical or mental violence, injury or abuse, neglect or negligent treatment, maltreatment or exploitation, including sexual abuse, while in the care of parent(s), legal guardian(s) or any other person who has the care of the child, including children residing in group homes and institutions.
- Children have a right to grow up in a family environment, in an atmosphere of happiness, love, and understanding.
- The several governments of the United States share a profound responsibility to ensure that children enjoy, at a minimum, such protection of their physical, sexual, and psychological security.
- The several governments of the United States bear a special duty to refrain from subjecting children in their care and custody to harm.
- Children have a right to be treated with respect as individuals, with due regard to cultural diversity and the need for culturally competent delivery of services in the child protection system.
- Children have a right to be provided the opportunity to be heard in any judicial and administrative proceedings affecting them, with ample opportunity for representation and for provision of procedures that comport with the child's sense of dignity.
- The duty to protect the integrity of children as persons implies a duty to prevent assaults on that integrity whenever possible.

There is an intimate and undeniable link between violence to the child and adult violence. If we desire a safer world, then we must stop harming children. In an interconnected world, abused children are too frequently weapons sent out into the world by troubled families, an unconscious way of generating world-destroying intergenerational revenge. As the psychohistorian, Lloyd DeMause has written, "Ultimately, of course, the ending of child assault, like the ending of wars and depressions, will only come when each adult has experienced enough love in their family of origin to make the use of children as poison containers unnecessary" (DeMause 1990).

The "Responsibility to Care" and the Bystander Effect

We may have civilized bodies and yet barbarous souls. We are blind to the real sights of this world; deaf to its voice; and dead to its death. And not till we know, that one grief outweighs ten thousand joys will we become what Christianity is striving to make us.

—Herman Melville

This "responsibility to care," as Harvard researcher Carol Gilligan has called it, is not a responsibility that stops with parenting (1982). We have fundamental responsibilities to care for others, as family members, as neighbors, as part of a community, as government leaders, as leaders of industry, in fact, in whatever capacity we serve in all of our human roles. This caring is not just an abstract concept. Every day, in virtually every situation in which there is a power imbalance, an injustice, a hurt person or hurt feeling, we are offered the opportunity to play one of three parts: the victim, the perpetrator, or the bystander. As the bystander we always are faced with a decision: Do we get involved, or do we stay silent? To understand the importance of such a choice we need to look at the work that has been done regarding the role of the bystander (Fogelman 1994; Staub 1989, 1992b, 1993).

In March, 1964, Kitty Genovese was brutally murdered in New York while thirty-eight of her neighbors watched from their apartment windows. Even though the attack lasted more than a half-hour, no one called the police until it was over. This became known as the "bystander effect." But, who is a bystander? If you are not a victim or a perpetrator, you are a bystander. Bystanders are the audience. They are all those present at the scene of an incident who provide or deny support for a behavior. Silence gives consent. The victim and perpetrator form a linked figure, and the bystanders form the ground against which perpetration is carried out or prevented.

Among many acts of perpetration that have been studied, the behavior of the bystanders determined how far the perpetrators went in carrying out their behavior. In this concept lies the key to interrupting the victim-perpetrator cycle of violence that is destroying our social safety. History attests to the fact that once violence is tolerated and supported as a group norm, an increasing number of bystanders become victims and/or perpetrators until it becomes increasingly difficult to make clear differentiations among the three groups. This describes the perilous situation in which we now find ourselves. Violence is no longer confined to the inner cities, to the poor, to the minority of our people. Violence now permeates every aspect of our social environment, wreaks its havoc on every stratum of our society.

The process of devaluation is the first and essential step in guaranteeing that bystanders will not act to stop perpetrators. Research indicates that when extremely negative statements are made about a group they affect basic attitudes toward that group even more than moderate statements. Thus, people will discredit the exact content of statements that, for instance, Jews murder babies, or African Americans have lower IQ's than whites, but will devalue Jews and African Americans in a general way in response to those statements more than they will devalue them in response to less extremely prejudicial statements. During World War II, countries in which anti-Semitism was highest in the general population were the countries in which most Jews were killed. This basic prejudice did not cause the Nazi destruction but instead, allowed it to happen. In countries where Jews were more highly valued, the Nazi destruction of the Jewish population was significantly less (Goldhagen 1996; Staub 1989). For the same reasons, we cannot now allow hate crimes or hate speech to be ignored, regardless of who the hate is directed at—children, women, blacks, the poor, Jews, homosexuals—hate is hate and it is infectious, and it influences action. Our influence upon each other is startlingly powerful. We can all bear witness to this responsibility by responding negatively to racist comments, sexist jokes, any remarks that are designed to hurt or humiliate others.

In social behavior, early intervention and prevention works best. As bystanders become increasingly passive in the face of abusive behavior, action becomes increasingly difficult. Just as there is a deteriorating spiral of perpetration in which each act of violence becomes increasingly easy to accomplish, so too is there a deteriorating cycle of passivity. As the perpetrators actively assume control over a system without any resistance on the part of bystanders, their power increases to the point that resistance on the part of bystanders becomes extremely difficult if not useless except to the extent that such behavior serves as an example for others.

Interestingly however, all it takes is for one bystander in a group to take some sort of positive action against perpetration and others will follow. There is much to be learned from the behavior of bystanders who *do* help because in any situation of perpetration, they define a different reality. Their actions provide an alternative way of relating, another example to the per-petrators, and would-be perpetrators, and victims, all of whom become locked into the cycle of violence and abuse.

The fundamental question is whether witnesses to the maltreatment of other people have an obligation to act. What is our moral responsibility to each other? Are we, in fact, "our brother's keeper?" Until quite recently in human history, the family group or the tribe were the only groups to which we felt the kind of loyalty that demands protective action. In the last two centuries, our sense of loyalty has expanded to our national groups. More recently, global ethnicity has been commanding fealty. But we have entered an age of such intense global interdependency that perpetration against one can be seen increasingly to effect the whole in an ever escalating cycle of violence and destruction.

The situation we find ourselves in cannot be remedied by law enforce-ment or by services to victims. The power to create safety lies with the masses of people who are currently neither victims, nor perpetrators. By our failure to act to protect our children, our neighbors, and even our ene-mies, we decide that the actions of the perpetrator are acceptable and they then have the room they need to move in. Bringing the perpetrator to justice after the fact, then, becomes a hollow sacrificial ritual, since we take no responsibility for the role we have played in providing a social atmosphere within which this conduct is permitted. It is time to turn our attention away from our exclusive preoccupation with the pathology of the victim and the pathology of the perpetrator and begin planning how to heal the pathology of the bystanders. We may never be able to eliminate the forces that produce violent perpetration but it is not too late to contain the violence. This con-tainment can happen, however, only if bystanders choose to become wit-nesses and rescuers, instead of silently colluding with the perpetrators.

Bearing Witness, Not Grudges

> I believe there are three major contributing factors responsible for the social injustices that cause poverty, powerlessness, and despair. One is class con-flict—the exploitation of the lower socioeconomic groups by the powerful elitist upper class; the second is the exploitation of females by males; the third is racism and ethnocentrism. . . . Standing directly in the path of reform is the chauvinistic, patriarchal male.
>
> —George W. Albee

We avoid other people's pain only to our peril. Our society is in a state of unhealth. It is not anyone's fault. There may indeed be a conspiracy of power brokers who enjoy generating death and destruction, but if so, they are another part of the symptom, not the cause, for all the damage they do. We cannot make significant strides forward in our social evolutionary growth unless we stop substituting blaming for problem solving. The cause of a problem is always systemic no matter what part of a system manifests the problem. This is a very different way of addressing problems, although it is a position that is occurring in businesses as changing trends in quality control. For every problem that exists we need to show compassion for the victim, to attempt to comprehend the perpetrator, and then to focus on fixing the problem, a practice that includes making amends to the victim and rehabilitating the perpetrator.

Bearing witness is a concept that is of vital importance particularly, right now, for men. The violence in our culture is perpetrated largely by men on women, children, the environment, and other men. Men still dominate in every culture. Men still run the world. Males in our culture are systematically conditioned for war, whether that war is to be on the battlefield, in the board room, or in the bedroom. This is carefully done by an insistence on emotional inhibition and encouragement of the brutalization of self and others that begins in early childhood. Male violence is supported, condoned, admired, and encouraged (Kokopeli and Lakey 1990, Koss et al. 1994, Miedzian 1991). This is a male problem that only men can fix. Just as women assumed responsibility for their own consciousness raising in the 1970s, so men must take responsibility for their unique problems and work to alter the behavior of and social norms for boys. Change can come about only in this way. As long as we continue to focus exclusively on the victims of violence while ignoring the pervasive male perpetration that creates those victims, there will be an unending stream of victims, as the testimony of this century bears out.

The concept of testimony comes out of the 1970s in Chile when psychologists collected testimonies from former political prisoners who had been tortured, and out of the social actions of the Holocaust survivors, who have created an archive of remembrance. This process became a therapeutic process by which a detailed account of their experiences reconnected the victims to a sense of meaning while providing the opportunity for a healing cathartic experience.

The objective of bearing witness is to tell the truth of one's experience, to expose one's helplessness, humiliation, pain, guilt, and shame and transform it into a political statement against malevolence. In this way, "The private pain is transformed into political or spiritual dignity" (Agger and Jenson 1990). This process of transformation is something that we can all do, even in the smallest ways, by just being willing to listen to our family, our friends, our neighbors, our colleagues without judging and without defensiveness. We each need to testify to the truth of our own pain, whatever that pain is. Bearing witness means breaking through the rigid wall of denial that keeps us from seeing the suffering that is all around us so that we thereby compound that suffering by our ignorance. When people are able to give testimony and to have it heard and respected, they are much less likely to carry grudges and seek revenge. It is far better to remember the pain, give it words, and be able to put it on the shelf than to pretend it doesn't exist and let it quietly dominate our existence.

Bearing witness means participating—going to school meetings, voting, running for city council, writing to the editor of the newspaper, speaking up in church meetings, calling in to radio talk shows, organizing a community watch, or doing any activity that reconnects us to other people, to meaning, and to our shared responsibility. Murder is the end point of a myriad of cruel and neglectful acts of conscious and unconscious violence. There is a downward spiral of corruption that gains momentum from every previous act of corruption. But this is a bidirectional spiral. Every act of involvement and protest is a victory of voice over silence that builds upon the previous act and powerfully influences the next. Our most pressing national problem today is not the growth of the criminal class. It is the silence, apathy, and passivity of the people in the middle, the settled, stable, caring, reasonable bunch who have become so easily manipulated by the vocal ends. This is the pathology of the bystander, to see what is wrong and to remain silent.

Creating Democracy

> Man's capacity for justice makes democracy possible, but man's inclination to injustice makes democracy necessary.
>
> —Reinhold Niebuhr

> The condition upon which God hath given liberty to man is eternal vigilance; which condition if he break, servitude is at once the consequence of his crime and the punishment of his guilt.
>
> —John Philpot Curran, Speech on the Right of Election of Lord Mayor of Dublin, July 10, 1790

As we have learned from the experience of our small community, democracy is better understood as a verb than a noun. It is a creative process that must be created and re-created constantly if it is to survive. The practice of democracy must begin in childhood, not when we are already adults. Normative behavior is instilled when we are children. Democracy requires the constant questioning of authority, the eternal vigilance and watchfulness that is required of liberty. These patterns must be established during the formative years in families and in schools if we are to rear good citizens. Through our patients, we have seen the deformations that occur if authority is hierarchical, arbitrary, and abusive. Such authority fails to induce a sense of personal and social responsibility and personal control that is so essential for the smooth operations of a democratic republic.

We have no right to a free and open democracy unless we are willing to maintain it and assume responsibility for it. Democracy requires a well-educated, involved, responsible, and mature populace. As a society, we have a long way to go before we can fulfill any of those four requirements. The increase of anarchic violence and hate crimes threatens our social stability and our democratic form of government along with it. But an even greater threat comes from corruption in business, in the justice system, in the military, in Congress.

THE CREATIVE LIFE AS SANCTUARY

Hearing the Voice of the Artist

In the haunted house of life, art is the only stair that doesn't creak.
—Tom Robbins, *Skinny Legs and All*

No psychiatric text or journal has been very helpful in explaining the process of what we do at *The Sanctuary* unit. When I read the literature of the past about the development of the therapeutic milieu, I have the same experience as when I read about similar new concepts emerging in education, the criminal justice system and business—there is a language problem. I suspect that relatively little is written about the process of creating and maintaining milieus because it is an essentially creative process, and creative endeavors are notoriously difficult to tie down with words. The best descriptions I have found derive from the theater and the arts, and the ongoing process of creation that exemplifies dramatic work.

Art has been present in the lives of men and women for as long as we have any history to report. Every human advance is heralded by a flowering of artistic achievement, a time in which art, in all its forms, is held in the highest esteem. It is no coincidence that the general improvement and artistic greatness go together. Knowing what we know now from our work with individual patients, it is entirely conceivable that artistic expression determines advancement, that it is vital for human progress to occur, and that without creative expression, a culture will involute and self-destruct.

The hallmark of trauma is dissociation, and dissociation is self-deception. Through dissociation we are able to convince ourselves that something that did happen did not, that we do not feel what we feel, that we do not remember what we remember, that we do not know what we know. The loss of integration, this separation into parts, has always been considered a signpost of disease. One word for the Devil is *Diabolos*—the divider, the splitter-into-fragments. Health, both mental and physical, individual and social, has traditionally been characterized by balance, when all the different parts are able to operate together harmoniously. If balance is lost, so too is health (Skynner and Cleese 1993).

Now, thanks to victims of trauma, we have been reminded, once again that illness is fragmentation and that health is balance and wholeness. Terror and physical pain deconstruct language. The victim experiences and remembers the trauma in nonverbal, visual, auditory, kinesthetic, visceral, and feeling modalities, but is not able to "think" about it or process the experience in any way. Our cognitive processes are dependent on language, and without words we cannot think. Trauma produces a disconnection syndrome, a "split-brain" in which the two hemispheres appear to function autonomously.

Traumatized people become possessed, haunted by the theaters in their minds. They cannot control the intrusive images, feelings, sensations that come into consciousness unbidden, terrifyingly vivid, producing a vicious cycle of helpless self-revictimization. Any efforts they took to protect themselves or others at the time of the trauma were a failure, and yet images of what they could have done—their "failed enactments"—obsess them. The victims of trauma are trapped within the silence of unwitnessed memory. To heal they must integrate the split-off, dissociated parts of their experience, the haunting fragments of memory and feeling that propel reenactment. They must speak, they must feel, and hearing the words, they must incorporate the experience into some kind of cognitive schema that allows them to make meaning and finally put the experience behind them so they can go on.

But the biological responses to trauma inhibit and prohibit such speech. The brain is disconnected from itself and perceives any attempt to reconnect as a dangerous threat to survival. So intrusive sensory experiences and negative feelings predominate and behavior becomes increasingly separated from the social meaning system. People disconnect from other people as they actively avoid listening or participating in a dialogue with the victims. Trapped in time, while the world moves on around them, they are neither alive nor dead. They cannot escape the trap alone: The biological reverberations have set up a snare that grabs at them and refuses to let go. So they do the only thing left to do—they speak in the only voice they have, in the language of the nonverbal brain. They act.

The act is a signal. The nonverbal brain signals its distress, but the verbal brain cannot see the signal. We are each other's mirror and we need other people from the time we are born, to mirror back to us messages from "the other side." But what happens when the other fails to respond to the signal? What happens when what is mirrored back is a partial or total misreading of the internal state? Is this not the way to madness?

Victims of trauma look mad because we have largely put aside our abilities to translate nonverbal messages into words. Our entire society is mad because it too has put aside the gifts that come from the gods, the emotional, artistic, holistic, relational, creative, expressive, nonverbal nondominant hemisphere language. Artists try to tell us how important this language is, how necessary it is to our individual and collective survival, but for the most part we fail to listen.

Victims of interpersonal violence illustrate ritual and performance run amok. Just as the capacity for dissociation is biologically based, so too is the response to dissociation—the ritual signal—and it too happens automatically, hard-wired into the brain chemistry itself. In earlier days, entire cultures provided for healing rituals in which trance was induced, the trauma could be relived and the pain integrated into a meaningful whole consistent with a larger mythical system. The ritual would involve music, dance, drama, and performance, and the entire social group would participate. In this way, cognitive, behavioral, and affect change and transformation could occur, social relations and subjective experience could be brought into harmony (Van der Hart 1983). Trauma and terror, pain and grief could be transmuted into the joy of performance, the creation of beauty, the healing rhythms of dance and song, story and poetry. Not forgotten, but changed and changed together. In place of the recurrent terrifying fantasies of a solitary victim, the trauma could be transformed into an addition to the culturally shared reality, another chapter in the culture's mythical system.

For the most part, we have lost our awareness of the true social nature of human existence, of tragic consciousness, of the "tragic sense of life" (De Unamuno 1954). Now we largely and erroneously choose to believe in a just world, where each individual person gets what he or she deserves, a world of inevitable progress in which the just are justly rewarded. Sickness is the problem of the individual, probably genetically and biologically based and the concern only of the medical and psychiatric experts assigned to ameliorate it or simply tolerate it. Poverty is the fault of the impoverished. Crime warrants punishment. Within our segregated, individualized, demystified, and fragmented lives we avoid resonating with the suffering of others. We are not our brother's keepers.

As a result, the victims signal their distress in the only way left open to them, through the repetitive, often ritualized, seemingly bizarre signal, antisocial, symbolic, and emotionally charged behavior of the nondominant hemisphere. One man tries to jump off a building, a woman repeatedly runs razor blades across her breasts, another buys an assault weapon and sprays bullets across a crowded street. These culminating acts of destruction are acts of desperation and helpless rage, the ultimate response to years of misunderstanding and misinterpretation on the part of the victim's social group. The play is performed over and over, often developing into such pervasive life themes that all that is apparent is pathology. Peter Brook, the great British director, has described the "Deadly Theater"—dull, repetitive, emotionally inauthentic, deceptive, self-destructive performance (1968). The "theater" of the victim often becomes truly deadly as their life force ebbs away, replaced only by dull repetition, the prisoner hammering on a locked door that no one ever opens.

In displaying a performance, traumatized people are doing what they are biologically evolved to do: engage their social group in a healing dialogue, a shared experience of pain. The problem does not lie with their body, which is just doing what it is supposed to do. The problem resides within the culture which has failed to serve its socializing function for the individual. It is the corporate body which has become impaired. It is the corporate body that refuses to hear the meanings in the messages, the cries for help and healing. We cannot afford to hear their cruel secrets or their guilty confessions because we would have to respond, we would have to resonate with their pain, we would have to help them find a way out of their prison, and perhaps worst of all, we would have to confront their perpetrators. Trapped within the tragic circumstances of their lives, the silenced victims of trauma are bereft of the shared experience of tragedy.

At The Sanctuary, the members of the staff and I are the directors in the staging of an ongoing play. We are faced with an endless procession of intense, dramatic moments in which the universal themes of Greek and Shakespearean tragedy and comedy are played out before us. But there is no script, there are no words that help to explain, transform, and affix the action to time, place, and setting. The course of our work is in the opposite direction from the work of the stage. We must direct our players towards the creation of a script that can then be altered, improvised, and redirected. When we begin, the scene is all action, well-rehearsed, compulsive, boring, dead—and speechless. We must help the actors find a narrative scripts that can begin to set them free from compulsive reenactment, so they can become the playwright of their own play.

Our job is to provide a space, direction, and opportunity for rehearsal of the play that has become the repetitive performance of the patient's life. Lacking an awareness of the script that accompanies their performance, they enter the inpatient unit and automatically create their scene. Over and over again, we rehearse them, challenging them, pushing them, encouraging them, bullying them—fulfilling many of the functions of any good theater director—into developing, interpreting, and altering their performance. But in the interaction with their directors, and the rest of the "cast", new seeds are being planted, just as they are for every actor during the creation of a new performance. Once the compulsive performance of the patient has been grounded, has been placed into a specific time, place, and setting and given a script, it can never be exactly the same performance again. It has changed. "Once word is made flesh, it becomes another thing" (Marowitz 1986).

The work of the theater is the work of process. It too is a verb, not a noun. In the world of the theater, in our therapeutic environment, and in any living organization, there are recurrent crises and we never know exactly how to resolve them until, collectively, we have resolved them. Any attempt to resolve them individually or linearly defeats the goal and creates more problems than it seeks to prevent. We see a problem emerge before our eyes—with an individual patient, with the patient community, with the staff community, or with the community as a whole. We focus on the problem with only a very hazy outline idea of what the desired outcome should be. In the process of focusing, we begin to understand the nature of the problem, and as reactions to that interpretation unfold, further action occurs. Only later, after we have found the right interpretation, the right resolution of the problem, will we be able to fully understand the problem. Susan Coles, in studying this directorial process in the theater has called it "the creative process in crisis . . . a kind of hermeneutic circle (Cole 1992).

In our present cultural milieu, we have more exposure to great works of art, literature, theater, music, and dance then ever before in the history of the human race. But there is probably less personal performance than ever before in history. Television discourages interaction, even interaction with other people in the house; people generally have less free time to pursue creative outlets; arts programs for the public are poorly funded and often the first to go whenever government budgets are cut. Arts programs in the schools are given the lowest funding priority. Creative expression of the artistically elite is grossly overvalued and creative expression of the general population is grossly undervalued. This is dangerous. The part of our beings that has no voice, perhaps our other hemisphere, needs a vehicle for expression. Without such a vehicle, expression is likely to come through action that is often violent and destructive instead of creative.

Over the years, many questions have arisen about the connection between creativity and madness, the artist and the madman. Both the artist and the madman speak a tongue that has become foreign to the rest of us. The mad person is to his or her family what the artist is to the culture, containing what is hidden, secret, denied, and dissociated and trying with more or less desperation to reveal the vital secrets to us all. The mad person—the person we would now call a victim of trauma—has always symbolically pointed out the discrepancies, inconsistencies, and lies in the family.

So too has there always been, within the practice of the arts, problem-posing aspects of artistic behavior. The artist frequently provokes a negative response from members of his social group because an essential role of the artist has been denied and dissociated by the larger social group. In many social groups the artist has been the provocateur, pointing out hidden, suppressed, and contradictory aspects of the culture, attempting to make conscious what is unconscious and denied. Art is meant to be an "investigation" (Becker 1994) to tell us something about our inner contradictions, to illuminate what is in darkness, to help us to integrate the split-off parts of our socially constructed consciousness. But in our modern culture, we resist facing these contradictions. We do not want to face up to the reality we have created. Art is acceptable only if it entertains and amuses. The social group does not always take kindly to the artist's tendency to reveal its inner contradictions, any more than the family responds well to the mad. In referring to the theater, which has historically been "the most dangerous of all arts" (Wickham 1985), the British playwright Howard Barker (1989) has written, "A theatre which dares to return the audience to its soul . . . will experience the hostility a wrecked ship feels for the gale."

Every culture joins together to distort and alter reality in a way that makes life bearable, and in doing so creates "positive illusions" that promote health (Taylor 1989). But sometimes the culture goes too far, or for too long, and distorts reality to the point of danger. The function of the artist is to stay in touch with the other truth, the truth of the less distorted, nonverbal, nonrationalized part of our consciousness, the part of us that still sees some vital importance in trees and animals and water and fish. The part of us that, despite deception, verbal gymnastics, elaborate rationalizations, and malignant propaganda, realizes that we are organic parts of an organic whole and that the whole cannot remain intact without all of its parts. The part of us that resists epidemic robopathology, the attempt to turn us all into machines (Yablonsky 1972). The part of us that always remains in touch with primary reality, no matter how much we distort our personal and cultural reality. Through their paintings, sculptures, photographs, poetry, drama, songs, music, and stories, artists attempt to remind us of what we are missing, what we fail to see, or have forgotten, or fear. "All drama is a political event: It either reasserts or undermines the code of conduct of a given society" (Eslin 1976).

If we are to survive as a viable species on a viable earth, then we must become grounded once again in the values of the earth. To do this, we must be willing to remember and feel our social past, just as victims of trauma must remember and feel their personal past. We must confess our wrongs, give voice to our sorrows, resolve our contradictions. Herbert Marcuse said that "if art cannot change the world, it can help to change the consciousness and drives of the men and women who would change the world" (Becker 1994). He said that the artist has a responsibility to help society deal with its hidden conflicts and contradictions and must embody hope in any way possible. To do this we must be able to share in a vision of what does not, but still could, exist.

Emergent Wholeness, Moral Safety, and Moral Integrity

I hope our wisdom will grow with our power, and teach us, that the less we use our power the greater it will be.

—Thomas Jefferson

Transcendence is the only alternative to extinction.

—Vaclav Havel, July 4 1994

Human evolution is not over but biological evolution, for the most part, has been supplanted by social evolution. Our individualistic, self-preoccupied, and disconnected point of reference has brought us to a biological, personal, social, economic, political, and spiritual dead-end. Our long-term survival on this planet is dependent on our species making a dramatic and rapid shift in our social evolution, a shift as dramatic, rapid, and creative as World War II, the Holocaust, and the nuclear bomb were destructive. We appear to be on the verge of a major transition, a movement which is emerging out of all areas of human endeavor. Walk into any bookstore and signs of this transition are all around. It begins with the connecting of ideas. Physicists are talking about theology, meaning, and ecology. Neuroscientists are discussing brains, and physics, anthropology, and philosophy. Business executives are discussing modern physics, creativity, spirituality, and stewardship of global ecology. Physicians are advocating for prayer and spiritual transformation. Psychologists are comparing the work of healing the mind

with the work of healing the earth. Transformational politics. Self-organiz-
ing systems. Complexity theory. The Gaia Hypothesis. Liberation theology.
Ecopsychology. Something really interesting is happening. And what all
these ideas have in common is connecting, building bridges, healing the
splits that for so long have kept us fragmented and dissociated. And all
bring meaning, purpose, and spirituality back into the world of science and
technology. In some way, each author is attempting to describe a new
vision, a vision of emergent wholeness.[8]

In this book I have been attempting to describe our piece of this vision,
our attempt at creating safe environments which can promote creativity,
rational thought, the expression of emotions, and, ultimately, wholeness.
Hints of how the process works are appearing sporadically here and there in
other settings as well, in a school here, a hospital there, for a moment in a
legislative body, for a day or a month in a factory, a church, a community
group, or a club meeting. By now, many people have had at least the momen-
tary experience of what it feels like to function in a setting within which they
have felt physically, psychologically, socially safe, a setting where they have
experienced themselves as an essential and unique part of a larger whole.

Thus far, however, our attempts are fairly bumbling and short-lived. We
are like children just learning to speak, only now and then able to say a
comprehensible word or a complete sentence before lapsing once again into
garbled nonsense. But we *are* learning. I have shared what my friends, colleagues, and I have learned thus far about the kind of environment that is
most likely to increase the likelihood that we will more rapidly learn this
new language. Out of the unintelligible syllables that make up the
phonemes of the tongue we have heard from our ancestors since birth, we
can invent a new way of talking, using many of the same sounds and words
but giving them added meaning, a new slant, a different dialect, a fuller
meaning. But just as children need a sense of safety and security within
which learning can occur and the brain can function properly, so too do we
all need safe environments if we are to adequately problem solve for today
and in service of tomorrow. This means we need to pay a great deal more
attention to what we value, how we define who we are and what we believe
in, and how consistently we behave in service of those values.

I have called this change at the level of meaning, the search for *moral
safety*. It is a search and a process, a seemingly never-ending quest. It is an
attempt to reduce the hypocrisy that is present, both explicitly and implicitly,
in our social systems. It is a fundamentally important quest for patients
who are victims of child abuse because their internal systems of meaning
and self are split, trapped within a world that says, among other things, that

children are valued, precious, and should be protected while it fails to value or protect those same children.

A morally safe environment struggles, in Sisyphean manner, with the issues of honesty and integrity. Our attempt to create a morally safe environment began with a self-evaluative look at our therapeutic presumptions, our training, our rationalizations, and our fixed beliefs, as well as our practice. We were forced to ask ourselves, "What is it that we are actually doing, and what are we trying to achieve?" "Will the means get us to the desired ends?" "Do the means *justify* the ends?" These were tough and embarrassing questions with answers that were, at times, noxious.

The larger systems problems are going to require a similar way of thinking, functioning, and problem solving *together*. We are being pushed and prodded to take the next step in growth and development, the step past adolescence into adult maturity, as individuals and as an entire social group. The tasks of adulthood are different from those of a child or an adolescent. Adults must learn how to get along with other people, establish reciprocal and intimate relationships, express their unique creativity, protect and nurture the next generation, and assume stewardship for the legacy of their elders, both the benefits and the liabilities. Adult development requires a development of a coherent and consistent moral system. I do not believe that everything is relative. As Ken Wilber has put it in his discussion of the various levels of truths, "These truths are the golden treasure of a collective humanity, hard won through blood and sweat and tears and turmoil in the face of falsity, error, deception, and deceit. Humanity has slowly and increasingly *learned* over a million year history, to separate truth from appearance, goodness from corruption, beauty from degradation, and sincerity from deception." (Wilber 1996). But none of these tasks of discernment can be accomplished alone. Just as mature moral beliefs emerge out of the integrated and synthesized adult development, environments of moral safety can only emerge out of the shared and realized commitment of many mature men and women who are devoted to the evolution of moral integrity.

Magic, The Mystical, and the Life of the Spirit

Every work of art points somewhere beyond itself; it transcends itself and its author; it creates a special force field around itself that moves the human mind and the human nervous system.

—Vaclav Havel

Anyone who is a theater-goer knows that sometimes, with the right cast, the right theater, the right play, the right audience, on the right night, something magic happens. The whole play comes together for a moment in time that will never be replicated. Magic is the word I think of when a process outside of the bounds of usual linear thinking is at work. Magic is what we say on our unit when the energy is present, when we are working in harmony together. When magic is present, transformative events occur. It does not matter whether the magic is on stage, in a movie, in a painting, a piece of music, a ballet, a poem, in school, a factory, a therapist's office, a day care center, or in a room full of people talking. Magic is the emergent quality that is bigger than the sum of the parts and cannot be explained by a simple addition of the parts. When we are awake to the possibility of wholeness and integration, then we know when the magic is present and we know when it is gone, even if we cannot put it into words. In the theater, the entire act of creation is aimed at providing a space and a time for the magic to happen.

Making the magic happen is just as important in any social setting as it is in the theater—magic really means the appearance of life, whether we call it the living theater, the living organization, the learning organization, living-learning situations, the free school, or *The Sanctuary*.

When I have spoken about our work to different audiences, there is often someone who approaches me at the end of my lecture and asks me where, in our work, is there a place for the spiritual? Discussing the spiritual can be a disconcerting task for a medically trained person and when I was first asked the question I felt some acute embarrassment because I had no ready answer. Looking back, I had no ready answer because I had always taken the answer for granted. Now, I would answer that the magic I have described *is* the spiritual, that the work itself is a spiritual practice, and that the life of the spirit, at least for me, emerges out of the wholeness of community. For me and for my colleagues, there is no question that we are serving a higher purpose, even a calling, that stretches way beyond our individual selves but which is connected to and emerges from our joined efforts.

This century has been astonishingly supportive of death. The question that faces us today, perhaps the most pressing question of human evolution, is how do we create and maintain environments now that are truly supportive to life? In awkward words, with slow and laborious efforts, fitful starts, and many stumbles there are people out there in every discipline who are struggling to find and define a new way of being, of learning, of acting, of working, of playing, of healing in the world. Now we need to reach out and find each other in order to create a community of care, of concern, of commitment—in order to create sanctuary.

Notes

INTRODUCTION

1. The Sanctuary, Friends Hospital, 4641 Roosevelt Boulevard, Philadelphia, PA 19124–2399. Joseph Foderaro, MSS, Program Director.
2. For an excellent appraisal of such a process see Seymour B. Sarason, 1972, *The Creation of Settings and Future Societies*. San Francisco: Jossey Bass.
3. For more information on the inpatient unit as laboratory see Tucker and Maxmen, 1973, and all of the works of Trigant Burrow.

CHAPTER ONE

1. The present criteria for Post-Traumatic Stress Disorder 309.81 from the *Diagnostic and Statistic Manual of Mental Disorders IV*

   A. The person has been exposed to a traumatic event in which both of following are present:
      • the person experienced, witnessed, or was confronted with an event or events that involved actual or threatened death or serious injury, or threat to physical integrity of self or others;
      • the person's response involved intense fear, helplessness, or horror. In children this may be expressed instead by disorganized or agitated behavior;
   B. The traumatic event is persistently reexperienced in one (or more) of the following ways:
      • recurrent and distressing recollections of the event, including images, thoughts, or perceptions. In young children, repetitive play may occur in which themes or aspects of the trauma are expressed;
      • recurrent distressing dreams of the event. In children, there may be frightening dreams without recognizable content;

- acting or feeling as if the traumatic event were recurring (includes a sense of reliving the experience, illusions, hallucinations, and dissociative flashback episodes, including those that occur on awakening or when intoxicated. In children, trauma-specific reenactment may occur;
- intense psychological distress at exposure to internal or external cues that symbolize or resemble an aspect of the traumatic event;
- physiological reactivity on exposure to internal or external cues that symbolize or resemble an aspect of the traumatic event.

C. Persistent avoidance of stimuli associated with the trauma and numbing of general responsiveness (not present before the trauma), as indicated by three (or more) of the following:
- efforts to avoid thoughts, feeling, or conversations associated with the trauma;
- efforts to avoid activities, places, or people that arouse recollections of the trauma;
- inability to recall an important aspect of the trauma;
- markedly diminished interest or participation in significant activities;
- feeling of detachment or estrangement from others;
- restricted range of affect (e.g. unable to have loving feelings);
- sense of foreshortened future (e.g. does not expect to have a career, marriage, children, normal life span).

D. Persistent symptoms of increased arousal (not present before the trauma) as indicated by two (or more) of the following:
- difficulty falling or staying asleep;
- irritability or outbursts of anger;
- difficulty concentrating;
- hypervigilance;
- exaggerated startle response;
- duration of the disturbance (symptoms in Criteria B, C, and D) is more than one month;
- the disturbance causes clinically significant distress or impairment in social, occupational, or other important areas of functioning.

Specify if:
- acute: If duration of symptoms is less than three months;
- chronic: If duration of symptoms is three months or more;
- with delayed onset: If onset of symptoms is at least six months after the stressor;

Diagnostic and Statistic Manual of Mental Disorders, Fourth Edition (DSM-IV). *Washington, D.C.: American Psychiatric Press.*

2. International Society for Traumatic Stress Studies (ISTSS), 60 Revere Drive, Suite 500, Northbrook, IL 60062. Phone: (847) 480–9028.

3. For a more complete exploration of traumatic vs. normal, "true" vs. "false" memories see: Alpert, J. L., Brown, L. S. and Courtois, C. A. 1996. *Symptomatic clients and memories of childhood abuse: What the trauma and child sexual abuse literature tells us.* In J. Alpert, L. S. Brown, S. J. Ceci, C. A. Courtois, E. F. Loftus and P. A. Ornstein, *Final report of the working group on investigation of memories of childhood abuse.* Washington, D.C.: American Psychological Association; Armstrong, L. 1994. *Rocking the cradle of*

sexual politics: What happened when women said incest. Reading, MA: Addison Wesley; Bremner, J. D., Randall, P. Scott, T. M., Bronen, R. A., Seibyl, J. P., Southwick, S. M., Delaney, R. C., McCarthy, G., Charney, D. S., and Innis, R. B. 1995. MRI-based measurement of hippocampal volume in patients with combat-related posttraumatic stress disorder. *American Journal of Psychiatry, 152, 973–981;* Christianson, A. (Ed). 1992. *The Handbook of Emotion and Memory: Research and Theory.* Hillsdale, New Jersey: Lawrence Erlbaum Associates; Elliott, D. and Briere, J. 1995. Post-traumatic stress associated with delayed recall of sexual abuse: A general population study. *Journal of Traumatic Stress* 8: 629–647; Freyd, J. 1996. *Betrayal trauma theory: The logic of forgetting abuse.* Cambridge: Harvard University Press; Pope, K. S. 1996. Memory, abuse and science: Question-ing claims about the false memory syndrome epidemic. *American Psychologist,* 51(9): 957–974; Pope, K. S. and L. S. Brown. 1996. *Recovered Memories of Abuse: Assessment, Therapy, Forensics.* Washington, D.C.: American Psychological Association; Whitfield, C. L. 1995. *Memory and Abuse: Remembering and Healing the Effects of Trauma.* Deerfield Beach, Florida: Health Communications, Inc.; Williams, L. M. 1994. Recall of childhood trauma: A prospective study of women's memories of child sexual abuse. *Journal of Consulting and Clinical Psychology, 62,* 1167–1176; Williams, L. M. 1995. Recovered memories of abuse in women with documented child sexual victimization histories. *Journal of Traumatic Stress* 8: 649–673.

CHAPTER THREE

1. More information on WWI and the effects of combat see Elaine Showal-ter's chapter on male hysteria in her book, *The Female Malady: Women, Madness and English Culture, 1830–1980,* New York: Penguin. An interest-ing fictional account, based on actual medical and literary characters is Pat Barker's trilogy, *Regeneration, The Eye in the Door,* and *The Ghost Road,* all published by Penguin.

2. There are many studies of comorbidity dating back to the late 1980s. For example, see: Barsky, A. J., C. Wool, M. C. Barnett, P. D. Cleary. 1994. His-tories of childhood trauma in adult hypochondriacal patients. *American Journal of Psychiatry* 151(3):397–401; Beck, J. C. and B. A. Van der Kolk. 1987. Reports of childhood incest and current behavior of chronically hos-pitalized psychotic women. *American Journal of Psychiatry,* 144, 1474–1476; Briere, J. 1988. Long-term clinical correlates to childhood sexual victimization. *Annals of the New York Academy of Sciences* 528: 327–334; Briere, J., and L.Y. Saidi. 1989. Sexual abuse histories and seque-lae in female psychiatric emergency room patients. *American Journal of Psychiatry,* 146, 1602–1606; Brown, A. and D. Finkelhor. 1986. Impact of child sexual abuse: A review of the literature. *Psychological Bulletin* 99: 66–77; Bryer, J. B., B. A. Nelson, J. B Miller, and P. A. Krol. 1987. Childhood

sexual and physical abuse as factors in adult psychiatric illness. *American Journal of Psychiatry*, 144, 1426–1430; Bulik, C. M., P. F. Sullivan, and M. Rorty. 1989. Childhood sexual abuse in women with bulimia. *Journal of Clinical Psychiatry*, 50, 460–464; David, D., A. Giron, T. A. Mellman. 1995. Panic-phobic patients and developmental trauma. *Journal of Clinical Psychiatry* 56: 113–117; Friedman, Matthew and Rachel Yehuda.1995. Post-traumatic stress disorder and comorbidity: Psychobiological approaches to differential diagnosis. In *Neurobiological and Clinical Consequences of Stress: From Normal Adaptation to Post-Traumatic Stress Disorder*. Matthew J. Friedman, Dennis S. Charney, and Ariel Y. Deutch, editors. Philadelphia: Lippincott Raven. Friedman, Matthew J. and Paula P. Schnurr.1995. The relationship between trauma, post-traumatic stress disorder, and physical health. In *Neurobiological and Clinical Consequences of Stress: From Normal Adaptation to Post-Traumatic Stress Disorder*. Matthew J. Friedman, Dennis S. Charney, and Ariel Y. Deutch, editors. Philadelphia: LippincottRaven; Goldman, S. J., E. J. D'Angelo, D. R. DeMaso, R. Mezzacappa. 1992. Physical and sexual abuse histories among children with borderline personality disorder. *American Journal of Psychiatry* 149: 1723–1726; Herman, J. L., Perry, J. C., and Van der Kolk, B. A. 1989. Childhood trauma in borderline personality disorder. *American Journal of Psychiatry*, 146, 490-495; Herman, J. L., Russell, D., and Trocki, K. 1986. Long-term effects of incestuous abuse in childhood. *American Journal of Psychiatry*, 143, 1293–1296; Mancini, C, M. Van Ameringen, and H. MacMillan. 1995. Relationship of childhood sexual and physical abuse to anxiety disorders. *Journal of Nervous and Mental Disorders* 183: 309–314; Morrison, J. 1989. Childhood sexual histories of women with somatization disorder. *American Journal of Psychiatry*, 146, 239–241; Shearer, S. L., Peters, C. P., Quaytman, M. S. and Ogden, R. L. 1990. Frequency and correlates of childhood sexual and physical abuse histories in adult female borderline inpatients. *American Journal of Psychiatry*, 147, 214–216; Schetky, D. H. 1990. A review of the literature on the long-term effects of childhood sexual abuse. In *Incest-Related Syndromes of Adult Psychopathology*. R. P. Kluft Editor. Washington, D.C.: American Psychiatric Press; Sierles, F. S., Chen, J. J., McFarland, R. E., Taylor, M. A. 1983. Posttraumatic stress disorder and concurrent psychiatric illness: A preliminary report. *American Journal of Psychiatry*, 140, 1177–1179; Swett, C., Surrey, J., Cohen, C. 1990. Sexual and physical abuse histories and psychiatric symptoms among male psychiatric oupatients. *American Journal of Psychiatry*, 147, 632–639; Walker, E., Katon, W., Harrop-Griffiths, J. 1988. Relationship of chronic pelvic pain to psychiatric diagnoses and childhood sexual abuse. *American Journal of Psychiatry*, 145, 75–80; Walker, E. A., Torkelson, N., Katon, W. J. and Koss, M. P. 1993. The prevalence rate of sexual trauma in a primary care clinic. *Journal of the American Board of Family Practice*, 6, 465–471; Yehuda R, B. Kahana, J. Schmeidler, S .M. Southwick, S. Wilson, E. L.Giller. 1995. Impact of cumulative lifetime trauma and recent stress on current posttraumatic stress disorder symptoms in holocaust survivors. *American Journal of Psychiatry* 152(12):1815–8.

CHAPTER FOUR

1. There is a growing recognition that the diagnosis of "post-traumatic stress disorder" does not adequately describe a number of people, particularly those who have been exposed to childhood trauma or the trauma of captivity. Field studies were conducted prior to the release of DSM-IV to see if these differences could be measured and it has become clear that these differences are real. Two alternative names have been offered: "complex PTSD" and "Disorders of Extreme Stress Not Otherwise Specified (DESNOS)." The following characteristics describe the proposed syndome:

   A. Alterations in regulating affective arousal
      1. chronic affect dysregulation
      2. difficulty modulating anger
      3. self-destructive and suicidal behavior
      4. difficulty modulating sexual involvement
      5. impulsive and risk-taking behavior
   B. Alterations in attention and consciousness
      1. amnesia
      2. dissociation
   C. Somatization
   D. Chronic characterological changes
      1. Alterations in self-perception: chronic guilt and shame; feelings of self-blame, of ineffectiveness, and of being permanently damaged
      2. Alterations in perception of perpetrator; adopting distorted beliefs and idealizing the perpetrator
      3. Alterations in relations with others
         a. an inability to trust or maintain relationships with others
         b. a tendency to be revictimized
         c. a tendency to victimize others
   E. Alterations in systems of meaning
      1. Despair and hopelessness
      2. Loss of previously sustaining beliefs

   For more detailed information about the ideas and research behind this proposed change in the diagnostic categories, please see Herman, J. L. 1992. *Trauma and Recovery.* New York: Basic and Van der Kolk, B. A. 1996a The complexity of adaptation to trauma. In Van der Kolk B. A., C. McFarlane and L. Weisaeth. *Traumatic Stress: The Effects of Overwhelming Experience on Mind, Body and Society.* New York: Guilford Press.

2. For more information about multiple personality disorder, see back issues of the journal *Dissociation,* a publication of the International Society for the Study of Dissociation, 4700 West Lake Avenue, Glenview, IL 60025–1485, 708–375–4718 or consult: Beahrs, J. O. 1983 *Unity and Mul-*

tiplicity: Multilevel Consciousness of Self in Hypnosis, Psychiatric Disorder, and Mental Health; Kluft, R. P. 1990. *Incest-related syndromes of adult psychopathology.* Washington: American Psychiatric Press; Kluft, R. P. and Fine, C. G. 1992. *Clinical perspective on multiple personality disorder.* Washington: American Psychiatric Press; Putnam, F.W. 1989. *Diagnosis and treatment of multiple personality disorder.* New York: Guilford Press; Ross, C. A. 1989. *Multiple personality disorder: Diagnosis, clinical features, and treatment.* New York: John Wiley and Sons; Spiegel, David, ed. 1994. *Dissociation: Culture, Mind and Body.* Washington, D.C.: American Psychiatric Press; Spiegel, David, ed. 1993. *Dissociative Disorders: A Clinical Review.* Lutherville, MD: The Sidran Press.

3. James Pennebaker and his colleagues have published important data on the positive effects of writing for anyone who has experienced an overwhelming life experience. See Pennebaker J. W. 1989. Confession, inhibition, and disease. *Advances in Experimental Social Psychology.* 22; 211–244; Pennebaker, J. W. and Beall, S. K. 1986. Confronting a traumatic event: Toward an understanding of inhibition and disease. *Journal of Abnormal Psychology,* 95, 274–281; Pennebaker, J. W. and Susman, J. R. 1988. Disclosure of traumas and psychosomatic processes. *Social Science and Medicine.* 26,3: 327–332; Pennebaker, J. W. 1993. Putting stress into words: health, linguistic, and therapeutic implications. *Behav. Res. Ther,* 31(6): 539–548.

4. Labeling theory has made an important contribution to the understanding of the social aspects of psychiatric care. For further reading please see Scheff, Thomas J. 1975. *Labeling Madness.* This edited volume contains several important and classic essays including several from the editor and another by David L. Rosenhan, "On Being Sane in Insane Places."

5. For further reading about fragmentation as it applies to social systems see Capra, F. 1996. *The Web of Life: A New Scientific Understanding of Living Systems.* New York: Anchor Books; and Wilber, K. 1996. *A Brief History of Everything.* Boston: Shambhala.

6. For examples of American discomfort with group ideas see Kovel, J. (1994). *Red hunting in the promised land: Anticommunism in the making of America.* New York: Basic Books and Sarason, Seymour B. 1981. *Psychology Misdirected.* New York: the Free Press.

7. According to Sarason (1972) this is a common finding, and that each time it occurs, the more fundamental issue of values conflict never gets addressed but is instead sidelined by the alleged personality issue.

CHAPTER FIVE

1. Government corruption is more pervasive than many of us realize. For an eye-opening education read current and back issues of *The Nation.* Some other recent books of interest: See Albeda, R., E. McCrate, E. Melendez, J. Lapidus. 1988. *Mink Coats Don't Trickle Down: The Economic Attack on Women and People of Color.* Boston: South End Press; Burnham, D. 1996.

Above the Law: Secret Deals, Political Fixes, and Other Misadventures of the U.S. Department of Justice. New York: Scribner's; Chomsky, N. 1988. *The Culture of Terrorism.* Boston: South End Press; Chomsky, N. 1993. *The Prosperous Few and the Restless Many.* Berkeley, CA: Odonian Press; Crossen, C. 1994. *Tainted Truth: The Manipulation of Fact in America.* New York: Simon and Schuster; Greider, W. 1992. *Who Will Tell the People: The Betrayal of American Democracy.* New York: Simon and Schuster; Hartung, W. D. 1994. *And Weapons For All.* New York: HarperCollins; Lapham, Lewis. 1995. *Hotel America: Scenes in the Lobby of the Fin-De-Siècle.* New York: Verso; Lewis, C. 1996. *The Buying of the President.* New York: Avon Books; Saul, J. R. 1992. *Voltaire's Bastard.* New York: Vintage Books; Zepezauer, M. 1994. *The CIA's Greatest Hits.* Tucson, AZ: Odonian Press.

2. A particularly innovative program has been created for this purpose in the Neshaminy School District, Langhorne, PA, Bernard Hoffman, Administrator Emeritus.

3. For more information about creating safety in the schools see Arbetter, Sandra. 1995. Violence—a growing threat. *Current Health* 2, 21(6):6–13; Brendtro, Larry and Nicholas Long. 1995. Breaking the cycle of conflict. *Educational Leadership* 52(5): 52–57. Clark, David. 1975. *Social Therapy in Psychiatry.* New York: Jason Aronson; Crouch, Elizabeth and Debra Williams. 1995. What cities are doing to protect kids. *Educational Leadership* 52(5): 60–3; Lantieri, Linda. 1995. Waging peace in our schools: beginning with the children. *Phil Delta Kappan* 76(5): 386–389; Lawry, John D. 1989. Caritas in the classroom: The opening of the American student's heart. *College Teaching* 38(3): 83–87; Mercogliano, Chris. 1995. *Making It Up As We Go Along: The Story of the (Albany) Free School.* Unpublished manuscript; O'Neil, John. 1995. On schools as learning organizations: a conversation with Peter Senge. *Educational Leadership* 52(7): 20–24; Sarason, Seymour. 1990. *The Predictable Failure of Educational Reform: Can We Change Course Befoer It's Too Late?* San Francisco: Jossey-Bass; Shanahan, Michael G. 1995. Solving campus-community problems. *The FBI Law Enforcement Bulletin* 64(2): 1–6; Watson, Robert. 1995. A guide to violence prevention. *Educational Leadership* 52(5): 57–60.

4. There is a growing body of literature on violence in the workplace, business and ethics. See Baron, S. A. (1993). *Violence in the Workplace: A Prevention and Management Guide for Businesses.* Ventura, California: Pathfinder Publishing of California; Bennis, Walter. 1993. A talk with Warren Bennis. *Psychology Today* 26(6): 30–2; Bovet, Susan Fry. 1994. Make companies more socially responsible. *Public Relations Journal* 50(8): 30–3; Caudron, Shari. 1994. Fight crime, sell products: Socially responsible companies that join the fight against crime may find new consumers in the process. *Industry Week* 243(20): 49–52; Dumain, Brian. 1994. Mr. Learning organization. *Fortune.* 130(8): 147–54; Duncan, T. Stanley. 1995. Death in the office: workplace homicides. *FBI Law Enforcement Bulletin* 64(4):

20–26; Frederick, William C. 1994 (reprint of classic paper from 1978) From CSR1 to CSR2: The maturing of business-and-society thought. *Business and Society* 33(2): 150–67; Garbarino, James. 1992. *Towards a Sustainable Society: An Economic, Social and Environmental Agenda for Our Children's Future.* Chicago: The Noble Press; Kohn, Alfie.1986. *No Contest: The Case Against Competition.* Boston: Houghton Mifflin Company; Labig, Charles E. 1995. Forming a violence response team. *HR Focus* 72(8): 15–17; Linden, Dana Wechsler. 1995. The mother of them all: early business management theorist Mary Parker Follett. *Forbes* 155(2): 75–77;Linton, Michael. 1993. Money and community economics. In Claude Whitmyer, Editor. *In the Company of Others: Making Community in the Modern World.* New York: Jeremy Tarcher; Shorris, Earl. 1994. *A Nation of Salesman: The Tyranny of the Market and the Subversion of Culture.* New York: W. W. Norton and Company; Van Buren III, Harry J. 1995. Business ethics for the new millenium. *Business and Society Review* 93:51–55; Will, Rosalyn. 1995. Corporations with a conscience. *Business and Society Review* 93:17–20.

5. The necessity for competition to insure success turns out to be another American myth. See Kohn, Alfie.1986. *No Contest: The Case Against Competition.* Boston: Houghton Mifflin Company.

6. For businesses who are trying to change this paradigm and create a "caring capitalism, see: Albelda, R, E. McCrate, E. Melendex, June 1988. *Mink Coats Don't Trickle Down: The Economic Attack on Women and People of Color.* Boston: South End Press; Barrentine, Pat, editor. 1993.*When The Canary Stops Singing.* San Francisco: Berrett-Koehler; Handy, Charles. 1994. *The Age of Paradox.* Boston: Harvard Business School Press; Hyman, Michael R. and Albert A. Blum. 1995. "Just" companies don't fail: the making of the ethical corporation. *Business and Society Review* 93: 48–50; Makower, Joel. 1994. *Beyond the Bottom Line: Putting Social Responsibility to Work for Your Business and the World.* New York: Simon and Schuster; Miller, William H. 1995. More than just making money: the last twenty-five years have seen industry assume a new mission: social responsibility. *Industry Week* 244(15): 91–96; Nirenberg, John. 1993. The Living Oranization: Transforming teams into workplace communities. *The Futurist* 27(6): 39–40; Ray, Michael and Alan Rinzler, editors. 1993. *The New Paradigm in Business.* New York: G. P. Putnam's Sons; Renesch, John, editor. 1992. *New Traditions in Business.* San Francisco: Berrett-Koehler; Scott, M and Rothman, H. 1994. *Twelve Companies With a Conscience.* New York: A Citadel Press Book. Senge, Peter. 1990. *The Fifth Discipline: The Art and Practice of the Learning Organization.* New York: Doubleday; Shaffer, Carolyn R. And Kristin Anundsen. 1993. *Creating Community Anywhere: Finding Support and Connection in a Fragmented World.* Los Angeles: Jeremy P. Tarcher.

7. For more information about therapeutic communities in prisons see Barr, Harriet. 1986. Outcome of drug abuse treatment in two modalities. In George DeLeon and James T. Ziegenfuss, Editors. *Therapeutic Communities*

For Addictions. Springfield, IL: Charles C. Thomas; Barthwell, A.G., P. Bokos, J. Bailey, M. Nisenbaum, J. Devereux, and E.C. Senay. 1995. Interventions/Wilmer: A continuum of care for substance abusers in the criminal justice system. *Journal of Psychoactive Drugs* 27(1): 39–47; Hinshelwood, R.D. and Nick Manning. 1979. *Therapeutic Communities: Reflections and Progress.* London: Routledge and Kegan Paul; Hooper, Robert M., Dorothy Lockwood, and James A. Inciardi. 1993. Treatment techniques in corrections-based therapeutic communities. *The Prison Journal* 73: 290–306;Jones, Maxwell. 1953. *The Therapeutic Community: A New Treatment Method in Psychiatry.* New York: Basic Books; Jones, Maxwell. 1968. *Social Psychiatry in Practice.* Middlesex, England: Penguin Books; Martin, S.S., C.A. Butzin, J.A. Inciardi. 1995. Assessment of a multistage therapeutic community for drug-involved offenders. *Journal of Psychoactive Drugs* 27(1): 109–16; Simpson, Dwayne D. 1986. Twelve-year follow-up: Outcomes of opioid addicts treated in therapeutic communities. In George DeLeon and James T. Ziegenfuss, Editors. *Therapeutic Communities For Addictions.* Springfield, IL: Charles C; Turner, Merfyn. 1972. Norman House. In Stuart Whiteley, Dennie Briggs, and Merfyn Turner. *Dealing with Deviants.* London: The Hogarth Press; Wexler, Harry K. 1986. Therapeutic communities within prisons. In George DeLeon and James T. Ziegenfuss, Editors. *Therapeutic Communities For Addictions.* Springfield, IL: Charles C. Thomas; Wexler, Harry K. 1995. The success of therapeutic communities for substance abusers in American prisons. *Journal of Psychoactive Drugs* 27 (1): 57–66; Wilmer, Harry. 1964. A living group experiment at San Quentin prison. *Corrective Psychiatry and Journal of Social Therapy* 10; Worth, Robert. 1995. A model prison. *Atlantic Monthly* November.

8. There is a rich body of material coming from every academic field of endeavor, broadly outlining the dimensions of this new reality. For further reading here are some suggestions: Capra, F. 1996. *The Web of Life: A New Scientific Understanding of Living Systems.* New York: Anchor Books; Darling, D. 1993. *Equations of Eternity.* New York: Hyperion; Davies, P. 1983. *God and the New Physics.* New York: A Touchstone Book; Dossey, L. 1993. *Healing Words: The Power of Prayer and the Practice of Medicine.* San Francisco: HarperSanFrancisco; Dyson, F. 1992. *From Eros to Gaia.* New York: Pantheon; Eisler, R. 1987. *The Chalice and the Blade: Our History and Our Future.* San Francisco: Harper; Freeman, W. J. 1995. *Societies of Brains: A Study in the Neuroscience of Love and Hate.* Hillsdale, NJ: Lawrence Erlbaum Associates; Johnson, G. 1996. *Fire in the Mind: Science, Faith, and the Search for Order.* New York: Alfred A. Knopf; Laszlo, E. 1994. *The Choice: Evolution or Extinction?* New York: G. P. Putnam's Sons; Lerner, M. 1996. *The Politics of Meaning: Restoring Hope and Possibility in an Age of Cynicism.* Reading, MA: Addison-Wesley; Maturana, H. R. and Varela, F. J. 1987. *The Tree of Knowledge: The Biological Roots of Human Understanding.*

Boston: Shambhala. Maynard, H. B. and Mehrtens, S. E. 1993. *The Fourth Wave: Business in the Twenty-first Century.* San Francisco: Berrett-Koehler; McLaughlin, C. and G. Davidson. 1994. *Spiritual Politics: Changing the World from the Inside Out.* New York: Ballantine Books; Montuori, A. and Conti, I. 1993. *From Power To Partnership: Creating The Future Of Love, Work, And Community.* San Francisco: Harper; Ray, M. and Rinzler, A. 1993. *The New Paradigm in Business: Emerging Strategies for Leadership and Organizational Change.* New York: G. P. Putnam's Sons; Roszak, T. Gomes, M. E. and Kanner, A. D. 1995. *Ecopsychology: Restoring the Earth, Healing the Mind.* San Francisco: Sierra Club Books; Talbot, M. 1991. *The Holographic Universe.* New York: Harper Collins; Wallis, J. 1994. *The Soul Of Politics.* New York: The New Press; Wilber, K. 1996. *A Brief History of Everything.* Boston: Shambhala; Santos, B. de S. 1995. *Toward a New Common Sense: Law, Science and Politics in the Paradigmatic Transition.* New York: Routledge.

References

Abroms, G. M. 1969. Defining milieu therapy. *Archives of General Psychiatry,* 21: 553–560.

Adorno, T. W., E. F. Frenkel-Brunswik, D. J. Levinson, and R. N. Sanford. 1982. *The Authoritarian Personality, Abridged Edition.* New York: W. W. Norton.

Agger, I., and S. B. Jenson. 1990. Testimony as ritual and evidence in psychotherapy for political refugees. *Journal of Traumatic Stress,* 3(1), January.

Ainsworth, M. 1991. Attachments and other affectional bonds across the life cycle. In *Attachment Across the Life Cycle,* edited by C. M. Parkes, J. Stevenson-Hinde, and P. Marris. London: Routledge.

Ainsworth, M., M.C. Blehar, E. Waters, and S. Wall. 1978. *Patterns of Attachment: A Psychological Study of the Strange Situation.* Hillsdale, NJ: Lawrence Erlbaum.

Alexander, F. G., and S. T. Selesnick. 1966. *The History of Psychiatry: An Evaluation of Psychiatric Thought and Practice From Prehistoric Times to the Present.* New York: New American Library.

Alexander, P. C. (1992). Application of attachment theory to the study of sexual abuse. *Journal of Consulting and Clinical Psychology,* 60 (2), 185–195.

Almond, R. 1974. *The Healing Community.* New York: Jason Aronson.

Anderson, B. J. 1995. Police trauma syndrome: Effects on officers and their families. Presented at Annual Meeting, International Society for Traumatic Stress Studies, *The Treatment of Trauma: Advances and Challenges,* November 2–6, Boston, MA.

Anderson, C. O., and W. A. Mason. 1978. Competitive social strategies in groups of deprived and experienced rhesus monkeys. *Journal of Comparative and Physiological Psychology,* 87: 681–690.

Anfuso, D. 1994. Deflecting workplace violence. *Personnel Journal,* 3(10): 66–78.

Arbetter, S. 1995. Violence—a growing threat. *Current Health 2*, 21(6): 6–13.

Åstedt-Kurki, Päivi and Arja Liukkonen. 1994. Humor in nursing care. *Journal of Advanced Nursing*, 20: 183–188.

Bandura A. 1982 Self-efficacy mechanism in human agency. *American Psychologist*, 37(2): 122–147.

Barker, H. 1989. *Arguments for a Theatre*. London: John Calder.

Barrier M. 1995a. The enemy within. *Nation's Business*, 83(2): 18–24.

Barrier, M. 1995b. Creating a violence-free company culture. *Nation's Business*, 83(2): 22–23.

Barlett, D. L., and Steele, J. B. 1992. *America: What Went Wrong?* Kansas City: Andrews and McMeel.

Barlett, D. L., and Steele, J. B. 1996. *America: Who Stole the Dream?* Kansas City: Andrews and McMeel.

Bastian, L. D. 1991. Bureau of Justice Statistics Bulletin: Crime and the Nation's Households. Washington, D.C.

Beahrs, J. O. 1983. *Unity and Multiplicity: Multilevel Consciousness of Self in Hypnosis, Psychiatric Disorder, and Mental Health*. New York: Brunner/Mazel.

Becker, C. 1994. Introduction: Presenting the problem. In *The Subversive Imagination: Artistis, Society, and Social Responsibility*, edited by C. Becker. New York: Routledge.

Becker, H. S. 1963. *Outsiders: Studies in the Sociology of Deviance*. New York: The Free Press.

Belenky, M. F., B.M. Clinchy, N.R.Goldberger, J. M. Tarule. 1986. *Women's Ways of Knowing: The Development of Self, Voice and Mind*. New York: Basic Books.

Bellah, R. N. 1973. Introduction. In *Emile Durkheim: On Morality and Society: Selected Writings*. Chicago: University of Chicago Press.

Benoit, D., C. H. Zeanah, C.H., and M. L. Varton. 1989. Maternal attachment disturbances in failure to thrive. *Infant Mental Health Journal*. 10(3): 185–202.

Bentovim, Arnon. 1992. *Trauma Organized Systems*. London: Karnac Books.

Berman, W. H., and M. B. Sperling, 1994. The structure and function of adult attachment. In M. B. Sperling, and W. H. Berman, Eds. *Attachment in Adults: Clinical and Developmental Perspectives*. New York: Guilford.

Bianchi, H. 1995. *Justice as Sanctuary: Toward a New System of Crime Control*. Bloomington: Indiana University Press.

Bion, W. R. 1991. *Experience in Groups*. London: Routledge.

Bloom, S. L. 1994a. The sanctuary model: Developing generic inpatient programs for the treatment of psychological trauma. In *Handbook of Post-Traumatic Therapy: A Practical Guide to Intervention, Treatment, and Research*, edited by M. B. Williams and J. F. Sommer. New York: Greenwood.

Bloom, S. L. 1994b. Creating sanctuary: Ritual abuse and complex PTSD. In *Treating Satanist Abuse Survivors: An Invisible Trauma*, edited by V. Sinason. London: Routledge.

Bloom, S. L. 1994c. Hearing the survivor's voice: Sundering the wall of denial. *Journal of Psychohistory*, 21(4): 461–477.

Bloom, S. L. 1995a. Creating sanctuary in the school. *Journal for a Just and Caring Education*, 1(4): 403–433.

Bloom, S. L. 1995b. When good people do bad things: Meditations on the "backlash." *Journal of Psychohistory*, 22(3): 273–304.

Bloom, S. L. 1996. Bridging the black hole of trauma: Victims, artists, and society. Presented at Annual Meeting, International Society for Traumatic Stress Studies, *Trauma and Controversy*, November 9–13, San Francisco, California.

Bloom, S.L. 1997. Every time history repeats itself the price goes up: The social reenactment of trauma. *Journal of Sexual Addiction and Compulsivity*, 3 (3): 161–194.

Bollerud, K. 1990. A model for the treatment of trauma-related syndromes among chemically dependent inpatient women. *Journal of Substance Abuse Treatment*, 7, 83.

Bowlby, J. 1979. *The Making and Breaking of Affectional Bonds*, London: Tavistock Publications.

Bowlby, J. 1982. *Attachment.* New York: Basic Books.

Breakey, G., and Pratt, B. 1991. Healthy growth for Hawaii's "healthy start": Toward a systematic statewide approach to the prevention of child abuse and neglect. *Bulletin of National Center for Clinical Infant Programs*, 11: 16–22.

Breiner, S. J. 1990. *Slaughter of the Innocents: Child Abuse Through the Ages and Today.* New York: Plenum Press.

Bremner, J. D., M. Davis, S. M. Southwick, J. H. Krystal, and D. S. Charney, 1993. Neurobiology of posttraumatic stress disorder. In *Review of Psychiatry: Volume 12*, edited by J. M. Oldham, M. B. Riba and A. Tasman. Washington, D. C.: American Psychiatric Press.

Bremner, J.D., J. H. Krystal, S. M. Southwick, and D. S. Charney. 1995. Functional neuroanatomical correlates of the effects of stress on memory. *Journal of Traumatic Stress*, 8: 527–553.

Brent, D.A., J. A. Perper, C. J. Allman, G. M. Moritz, M. E. Wartella, and J. P. Zelenak. 1991. The presence and accessibility of firearms in the homes of adolescent suicides, a case control study. *Journal of the American Medical Association*, 266(21): 2989–2995.

Breslau, N., G. C. Davis, P Andreski, and E. Peterson. 1991. Traumatic events and post-traumatic stress disorder in an urban population of young adults. *Archives of General Psychiatry*, 48: 216–222.

Brill, N. Q. 1993. *America's Psychic Malignancy.* Springfield, IL: Charles C. Thomas.

Brody, E. B. 1973. *The Lost Ones: Social Forces and Mental Illness in Rio De Janeiro.* New York: International Universities Press.

Brook, P. 1968. *The Empty Space.* New York: Atheneum.

Brown, D. 1993. Stress and emotion: Implications for illness development and wellness. In *Human Feelings: Explorations in Affect, Development and Meaning,* edited by S. L. Ablon, D. Brown, E. J. Khantzian, and J. E. Mack. Hillsdale, NJ: The Analytic Press.

Brzezinski, Zbigniew. 1993. *Out of Control: Global Turmoil on the Eve of the Twenty-First Century.* New York: Scribner.

Bureau of Justice Statistics Bulletin. 1985. The crime of rape. Washington, D.C.

Burrow, T. 1926. The laboratory method in psychoanalysis: Its inception and development. *The American Journal of Psychiatry,* 5: 345–55.

Burrow, T. 1927. *The Social Basis of Consciousness.* New York: Harcourt, Brace and Company.

Burrow, T. 1950. Prescription for peace: The biological basis of man's ideological conflicts. In *Explorations in Altruistic Love and Behavior* edited by P.A. Sorokin. Boston: The Beacon Press.

Burrow, T. 1953. *Science and Man's Behavior: The Contribution of Phylobiology.* Edited by W. E. Galt. New York: Philosophical Library.

Burrow, T. 1984. *Toward Social Sanity and Human Survival: Selections from His Writings.* Edited by A. S. Galt. New York: Horizon Books.

Busfield, J. 1986. *Managing Madness: Changing Ideas and Practice.* London: Unwin Hyman.

Caldwell, M. F. 1992. Incidence of PTSD among staff victims of patient violence. *Hospital and Community Psychiatry,* 43(8).

Callahan, C. M., and F. P. Rivara. 1992. Urban high school youths and handguns, a school based survey. *Journal of the American Medical Association,* 267: 3038.

Callahan, S. 1991. *In Good Conscience: Reason and Emotion in Moral Decision Making.* San Francisco: HarperSanFrancisco

Campbell, J. 1995. *Understanding John Dewey: Nature and Cooperative Intelligence.* Chicago: Open Court.

Cannon, W. B. 1939. *The Wisdom of the Body,* 2nd ed. New York: W. W. Simon.

Caplan, G. 1964. *Principles of Preventive Psychiatry.* New York: Basic Books.

Caplan, G. 1974. *Support Systems and Community Mental Health.* New York: Behavioral Publications.

Capra, F. 1996. *The Web of Life: A New Scientific Understanding of Living Systems.* New York: Anchor Books.

Carleton, J. L., and U. R. Mahlendorf. 1979. *Dimensions of Social Psychiatry.* Princeton, N. J.: Science Press.

Cassel, J. 1976. The contribution of the social environment to host resistance. *American Journal of Epidemiology,* 104: 107–123.

Caudill, W. 1958. *The Psychiatric Hospital as a Small Society.* Cambridge, MA: Harvard University Press.

Centerwall, B.S. 1992. Television and violence. The scale of the problem and where to go from here. *Journal of the American Medical Association,* 267: 3059–3063.

Chesler, P. 1972. *Women and Madness.* New York: Doubleday.

Chodorow, N. 1978. *The Reproduction of Mothering: Psychoanalysis and the Sociology of Gender.* Berkeley: University of California Press.

Cicchetti, D and J. White. 1990. Emotion and developmental psychopathology. In *Psychological and Biological Approaches to Emotion,* edited by N. Stein, B. Leventhal, and T. Trebasso. Hillsdale, NJ: Lawrence Erlbaum.

Cicchetti, D and M. Lynch. 1995. Failures in the expectable environment and their impact on individual development: The case of child maltreatment. In *Developmental Psychopathology, Volume 2 Risk, Disorder, and Adaptation,* edited by D. Cicchetti and D. J. Cohen. New York: Wiley.

Clastres, P. 1987. *Society Against the State.* New York: Zone Books.

Coates, D., C. B. Wortman, and A. Abben. 1979. Reactions to victims. In *New Approaches to Social Problems,* edited by I.H. Frieze, D. Bar-Tal, and J.S. Carroll. San Francisco: Jossey Bass.

Cole, S. L. 1992. *Directors in Rehearsal.* New York: Routledge.

Collier, G., H. L. Minton, and G. Reynolds. 1991. *Currents of Thought in American Social Psychology.* New York: Oxford University Press.

Conrad, P and J. Schneider. 1980. *Deviance and Medicalisation, from Badness to Sickness.* St. Louis, MO: C.V. Mosby.

Cooley, C. H. 1967. Primary groups. In *Small Groups: Studies in Social Interaction,* edited by P. Hare, E. F. Borgatta and R. F. Bales. New York: Knopf.

Cousins, N. 1976. Anatomy of an illness. *New England Journal of Medicine,* 295: 1485–1463.

Crewdson, J. 1988. *By Silence Betrayed: Sexual Abuse Of Children In America.* Boston: Little, Brown, and Co.

Cumming, J., and E. Cumming. 1962. *Ego and Milieu.* Hawthorne, NY: Aldine.

D'Aquili, E. G., and C. D. Laughlin, Jr. 1979. The neurobiology of myth and ritual. In *The Spectrum of Ritual: A Biogenetic Structural Analysis* edited by E. G. D'Aquili, C. D. Laughlin Jr., and J. McManus, J New York: Columbia University Press.

Danielli, Y. 1985. The treatment and prevention of long-term effects and intergenerational transmission of victimization: A lesson from Holocaust survivors and their children. In *Trauma and Its Wake: The Study and Treatment of Post-Traumatic Stress Disorder,* edited by C. R. Figley. New York: Brunner/Mazel.

De Bono, E. 1990. *Daily Mail.* London, January 29.

Dellums, R. V. 1995. Stealth bombing America's future. *The Nation* 261(10): 350–353.

DeMause, L. 1982. The evolution of childhood. In *Foundations of Psychohistory.* New York: Creative Roots.

DeMause, L. 1990. The history of child assault. *The Journal of Psychohistory,* 18 (1): 1–30.

DeMause, L. 1993. A proposal to President Clinton on behalf of America's children. *Journal of Psychohistory,* 21(1)1–5.

De Unamuno, M. 1954. *Tragic Sense of Life.* New York: Dover.

De Zulueta, F. 1993. *From Pain to Violence: The Traumatic Roots of Destructiveness.* London: Whurr.

Dilworth, D. D. 1994. 1 million victimized at work annually. *Tria,* 30(10): 109–111.

Dissanayake, E. 1992. *Homoaestheticus: Where Art Comes From and Why.* New York: Free Press.

Dolinskas, C. 1995. Bullets as pathogens. Slide presentation. *Physicians for Social Responsibility,* Philadelphia Chapter.

Donald, M. 1991. *Origins of the Modern Mind: Three Stages in the Evolution of Culture and Cognition.* Cambridge, MA: Harvard University Press.

Douglas, T. 1986. *Group Living: The Application of Group Dynamics in Residential Settings.* London: Tavistock.

Driver, T. F. 1991. *The Magic of Ritual: Our Need for Liberating Rites That Transform Our Lives and Our Communities.* San Francisco: HarperSan Francisco.

Duncan, T. S. 1995. Death in the office: workplace homicides. *FBI Law Enforcement Bulletin* 64(4): 20–26.

Durkheim, E. 1951. *Suicide.* Glencoe, IL: Free Press

Dutton, D., and S. L. Painter. 1981 Traumatic bonding: The development of emotional attachments in battered women and other relationships of intermittent abuse. *Victimology: An International Journal,* 6: 139–155.

Dwyer, E. 1987. *Homes For the Mad.* New Brunswick, N.J.: Rutgers University Press.

Edelman, M. W. 1987. *Families in Peril: An Agenda for Social Change.* Cambridge: Harvard University Press.

Edelman, S. E. 1978. Managing the violent patient in a community mental health center. *Hospital and Community Psychiatry,* 29(7).

Ehrenreich, B., and D. English. 1978. *For Her Own Good: 150 Years of the Experts' Advice to Women.* New York: Anchor.

Eibl-Eibesfeldt, I. 1989. *Human Ethology.* New York: Aldine de Gruyter.

Erikson, K. 1994. *A New Species of Trouble: The Human Experience of Modern Disasters.* New York: W. W. Norton.

Eslin, M. 1976. *The Anatomy of Drama.* New York: Hill and Wang.

Etzioni, A. 1993. *The Spirit Of Community: Rights Responsibilities And The Communitarian Agenda.* New York: Crown.

Figley, Charles R. 1995. *Compassion Fatigue: Coping With Secondary Traumatic Stress Disorder in Those Who Treat the Traumatized.* New York: Brunner/Mazel.

Figley, C. R., and Sprenkle, D. H. 1978. Delayed stress response syndrome: Family therapy indications. *Journal of Marital and Family Therapy,* 4: 53–60.

Fingerhut, L. A and J. C. Kleinman. 1990. International and interstate comparisons of homicide among young males. *Journal of the American Medical Association,* 263: 3292–3295.

Fish-Murray, C. C., E. V. Koby, and B. A. Van der Kolk, B.A. 1987. Evolving ideas:

the effect of abuse on children's thought. In *Psychological Trauma*, edited by Bessel A. Van der Kolk. Washington, D. C.: American Psychiatric Press.

Flannery, R. B. 1990. *Becoming Stress-Resistant: Through the Project SMART Program.* New York: Continuum.

Flannery, R. B., P. Fulton, J. Tausch, A.Y. DeLoffi. 1991. A program to help staff cope with psychological sequelae of assaults by patients. *Hospital and Community Psychiatry.* 42(9): 935–938.

Foderaro, J. F. 1989. Personal communication.

Foderaro, J.F. 1996. Position statement on suicide and suicidal ideation. *The Sanctuary*, Friends Hospital, Philadelphia, PA.

Fogelman, E. 1994. *Conscience and Courage: Rescuers of Jews During the Holocaust.* New York: Anchor.

Forer, L. 1994. *The Rage to Punish.* New York: W.W. Norton

Forsyth, D. R. 1990. *Group Dynamics, Second Edition.* Pacific Grove: CA: Brooks/Cole.

Foucault, M. 1965. *Madness and Civilization: A History of Insanity in the Age of Reason.* New York: Vintage

Foulkes, S. H. 1964. *Therapeutic Group Analysis.* London: Allen and Unwin.

Foulkes, S. H., and G. S. Prince. 1969. *Psychiatry in a Changing Society.* London: Tavistock.

Frank, J. 1976. New Therapeutic Roles. In *Further Explorations in Social Psychiatry Further Explorations in Social Psychiatry Further Explorations in Social Psychiatry* edited by B. H. Kaplan, R. N. Wilson, and A. H. Leighton. New York: Basic Books.

Freedman, J. 1993. *From Cradle to Grave: The Human Face of Poverty in America.* New York: Atheneum.*41: 101–116.*

Freyberg, J. 1980. Difficulties in separation-individuation as experienced by off-spring of Nazi Holocaust survivors. *American Journal of Orthopsychiatry*

Freyd, J. 1996. *Betrayal Trauma Theory: The Logic of Forgetting Abuse.* Cambridge: Harvard University Press.

Friedman, M. J. 1990. Interrelationships between biological mechanisms and pharmacotherapy of posttraumatic stress disorder. In *Posttraumatic Stress Disorder: Etiology, Phenomenology and Treatment,* edited by M.E. Wolf and A.D. Mosnaim. Washington, D.C.: American Psychiatric Press.

Friedman, M. J., and P. Schnurr. 1995. The relationship between trauma, post-traumatic stress disorder, and physical health. In *Neurobiological and Clinical Consequences of Stress: From Normal Adaptation to PTSD,* edited by M. J. Friedman, D. S. Charney, and A. Y. Deutch. Philadelphia: Lippincott-Raven.

Fromm, E. 1956. *The Sane Society.* London: Routledge and Kegan Paul, Ltd.

Fullilove, M. T., R. S. Fullilove, M. Smith, K. Winkler, C. Michael, P. G. Panzer, and R. Wallace. 1993. Violence, trauma, and post-traumatic stress disorder among women drug users. *Journal of Traumatic Stress,* 6: 533–543.

Garbarino, J., N. Dubrow, K. Kostelny, and C. Pardo. 1992. *Children in Danger: Coping with the Consequences of Community Violence.*

Gelles, R. J., and D. R. Loseke, editors. *Current Controversies on Family Violence.* Newbury Park: Sage.

Gelles, R. J., and M. A. Straus, M.A. 1988. *Intimate Violence: The Definitive Study of the Causes and Consequences of Abuse in the American Family.* New York: Simon and Schuster.

Gerbner, G. 1993. Violence on Television Challenging Media *Images of Women,* 5(2): 1, 4, 8.

Gerbner, G. 1994. Television violence. The art of asking the wrong question. *The World and I,* July: 385–392.

Gersons, B. 1989. Patterns of PTSD among police officers following shooting incidents: A two-dimensional model and treatment implications. *Journal of Traumatic Stress,* 2(3): 247–257.

Gilligan, C. 1982. *In a Different Voice: Psychological Theory and Women's Development.* Cambridge, MA: Harvard University Press

Gilligan, J. 1996. *Violence: Our Deadly Epidemic and Its Causes.* New York: G.P. Putnam's Sons.

Glaser, D. 1971. *Social Deviance.* Chicago: Markham.

Glover, H. 1992. Emotional numbing: A possible endorphin-mediated phenomenon associated with post-traumatic stress disorders and other allied psychopathologic states. *Journal of Traumatic Stress* 5(4): 643–676.

Goldhagen, D. J. 1996. *Hitler's Willing Executioners: Ordinary Germans and the Holocaust.* New York: Knopf.

Goleman, D. 1995. *Emotional Intelligence.* New York: Bantam Books.

Gray, W., F. J. Duhl and N. D. Rizzo, eds. 1969. *General Systems Theory and Psychiatry.* Boston: Little Brown.

Green, A. 1993. Childhood sexual and physical abuse. In *International Handbook of Traumatic Stress Syndromes* edited by J.P. Wilson & B. Raphael. New York: Plenum Press.

Green, B. L., J. D. Lindy, M. C. Grace, G. C. Gleser, A. C. Leonard, M. Korol, and C. Winget. 1990. Buffalo Creek survivors in the second decade: Stability of stress symptoms. American Journal of Orthopsychiatry, 60(1): 43–54.

Green, B. L. 1994. Psychosocial research in traumatic stress: An update. *Journal of Traumatic Stress Studies,* 7(3): 341–362.

Greenblatt M., R. M. Becerra, and E. A. Serafetinides. 1982. *Social Networks and Mental Health: An Overview.* American Journal of Psychiatry 139: 977–984

Greenblatt, M., D. J. Levinson, and R. H. Williams, editors. 1957. *The Patient and the Mental Hospital: Contributions of Research in the Science of Social Behavior.* Glencoe, IL: Free Press.

Grinker, R. R., and J. P. Spiegel. 1945. *Men Under Stress.* Philadelphia: Blakiston.

Grob, G. N. 1991. *From Asylum to Community: Mental Health Policy in Modern America.* Princeton, N.J.: Princeton University Press.

Grossman, K. E., and K. Grossman. 1991. Attachment quality as an organizer of emotional and behavioral responses in a longitudinal perspective. In *Attachment Across the Life Cycle*, edited by C. M. Parkes, J. Stevenson-Hinde, and P. Marris. London: Routledge.

Guyer, B., I. Lescohier, S. Gallagher, A. Hausman, and C. V. Azzara. 1989. Intentional injuries among children and adolescents in Massachusetts. *The New England Journal of Medicine*, 321: 1584–1589.

Harber, K. D., and J. W. Pennebaker. 1992. Overcoming traumatic memories. In *The Handbook of Emotion and Memory: Research and Theory* edited by S.A. Christianson. Hillsdale, N.J.: Lawrence Erlbaum. pp. 359–387.

Harkness, L. L. 1993. Transgenerational transmission of war-related trauma. In *International Handbook of Traumatic Stress Syndromes*, edited by J. P. Wilson & B. Raphael. New York: Plenum

Harlow, H. F. 1962. The heterosexual affectional system in monkeys. *American Psychologist*, 17: 1–9.

Harlow, H. F. 1974. *Learning to Love, 2nd ed.* New York: Aronson.

Harlow, H. F., and Mears, C. 1979. *Primate Perspectives.* New York: Wiley.

Hartung, W. D. 1995. Notes from the underground; an outsider's guide to the defense budget debate. *World Policy Journal* 12(3): 15–19.

Hatfield, E., J. T. Cacioppo, R. L. Rapson. 1994. *Emotional Contagion*. Paris: Cambridge University Press.

Havel, V. 1990. *Disturbing the peace: Conversations with Karel Hvizdala*. New York: Knopf.

Heath, L., L. B. Bresolin, and R. C. Rinaldi, 1989. Effects of media violence on children. *Archives of General Psychiatry*, 46: 376–379.

Helgesen, S. 1990. *The Female Advantage: Women's Ways of Leadership*. New York: Doubleday.

Henry, J. 1965. *Pathways to Madness*. New York: Random House.

Herbert, B. 1995. What special interest? *New York Times*, March 22, p. A19.

Herman, J. L., 1981. *Father-Daughter Incest*. Cambridge, MA: Harvard University Press.

Herman, J. L. 1992. *Trauma and Recovery*. New York: Basic Books.

Herman, J. L., J. C. Perry, and B. A. Van der Kolk. 1989. Childhood trauma in borderline personality disorder. *American Journal of Psychiatry*, 146: 490–495.

Herzog, J. 1982. World beyond metaphor: thoughts on the transmission of trauma. In *Generations of the Holocaust*, edited by M.S. Bergmann and M.E. Jucovy. New York: Basic Books.

Hewstone, M., W. Stroebe, J. Codol, and G. M. Stephenson. 1989. *Introduction to Social Psychology*. Oxford, England: Basil Blackwell.

Hilgard, E. R. 1986. *Divided Consciousness: Multiple Controls in Human Thought and Action*. New York: John Wiley

Hirsch, H. 1995. *Genocide and the Politics of Memory: Studying Death to Preserve Life*. Chapel Hill: University of North Carolina Press.

Holland, J. H. 1995. *Hidden Order: How Adaptation Builds Complexity.* Reading, MA: Addison-Wesley.

Holmes, T.H., and R. H. Rahe. 1967. The social readjustment rating scale. *Journal of Psychosomatic Research* II: 213–218.

Horney, K. 1937. *The Neurotic Personality of Our Time.* London: Routledge and Kegan Paul.

Inkeles, A. 1997. *National Character: A Psycho-Social Perspective.* New Brunswick, NJ: Transaction.

Itzen, C. 1992. Pornography and the social construction of sexual inequality. In *Pornography: Women, Violence and Civil Liberties,* edited by C. Itzin. New York: Oxford University Press.

Jackson, D. 1969. The individual and the larger Contexts. In *General Systems Theory and Psychiatry* edited by W. Gray, F. J. Duhl and N. D. Rizzo. Boston: Little Brown.

Jacobs, R. C., and D. T. Campbell. 1965. The perpetuation of an arbitrary tradition through several generations of a laboratory microculture. In *Small Groups: Studies in Social Interaction* edited by A. P. Hare, E. F. Borgatta, and R. F. Bales. New York: Knopf.

Jacobson, A., and C. Herald. 1990. The relevance of childhood sexual abuse to adult psychiatric inpatient care. *Hospital and Community Psychiatry,* 41: 154–156.

Jacobson, A., J. E. Koehler, and C. Jones-Brown. 1987. The failure of routine assessment to detect histories of assault experienced by psychiatric patients. *Hospital and Community Psychiatry,* 38: 386–389.

Jacobson, A., and B. Richardson. 1987. Assault experiences of 100 psychiatric inpatients: Evidence of the need for routine inquiry. *American Journal of Psychiatry* 144(7): 908–913.

James, B. 1989. *Treating Traumatized Children: New Insights and Creative Interventions.* New York: Lexington Books.

James, B. 1994. *Handbook for Treatment of Attachment Trauma Problems in Children.* New York: Lexington Books.

Janis, I. L. 1972. *Victims of Groupthink.* Boston: Houghton Mifflin.

Janis, I. L. 1982. Decision making under stress. In *Handbook of Stress: Theoretical and Clinical Aspects* edited by L. Goldberger and S. Breznitz. New York: Free Press.

Janis, I. L., and L. Mann. 1977. *Decision Making.* New York: Free Press

Janoff-Bulman, R. 1992. *Shattered Assumptions: Towards a New Psychology of Trauma.* New York: Free Press.

Jenkinson, W.R. 1993. Attacks on postmen in Northern Ireland. What features of the attack are associated with prolonged absence from work? *Occupational Medicine* 43: 39–42.

Johnson, D. W., and R. T. Johnson. 1995. Why violence prevention programs don't work—and what does. *Educational Leadership* 52(5): 63–69.

Jones, B. 1983. Healing factors in psychiatry in light of attachment theory. *American Journal of Psychotherapy,* 37(2): 235–244.

Jones, M. 1953. *The Therapeutic Community: A New Treatment Method in Psychiatry.* New York: Basic Books.

Jones, M. 1968a. *Social Psychiatry in Practice.* Middlesex, England: Penguin.

Jones, M. 1968b. *Beyond the Therapeutic Community: Social Learning and Social Psychiatry.* New Haven, CT: Yale University Press.

Joseph, R 1992. *The Right Brain And The Unconscious: Discovering The Stranger Within.* New York: Plenum.

Katz, M. 1989. *The Undeserving Poor: From the War on Poverty to the War on Welfare.* New York: Pantheon.

Kellerman, A. L., and D. T. Reay. 1986. Protection or peril? An analysis of firearm-related deaths in the home. *New England Journal of Medicine,* 314: 1557.

Kelly, L. 1992. Pornography and child sexual abuse. In *Pornography: Women, Violence and Civil Liberties* edited by C. Itzian. New York: Oxford University Press.

Kestenberg, J. 1980. Psychoanalysis of children of survivors from the Holocaust: Case presentations and assessment. *Journal of the American Psychoanalytic Association,* 28: 775–804.

Kilpatrick, D. G., C. N. Edmunds, and A. K. Seymour. 1992. *Rape in America: A Report to the Nation.* Arlington, VA: National Victim Center.

Kilpatrick, D. G., and H. S. Resnick. 1993. PTSD associated with exposure to criminal victimization in clinical and community populations. In *Post-traumatic Stress Disorder: DSM IV and Beyond,* edited by J. R. T. Davidson and E. B. Foa. Washington, D.C.: American Psychiatric Press.

Kimmel, M. S. 1990. *Men Confront Pornography.* New York: Crown.

King, S. 1995. *Rose Madder.* New York: Viking.

Kirshner, L. A., and L. Johnston. 1982. Current status of milieu psychiatry. *General Hospital Psychiatry,* 4: 75–80

Kittrie, N. N. 1971. *The Right to Be Different: Deviance and Enforced Therapy.* Baltimore, MD: Johns Hopkins University Press.

Kluft, R.P. 1996. Dissociative identity disorder. In *Handbook of Dissociation: Theoretical, Empirical, and Clinical Perspectives* edited by L.K. Michelson and W.J. Ray. New York: Plenum Press.

Kokopeli B., and G. Lakey. 1990. More power than we want. In *Men and Intimacy.* Edited by F. Abbott. Freedom, CA: Crossing Press.

Koss, M. P., P. G. Koss, and W. J. Woodruff. 1991. Deleterious effects of criminal victimization on women's health and medical utilization. *Archives of Internal Medicine* 151: 342–347.

Koss, M. P., L. A. Goodman, A. Browne, L. F. Fitzgerald, G. P. Keita, N. F. Russo, 1994. *No Safe Haven: Male Violence Against Women at Home, at Work, and in the Community.* Washington, D. C.: American Psychological Association Press.

Kraemer, G. W. 1985. Effects of differences in early social experiences on primate neurobiological-behavioral development. In *The Psychobiology of Attachment and Separation* edited by M. Reite and T. Fields. Orlando, FL: Academic Press.

Kroll-Smith, J. S., and S. R. Couch. 1993. Technological hazards: Social responses as traumatic stressors. In *International Handbook of Traumatic Stress Syndromes,* edited by J. P. Wilson & B. Raphael. New York: Plenum.

Krystal, H. 1978. Trauma and affects. *Psychoanalytic Study of the Child,* 33: 81–116.

Kuhn, T. 1970. *The Structure of Scientific Revolutions,* 2nd ed. Chicago: University of Chicago Press.

Laing, R. D. 1967. *The Politics of Experience.* New York: Pantheon.

Lansky, M. R., and C. R. Bley. 1995. *Posttraumatic Nightmares: Psychodynamic Explorations.* Hillsdale, NJ: The Analytic Press.

Larson, E. 1993. The story of a gun. *Atlantic Monthly,* January.

Lasch, C. 1977. *Haven in a Heartless World: The Family Besieged.* New York: Basic Books.

Laub, J. H., and J. L. Lauritsen. 1995 Violent criminal behavior over the life course: A review of the longitudinal and comparative research. In *Interpersonal Violent Behaviors: Social and Cultural Aspects* edited by. R. B. Ruback and N.A. Weiner. New York: Springer Publishing.

Laughlin Jr., C. D., J. McManus, and E. G. d'Aquili. 1979. Introduction. In *The Spectrum of Ritual: A Biogenetic Structural Analysis* edited by E. G. D'Aquili, C. D. Laughlin Jr., and J. McManus. New York: Columbia University Press.

Lazarus, R. S. 1991. *Emotion and Adaptation.* New York: Oxford University Press.

LeDoux, J. E. 1992. Emotion as memory: Anatomical systems underlying indelible neural trances. In *The Handbook of Emotion and Memory: Research and Theory* edited by S.A. Christianson. Hillsdale, NJ: Lawrence Erlbaum Associates

LeDoux, J. E. 1994. Emotion, memory, and the brain. *Scientific American* 270: 50–57.

Leeman, C.P. 1986. The therapeutic milieu and its role in clinical management. In *Inpatient Psychiatry* edited by L. I. Sederer. Baltimore: Williams and Wilkins.

Leeman, C. P., and S. Autio. 1978. Milieu therapy: The need for individualization. *Psychotherapy and Psychosomatics* 29: 84–92.

Leighton, A. H. 1960. *An Introduction to Social Psychiatry.* Springfield, IL: Charles C. Thomas

Lerner, M. J. 1980. *The Belief in a Just World.* New York: Plenum.

Lewin, K. 1943. Forces behind food habits and methods of change. *Bulletin of the National Research Council,* 108, 35–65.

Lewin, T. 1995. Parents poll shows child abuse to be more common. *New York Times,* December 7.

Lex, B. 1979. The neurobiology of ritual traunce. In E.G. D'Aquili, C.D. Laughlin Jr., and J. McManus, editors. *The Spectrum of Ritual: A Biogenetic Structural Analysis.* New York: Columbia University Press.

Linden, K., and R. B. McFarland. 1993. Community parenting centers in Colorado. *Journal of Psychohistory,* 21(1): 7–19.

Lindquist, B., and A. Molnar. 1995. Children learn what they live. *Educational Leadership* 52(5): 50–52.

Linton, M. 1993. Money and community economics. In *In the Company of Others: Making Community in the Modern World* edited by C. Whitmyer. New York: Jeremy Tarcher.

Loring, M. T. 1994. *Emotional Abuse*. New York: Lexington Books.

Macalpine, I., and R. Hunter. 1993. *George III and the Mad-Business*. London: Pimlico.

Main, M., and R. Goldwyn. 1984. Predicting rejecting of her infant from mother's representation of her own experience: Implications for the abused-abusing intergenerational cycle. *Child Abuse and Neglect*, 8: 203–217.

Main, M., and E. Hesse. 1990. Parents' unresolved traumatic experiences are related to infant disorganized attachment status: Is frightened and/or frightening parental behavior the linking mechanism? In *Attachment in the Preschool Years: Theory, Research, and Intervention* edited by M.T. Greenberg, D. Cicchetti, and E.M. Cummings. Chicago: University of Chicago Press.

Main, M., N. Kaplan, and J. Cassidy. 1985. Security in infancy, childhood, and adulthood: A move to the level of representation. In *Growing Points of Attachment Theory and Research* edited by I. Bretherton and E. Waters. *Monography of the Society for Research in Child Development* 50: 66–104.

Main, T. 1989. *The Ailment and Other Psychoanalytic Essays*. London: Free Association Books.

Main, T. F. 1946. The hospital as a therapeutic institution. *Bulletin of the Menninger Clinic,* 10(3): 66–70.

Mainellis, K. A. 1996. How bad is violence in hospitals? *Safety and Health* 153(1): 50–55.

Maloney, J. C. 1949. *The Magic Cloak: A Contribution to the Psychology of Authoritarianism*. Wakefield, MA: Montrose Press.

Manning, N. 1989. *The Therapeutic Community Movement: Charisma and Routinization*. New York: Routledge.

Marowitz, C. 1986. *Directing the Action: Acting and Directing in the Contemporary Theatre*. New York: Applause Books.

Mason, W. A. 1968. Early social deprivation in the nonhuman primates: Implications for human behavior. In *Environmental Influences: Proceedings of a Conference Under the Auspices of Russell Sage Foundation and The Rockefeller University* edited by D. C. Glass. New York: Rockefeller University Press.

Matsakis, A. 1988. *Vietnam Wives: Women and Children Suriving Life with Veterans Suffering Posttraumatic Stress Disorder*. Kensington, MD: Woodbine House.

Matsakis, A. 1994. *Post-Traumatic Stress Disorder: A Complete Treatment Guide*. Oakland, CA: New Harbinger Publications.

May, E. T. 1991. Myths and realities of the American family. In *A History of Private Life: Riddles of Identity in Modern Times,* edited by A. Prost and G. Vincent. Cambridge: Belknap.

McCann, I. L., and L. A. Pearlman. 1990. Vicarious traumatization: A framework for understanding the psychological effects of working with victims. *Journal of Traumatic Stress*, 3: 131–147.

McDougall, W. 1920. *The Group Mind*. London: Cambridge University Press.

McGovern, C. M. 1985. *The Masters of Madness: Social Origins of the American Psychiatric Profession*. Hanover, NH: University Press of New England.

McLennan, K. J. 1996. *Nature's Ban: Women's Incest Literature*. Boston: Northeastern University Press.

Mead, G. H. 1934. *Mind, Self, and Society*. Chicago: University of Chicago Press.

Meichenbaum, D. 1994. *A Clinical Handbook: Practical Therapist Manual*. Ontario, Canada: Institute Press.

Menninger, W. C. 1945. Psychiatry and the war. *Atlantic Monthly* 176: 107–114.

Menzies, I. E. P. 1975. A case-study in the functioning of social systems as a defense against anxiety. In *Group Relations Reader 1* edited by A. D. Colman and W. H. Bexton. Washington, D. C.: Rice Institute Series.

Mercogliano, C. 1995. *Making It Up As We Go Along: The Story of the (Albany) Free School*. Unpublished manuscript.

Mercy, J. A., and V. N. Houk 1988. Firearm injuries: a call for science. *New England Journal of Medicine*, 319: 1283.

Miedzian, M. 1991. *Boys Will Be Boys: Breaking The Link Between Masculinity and Violence*. New York: Doubleday.

Milgram, S. 1974. *Obedience to Authority*. New York: Harper Colophon.

Miller, A. 1983. *For Your Own Good: Hidden Cruelty in Child-Rearing and the Roots of Violence*. New York: Farrar, Straus, and Giroux.

Miller, J. B. 1973. *Psychoanalysis and Women: Contributions to New Theory and Therapy*. New York: Brunner/Mazel.

Miller, J.B. 1976. *Toward A New Psychology of Women*. Boston: Beacon.

Mitchell, J. T., and Dyregrov, A. 1993. Traumatic stress in disaster workers and emergency personnel: Prevention and intervention. In *International Handbook Of Traumatic Stress Syndromes* edited by J. P. Wilson and B. Raphael. New York: Plenum.

Moreno, J. L. 1953. *Who Shall Survive?: Foundations of Sociometry, Group Psychotherapy and Sociodrama*. Beacon, NY: Beacon House.

Moses, R. 1989. Denial in political process. In *Denial: A Clarification Of Concepts And Research* edited by E. L. Edelstein, D. L. Nathanson, and A.M. Stone. New York: Plenum.

Moyers, B. 1993. *Healing and the Mind*. New York: Doubleday.

Muller, R. T., J. E. Hunter, and G. Stollak. 1995. The intergenerational transmission of corporal punishment: A comparison of social learning and temperament models. *Child Abuse and Neglect*, 19(11): 1323–35.

Nathanson, D. L. 1992. *Shame and Pride: Affect, Sex, and the Birth of the Self*. New York: W.W. Norton.

National Television Violence Study. 1996. http://www.igc.apc.org/mediascope/ntvs.html#3

National Victim Center. 1993. *Crime and Victimization in America: Statistical Overview.* Arlington, VA: National Victim Center.

Nichols, W. D. 1995. Violence on campus: The intruded sanctuary. *The FBI Law Enforcement Bulletin* 64(6): 1–6.

Norris, F .H. 1992. Epidemiology of trauma: frequency and impact of different potentially traumatic events on different demographic groups. *Journal of Consulting and Clinical Psychology* 60(3): 409–418.

Oldenquist, A. 1986. *The Nonsuicidal Society.* Bloomington: Indiana University Press.

Oliver, J. E. 1993. Intergenerational transmission of child abuse: Rates, research, and clinical implications. *American Journal of Psychiatry,* 150(9): 1315–1324.

Omar, D. 1996. Introduction by the Minister of Justice, Mr. Dullah Omar. *Truth Commission Web Site.* Www.truth.org.za.

Orbach, S. 1993. Personal communication.

Packard, E. P. W. 1882. *Modern Persecution or Married Woman's Liabilities.* Hartford: Case, Lockwood and Brainard.

Pearlman, L. A., and K. W. Saakvitne. 1995. *Trauma and the Therapist: Countertransference and Vicarious Traumatization in Psychotherapy with Incest Survivors.* New York: Norton.

Pennebaker J. W. 1989. Confession, inhibition, and disease. *Advances in Experimental Social Psychology.* 22; 211–244.

Pennebaker, J. W. 1995. *Emotion, Disclosure, and Health.* Washington D.C.: American Psychological Association.

Perry, B. D. 1994. Neurobiological sequelae of childhood trauma: PTSD in children. In *Catecholamine Function in Posttraumatic Stress Disorders: Emerging Concepts* edited by M. M. Murburg. Washington, D. C.: American Psychiatric Press.

Perry, B. D., and J. E. Pate. 1994. Neurodevelopment and the psychobiological roots of post-traumatic stress disorder. In *The Neuropsychology of Mental Disorders: A Practical Guide* edited by L.F. Koziol and C.E. Stout. Springfield: Charles C. Thomas.

Perry, J. C., J. L. Herman, B. A. Van der Kolk, and L. A. Hoke, 1990. Psychotherapy and psychological trauma in borderline personality disorder. *Psychiatric Annals,* 20: 33–43.

Peterson, K. C., K. C. Prout, R. A. Schwarz, 1991. *Post-traumatic Stress Disorder: A Clinician's Guide.* New York: Plenum.

Pilisuk, M., and S. H. Parks. 1986. *The Healing Web: Social Networks and Human Survival.* Hanover, NH: University Press of New England.

Pitman, R. K., and S. Orr, 1990. The black hole of trauma. *Biological Psychiatry,* 27: 469–471.

Porter, R. 1987. *A Social History of Madness: The World Through the Eyes of the Insane.* New York: Weidenfeld and Nicolson.

Portnoy, I. The School of Karen Horney. In *American Handbook of Psychiatry, Second Edition, Volume One: The Foundations of Psychiatry* edited by S. Arieti. New York: Basic Books.

Putnam, F. W. 1990. Disturbances of "self" in victims of childhood sexual abuse. In *Incest-Related Syndromes Of Adult Psychopathology* edited by R. P. Kluft. Washington, D. C.: American Psychiatric Press.

Rapoport, R. N. 1960. *Community as Doctor.* Springfield, IL: Charles C. Thomas.

Rauch, S. L., B. A. Van der Kolk, R. E. Fisler, N. M. Alpert, S. P. Orr, C. R. Savage, A. J. Fischman, M. A. Jenike, and R. K. Pitman. 1996. A symptom provocation study of posttraumatic stress disorder using positron emission tomography and script-drive imagery. *Archives of General Psychiatry,* 53: 380–387.

Rees, J. R. 1945. *The Shaping of Psychiatry By War.* New York: W.W. Norton.

Reite, M., and Boccia, M. L. 1994. Physiological aspects of adult attachment. In *Attachment in Adults: Clinical and Developmental Perspectives* edited by M. B. Sperling and W. H. Berman. New York: Guilford.

Richardson J. S., W. A. Zaleski. 1983 Naloxone and self-mutilation. *Biological Psychiatry* 18: 99–101.

Rosen, G. 1959. Social stress and mental disease from the 18th century to the present: Some origins of social psychiatry. *Milbank Memorial Fund Quarterly* 37: 5–32.

Rosenheck, R. 1986. Impact of post-traumatic stress disorder of World War II on the next generation. *Journal of Nervous and Mental Disease* 174(6): 319–327.

Rothman, D. J. 1980. *Conscience and Convenience.*Glenview, IL: Scott, Foresman.

Ruppenthal, G. C., H. F. Harlow, G. P. Sackett, and S. J. Suomi. 1976. A ten-year perspective of motherless mother monkey behavior. *Journal of Abnormal Psychology,* 85: 341–349.

Russell, D.1993. *Philadelphia Daily News,* 3.

Russell, D. 1992a. Pornography and rape: A causal model. In *Pornography: Women, Violence and Civil Liberties* edited by C. Itzen. New York: Oxford University Press.

Russell, P. 1992b. *The White Hole in Time: Our Future Evolution and the Meaning of Now.* San Francisco: Harper San Francisco.

Salasin, S. E., and R. F. Rich. 1993. Mental health policy for victims of violence: The case against women. In *International Handbook of Traumatic Stress Syndromes* edited by J.P. Wilson and B. Raphael. New York: Plenum.

Sanford, N. 1966. *Self and Society: Social Change and Individual Development.* New York: Atherton.

Sarason, S. B. 1972. *The Creation of Settings and the Future Societies.* San Francisco: Jossey-Bass.

Sarason, S. B. 1981. *Psychology Misdirected.* New York: Free Press.

Sashin, J. I. 1993 Duke Ellington: The creative process and the ability to experience and tolerate affect. In *Human Feelings: Explorations in Affect Development and Meaning* edited by S L. Ablon, D. Brown, E. J. Khantzian, and J. E. Mack. Hillsdale, NJ: The Analytic Press.

Saul, J. R. 1992. *Voltaire's Bastard.* New York: Vintage Books.

Scheff, T. J. 1975. *Labeling Madness.* Englewood Cliffs, N.J.: Prentice-Hall.

Scheff, T. J. 1984. *Being Mentally Ill: A Sociological Theory, 2nd ed.* New York: Aldine.

Schetky, D. 1990. A review of the literature on the long-term effects of childhood sexual abuse. In *Incest-Related Syndromes of Adult Psychopathology* edited by R. P. Kluft. Washington, D.C.: American Psychiatric Press.

Schindler, C., and G. Lapid. 1989. *The Great Turning: Personal Peace, Global Victory.* Santa Fe, NM: Bear Press.

Schmookler, A.B. 1983. *The Parable of the Tribes: The Problem of Power in Social Evolution.* Boston: Houghton Mifflin.

Schore, A. N. 1994. *Affect Regulation and the Origin of the Self: The Neurobiology of Emotional Development.* Hillsdale, N.J.: Lawrence Erlbaum.

Schumaker, J. F. 1995. *The Corruption of Reality: A Unified Theory of Religion, Hypnosis, and Psychopathology.* Amherst, N.Y.: Prometheus Books

Schwab, C. W. 1993. Presidential address, 6th Scientific Assembly of the Eastern Association for the Surgery of Trauma. January 14.

Schwarz, D. F., J. A. Grisso, C. G. Miles, J. H. Holmes, R. L. Wishner, and R. L. Sutton. 1994. A longitudinal study of injury morbidity in an African American population. *Journal of the American Medical Association,* 271: 755.

Sedlak, A. J., and D. D. Broadhurst. 1996. Executive summary of the Third National Incidence Study of Child Abuse and Neglect. U.S. Department of Health and Human Service, Administration for Children and Families, Administration on Children, Youth and Families, and National Center on Child Abuse and Neglect.

Seligman, M. E. P. 1992. *Helplessness: On Development, Depression and Death.* New York: Freeman

Selye, H. 1982. History and present status of the stress concept. In *Handbook of Stress: Theoretical and Clinical Aspects* edited by L. Goldberger and S. Breznitz. New York: Free Press.

Sewell J. D. 1993. Traumatic stress of multiple murder investigations. *Journal of Traumatic Stress,* 6(1): 108–118.

Shavit, Y. 1991. Stress-induced immune modulation in animals: Opiates and endogenous opioid peptides. In Psychoimmunology, 2nd ed. Edited by R. Ader, D. L. Felten, E. N. Cohen. San Diego: Academic Press.

Shay, J. 1994. *Achilles in Vietnam: Combat Trauma and the Undoing of Character.* New York: Atheneum.

Shay, J. 1995a. No escape from philosophy in trauma treatment and research. In *Secondary Traumatic Stress: Self Care Issues for Clinicians, Researchers, and Educators* edited by B. H. Stamm. Lutherville, MD: Sidran Press.

Shay, J. 1995b. The Greek tragic theater and a contemporary theater of witness. Presentation at *The Treatment of Trauma: Advances and Challenges, International Society for Traumatic Stress Studies, Annual Meeting.* Boston, November 2–6.

Shengold, L. 1989. *Soul Murder: The Effects of Childhood Abuse and Deprivation.* New Haven: Yale University.

Sigal, J. J., and M. Weinfeld. 1989. *Trauma and Rebirth: Intergenerational Effects of the Holocaust.* New York: Praeger.

Silver, S. M. 1986. An inpatient program for post-traumatic stress disorder: Context as treatment. In *Trauma And Its Wake, Volume II: Post-Traumatic Stress Disorder: Theory, Research And Treatment* edited by C. R. Figley. New York: Brunner/Mazel.

Skynner, R., and Cleese, J. 1993. *Life and How To Survive It.* London: Methuen.

Sloan, J. H., A. L. Kellermann, D. T. Reay, J. A. Ferris, T. Koepsell, F. P. Rivara, C. Rice, L. Gray and J. LoGerfo. 1988. Handgun regulations, crime, assaults and homicide: A tale of two cities. *New England Journal of Medicine,* 319: 1256.

Solomon, J., and George, C. 1996. Defining the caregiving system: Toward a theory of caregiving. *Infant Mental Health Journal,* 17(3): 183–197.

Southard, E. E., and M C. Jarrett. 1922. *The Kingdom of Evils.* New York: Macmillan.

Southwick S. M., R. Yehuda, and E. L.Giller. 1993. Personality disorders in treatment-seeking combat veterans with posttraumatic stress disorder. *American Journal of Psychiatry,* 150: 1020–1023.

Southwick, S. M., D. Bremner, J. H. Krystal, and D. S. Charney. 1994. Psychobiologic research in post-traumatic stress disorder. In *Psychiatric Clinics of North America,* 17(2) edited by D. A. Tomb. Philadelphia: W. B. Saunders.

Spitz, R. A. 1945. Hospitalism: An inquiry into the genesis of psychiatric conditions of early childhood. *Psychoanalytic Study of the Child,* 1: 53–74.

Squire, L. 1987. *Memory and Brain.* New York: Oxford University Press.

Sroufe, L. A. 1985. Attachment classification from the perspective of infant-caregiver relationships and infant temperament. *Child Development* 56: 1–14.

Sroufe, L. A., and E. Waters. 1977. Attachment as an organizational construct. *Child Development* 48: 1184–1199.

Stamm, B. H. (ed). 1995. *Secondary Traumatic Stress: Self Care Issues for Clinicians, Researchers, and Educators.* Lutherville, MD: Sidran Press.

Stanton, A. H., and M. S. Schwartz. 1954. *The Mental Hospital: A Study of Institutional Participation in Psychiatric Illness and Treatment.* New York: Basic Books.

Starer, D. 1995. *Hot Topics.* New York: Touchstone.

Staub, E. 1989. *The Roots of Evil: The Origins of Genocide and Other Group Violence.* New York: Cambridge University Press.

Staub, E. 1992a. The origins of caring, helping, and nonaggression: parental socialization, the family system schools, and cultural influence. In *Embracing*

The Other: Philosophical, Psychological, and Historical Perspectives on Altruism edited by P. M. Oliner, S. P. Oliner, L. Baron, L. A. Blum, D. L. Krebs, and M. Z. Smolenska. New York: New York University Press.

Staub, E. 1992b. Transforming the bystanders: Altruism, caring and social responsibility. In *Genocide Watch* edited by H. Fein. New Haven: Yale University Press.

Staub E. 1993. Individual and group selves: Motivation, morality, and evolution. In G. G Noam and T. E. Wren. *The Moral Self.* Cambridge, MA: MIT Press.

Steiner, G. 1961. *The Death of Tragedy.* London: Faber and Faber

Stern, D. 1985. *The Interpersonal World of the Infant: A View From Psychoanalysis and Developmental Psychology.* New York: Basic Books.

Straus, M. A. 1994. *Beating the Devil Out of Them: Corporal Punishment in American Families.* New York: Lexington Book.

Suomi, S. J., and Harlow, H. F. 1972. Social rehabilitation of isolate-reared monkeys. *Developmental Psychology*, 6: 487–496.

Suomi, S. J., H. F. Harlow, and M. A. Novak. 1974. Reversal of social deficits produced by isolation rearing in monkeys. *Journal of Human Evolution* 3: 527–534.

Suomi, S. J., and Ripp, C. 1983. A history of motherless mother monkey mothering at the University of Wisconsin Primate Laboratory. In *Child Abuse: The Non-human Primate Data,* edited by M. Reite and N. Caine.

Tate, T. 1992. The child pornography industry: International trade in child sexual abuse. In *Pornography: Women, Violence and Civil Liberties* edited by C. Itzen. New York: Oxford University Press.

Taylor, S. 1989. *Positive Illusions: Creative Self-Deception and the Healthy Mind.* New York: Basic Books.

Tedeschi, R. G., and L. G. Calhoun. 1995. *Trauma and Transformation: Growing in the Aftermath of Suffering.* Thousand Oaks: Sage.

Teicher, M. H., C. A. Glod, J. Surrey, C. Swett. 1993. Early childhood abuse and limbic system ratings in adult psychiatric outpatients. *Journal of Neuropsychiatry and Clinical Neurosciences*, 5(3): 301–306.

Tierney, P. 1989. *The Highest Altar: Unveiling the Mystery of Human Sacrifice.* New York: Penguin.

Terr, L. 1990. *Too Scared to Cry: Psychic Trauma in Childhood.* New York: Harper and Row.

Tichener, J. L. 1986. Post-traumatic decline: A consequence of unresolved destructive drives. In *Trauma and Its Wake, Volume 2,* edited by C. Figley. New York: Brunner/Mazel

Tinnin, L. 1990. Mental Unity, Altered States of Consciousness and Dissociation. *Dissociation* III(3): 154–159.

Tinnin, L., and L. Bills. 1994. *Time-Limited Trauma Therapy.* Bruceton Mills, WV: Gargoyle Press.

Toch, T., and M. Silver. 1993. Violence in schools. *U.S. News and World Report* 115(18): 30–6.

Tucker, G., and J. Maxmen. 1973. The practice of hospital psychiatry: A formulation. *American Journal of Psychiatry*, 130: 887–891.

Turnbull, C.M. 1972. *The Mountain People*. New York: Simon and Schuster.

U. S. Advisory Board on Child Abuse and Neglect. 1993. *Neighbors Helping Neighbors: A New National Strategy for the Protection of Children*. Washington, D.C.: U. S. Government Printing Office.

Ullman, M. 1969. A unifying concept linking therapeutic and community process. In *General Systems Theory and Psychiatry*, edited by W. Gray, F. J. Duhl and N. D. Rizzo. Boston: Little Brown.

USA Today. 1995. Company programs can prevent violence. *USA Today Magazine* 124(2607): 6–8.

Van der Hart, O. 1983. *Rituals in Psychotherapy: Transition and Continuity*. New York: Irvington.

Van der Kolk, B. A. 1987a. *Psychological Trauma*. Washington, D. C.: American Psychiatric Press.

Van der Kolk, B. A. 1987b. The separation cry and the trauma response: developmental issues in the psychobiology of attachment and separation. In *Psychological Trauma* edited by B. A. Van der Kolk. Washington, D.C.: American Psychiatric Press.

Van der Kolk, B. A. 1989. The compulsion to repeat the trauma: reenactment, revictimization, and masochism. *Psychiatric Clinics Of North America, Volume 12, Treatment of Victims of Sexual Abuse*. Philadelphia: W.B. Saunders.

Van der Kolk, B. A. 1994. The body keeps the score: Memory and the evolving psychobiology of posttraumatic stress. *Harvard Review of Psychiatry*, 1: 253–265.

Van der Kolk, B. A. 1996a. The complexity of adaptation to trauma. In Van der Kolk B. A., C. McFarlane and L. Weisaeth. *Traumatic Stress: The Effects of Overwhelming Experience on Mind, Body and Society*. New York: Guilford Press.

Van der Kolk, B. A. 1996b. The body keeps the score: Approaches to the psychobiology of posttraumatic stress disorder. In B. A. Van der Kolk, C. McFarlane, and L. Weisaeth. *Traumatic Stress: The Effects of Overwhelming Experience on Mind, Body and Society*. New York: Guilford Press.

Van der Kolk, B. A. 1996c. Trauma and memory. In Van der Kolk B. A., C. McFarlane and L. Weisaeth. *Traumatic Stress: The Effects of Overwhelming Experience on Mind, Body and Society*. New York: Guilford Press.

Van der Kolk, B. A. in press. The psychobiology of traumatic memory: Clinical implications of neuroimaging studies. *Annals New York Academy of Sciences*.

Van der Kolk, B. A., and R. Fisler. 1995. Dissociation and the fragmentary nature of traumatic memories: Overview and exploratory study. *Journal of Traumatic Stress* 8: 505–525.

Van der Kolk, B. A., and C. P. Ducey. 1989. The psychological processing of traumatic experience: Rorschach patterns in PTSD. *Journal of Traumatic Stress*, 2: 259–274.

Van der Kolk, B. A., and M. S. Greenberg. 1987. The psychobiology of the trauma response: Hyperarousal, constriction, and addiction to traumatic reexposure. In *Psychological Trauma* edited by B. A. Van der Kolk. Washington, D.C.: American Psychiatric Press.

Van der Kolk, B. A., M. Greenberg, H. Boyd, and J. Krystal. 1985. Inescapable shock, neurotransmitters, and addiction to trauma: Toward a psychobiology of post traumatic stress. *Biological Psychiatry* 20: 314–325.

Van der Kolk, B. A., M. S. Greenberg, S. P. Orr. 1989. Endogenous opioids, stress induced analgesia, and posttraumatic stress disorder. *Psychopharmacol Bull* 25: 417–42

Van der Kolk, B. A., and A. C. McFarlane. 1996. The black hole of trauma. In B. A. Van der Kolk, C. McFarlane, and L. Weisaeth. *Traumatic Stress: The Effects of Overwhelming Experience on Mind, Body and Society.* New York: Guilford Press.

Van der Kolk, B. A., and O. Van der Hart. 1989. Pierre Janet and the breakdown of adaptation in psychological trauma. *American Journal of Psychiatry,* 146: 1530–1540.

Van der Kolk, B. A., and O. Van der Hart. 1991. The intrusive past: The flexibility of memory and the engraving of trauma. *American Imago,* 48(4): 425–454.

Vaux, A. 1988. *Social Support: Theory, Research, and Intervention.* New York: Praeger.

Vogel, J. 1994. Creative arts therapies on a Sanctuary voluntary inpatient unit. In *Handbook of Post-traumatic Therapy* edited by M. B. Williams and J. F. Sommer Jr. Westport, CN: Greenwood.

Volavka, J. 1995. *Neurobiology of Violence.* Washington, D.C.: American Psychiatric Press.

Von Bertalanffy, L. 1967. *Robots, Men and Minds: Psychology in the Modern World.* New York: George Braziller.

Von Bertalanffy, L. 1974. General systems theory and psychiatry. In *Volume One: The Foundations of Psychiatry; American Handbook of Psychiatry* edited by S. Arieti. New York: Basic Books.

Wakin, E. 1977. *The Immigrant Experience: Faith, Hope and the Golden Door.* Huntington, IN: Our Sunday Visitor.

Wallis, S. 1995. Discipline and civility must be restored to America's public schools. *USA Today Magazine* 124(2606): 32–35.

Watson, L. 1995. *Dark Nature: A Natural History of Evil.* New York: Harper Collins.

Weiss, R. S. 1991. The attachment bond in childhood and adulthood. In *Attachment Across the Life Cycle* edited by C. M. Parkes, J. Stevenson-Hinde and P. Marris. London: Routledge.

Wheeler, E. D., and S. A. Baron. 1994. *Violence in Our Schools, Hospitals, and Public Places: A Prevention and Management Guide.* Ventura, CA: Pathfinder Publishing of California.

White, W. A. 1919. *Thoughts of a Psychiatrist on the War and After.* New York: Paul Hoeber.

Wickham, G. 1985. *A History of the Theatre, 2nd Ed.* London: Phaidon.

Wilber, K. 1996. *A Brief History of Everything.* Boston: Shambhala

Williams, H. 1986. Humour and healing. Therapeutic effects in geriatrics. *Gerontion* 1(3): 14–17.

Williams, R. B. 1995. Somatic consequences of stress. In *Neurobiological and Clinical Consequences of Stress: From Normal Adaptation to PTSD,* edited by M. J. Friedman, D. S. Charney, and A. Y. Deutch. Philadelphia: Lippincott-Raven.

Wilmer, H. A. 1958. *Social Psychiatry In Action: A Therapeutic Community.* Springfield, IL: Charles C. Thomas.

Wilmer, H. 1981. Defining and understanding the therapeutic community. *Hospital and Community Psychiatry* 32: 95–99.

Wilson, J. Q. 1993. *The Moral Sense.* New York: Free Press

Wolin, S. J., and S. Wolin. 1993. *The Resilient Self.* New York: Villard.

Worth, R. 1995. A model prison. *Atlantic Monthly* November.

Wright, R. 1994. *The Moral Animal.* New York: Pantheon.

Wuthnow, R. 1991. *Acts of Compassion.* Princeton: Princeton University Press.

Yablonsky L. 1972. *Robopaths: People As Machines.* New York: Bobbs-Merrill.

Yarborough, M. H. 1994. Securing the American workplace. *HR Focus* 71(9): 1–4.

Yehuda, R., B. Kahana, K. Binder-Byrnes, S. Southwick, J. Mason, and E. L. Giller. 1995. Low urinary cortisol excretion in Holocaust survivors with posttraumatic stress disorder. *American Journal of Psychiatry,* 152: 982–986.

Yehuda, R., and H. Harvey. in press. Relevance of neuroendocrine alteration in PTSD to cognitive impairments of trauma survivors. In *Recollections of Trauma: Scientific Research and Clinical Practice: Proceedings of the 1996 NATO Conference on Trauma and Memory in Port Bourgenay, France.* New York: Plenum.

Yuille, J. C., and Cutshall, J. L. 1989. Analysis of the statements of victims, witnesses and suspects. In *Credibility Assessment* edited by J. C. Yuille. Norwell, MA: Kluwer Academic.

Zahn, T. P., R. Moraga, and W. J. Ray. 1996. Psychophysiological assessment of dissociative disorders. In *Handbook of Dissociation: Theoretical, Empirical, and Clinical Perspectives* edited by L. K. Michelson and W.J. Ray. New York: Plenum.

Zeanah C. H., and Zeanah P. D. 1989. Intergenerational transmission of maltreatment: Insights from attachment theory and research. *Psychiatry* 52: 177–196.

Zimring, F. E., and G. Hawkins. 1987. *The Citizen's Guide to Gun Control.* New York: Macmillan.

Subject Index

Author Index